Healing
the
Vegan Way

Healing the Vegan Way

plant-based eating for optimal health and wellness

MARK REINFELD

WITH CONTRIBUTIONS FROM

MICHAEL KLAPER M.D., MICHAEL GREGER M.D., HANS DIEHL M.D.,

JOEL KAHN M.D., JULIEANNA HEVER R.D, BRENDA DAVIS R.D.,

ROSINA PELLERANO, M.D., AND ASHLEY BOUDET N.D.

Da Capo
LIFE
LONG

Da Capo Lifelong Books

Copyright © 2016 by Mark Reinfeld

Recipe credits: Basic Nut or Seed Milk (page 104) first appeared in *The 30-Minute Vegan;* Ethiopian Spice Mix (page 106) first appeared in *The 30-Minute Vegan: Soup's On!;* Herbes de Provence Spice Mix (page 106) first appeared in *The 30-Minute Vegan's Taste of Europe*

Excerpt on page 7 reprinted from *The Plant-Powered Diet*, by Sharon Palmer, RD, copyright © 2012 Sharon Palmer. Reprinted with the permission of The Experiment, LLC.

All photos by Mark Reinfeld, except as noted. Elizabeth Arraj: Rainbow Fruit and Crème, Simple One-Pot Meal, Grilled Eggplant Towers with Cashew Ricotta, Raw Chocolate Pudding, Crunchy Chocolate Buckwheat Clusters. Ami Lawson: Garden Veggie Scramble and Herb-Roasted Potatoes. Erik Rudolph: Curried Garbanzo Cakes with Poppy Seeds, Veggie Lettuce Boats, Grilled Plaintain Kebabs, Watermelon Gazpacho, Raw Carrot Brazil Nut Soup, Raw Coconut Curry Vegetables, Mushroom Cauliflower Tacos, Raw Carrot Ginger Cake. Suzanne Rudolph: Avocado Mousse–Stuffed Tomatoes

First Da Capo Press edition 2016

Published by Da Capo Press
An imprint of Perseus Books, a division of PBG Publishing, LLC,
a subsidiary of Hachette Book Group, Inc.
www.dacapopress.com

Library of Congress Control Number: 2016014780
ISBN 978-0-7382-1777-2 (paperback)
ISBN 978-0-7382-1778-9 (e-book)

Editorial production Christine Marra by *Marra*thon Production Services. www.marrathon.net

Book design by Jane Raese
Set in 10.5-point Archer

To my son Sage Martin Mahalo Reinfeld,
who has motivated me even more to help create
a more peaceful and sustainable world.

To Daniel Rhoda, whose friendship, kindness, and support
have propelled me on my path as an author.

And to Lisa Shapiro, whose tireless activism continues to inspire me.

Let thy food be thy medicine and thy medicine thy food.
—HIPPOCRATES, FATHER OF MODERN MEDICINE

Contents

Foreword by Dr. Michael Klaper, MD   xi

Bite by Bite, Bowl by Bowl:
A Recipe for Healing   xiv

How to Use This Book   xv

part one
THE HEALING

1. Preventable Health Challenges   3

2. A Cornucopia of Nutritional Theories:
Which is right for you?   22

3. The Pillars of the Plant Kingdom:
Nutrient dense foods for optimal health   44

4. The Extraordinary Health Benefits
of Raw Whole Foods   63

5. Putting It into Practice: Meal Plans   70

part two
THE RECIPES:
200 RECIPES for EVERY SEASON

6. Preparing Your Kitchen   81

Kitchen Gear, 81
The Vegan Pantry, 83
Natural Sweeteners, 88

7. How One Recipe Can Equal Thousands
+ Easy Cooking Techniques   91

Top Ten Tips for Efficient Food
    Preparation, 91

About the Recipes and Vegan Fusion
    Cuisine, 92
About the Template Recipes, 93
The Monk Bowl, 94
Storage of Prepared Foods, 94
Techniques, 95

8. Easy Pantry Basics   103

Brazil Nut Milk, 104
TEMPLATE: Plant-Based Milk, 104
Gluten-Free Flour Mix, 105
Ethnic Spice Blends, 105
    Italian Spice Mix, 105
    Indian Spice Mix, 106
    Mexican Spice Mix, 106
    Moroccan Spice Mix, 106
    Ethiopian Spice Mix, 106
    Herbes de Provence Spice Mix, 106
Marinades, 107
    Maple Balsamic Marinade, 107
    Lemon Dijon Marinade, 107
Soup Stock, 108
Condiments and Accompaniments, 108
    Salt-free Seasoning, 108
    Balsamic Reduction, 109
    Turmeric Hot Sauce, 109
    Homemade Catsup, 110
    Raw Brazil Nut Parmesan, 111
    Herb Croutons, 111
    Coco Bacon, 112
    Vegan Sour Cream, 112
    Raw Cashew Sour Cream, 113
    Vegan Mayonnaise, 113
    Roasted Garlic Spread, 114

9. Breakfast   116

Simple Breakfast Chia Pudding, 117
TEMPLATE: Chia Pudding, 117
Rainbow Fruit and Crème, 118
Sunflower Seed Fig Puree, 118
TEMPLATE: Raw Breakfast Seed and
   Fruit Puree, 119
Raw Pumpkin Seed and Sunseed Yogurt,
   119
Açai Power Bowl, 120
Trifecta Stewed Dried Fruit, 121
Raw Apricot Fennel Granola, 121
Banana Date Breakfast Muffins, 122
Lemon Blueberry Pancakes, 123
Pepita Pecan Granola, 124
TEMPLATE: Homemade Granola, 126
Multigrain Grits, 126
Iron-Rich Morning Glory Steel Cut Oats,
   127
Garden Veggie Scramble, 128
TEMPLATE: Garden Scramble, 128
Sun-Dried Tomato Fennel Breakfast Tart,
   129
Purple Potato Tempeh Hash, 130

10. Teas, Juices, Elixirs, and Smoothies   132

Digestive Tea, 133
Warming Herbal Chai, 133
Ultimate Hangover Cure, 135
Galactic Green Juice, 135
TEMPLATE: Green Juices, 136
Rehydrating Watermelon Chiller, 136
Digest Aid Juice, 136
Sunrise Carrot Juice, 137
Citrus Magic, 137
Green Master Cleanse, 138
Ginger Turmeric Shooter, 140
Flu Buster, 140

Basil Rosemary Lemonade, 141
Açai Spritzer, 142
Kale Kolada, 143
Quinoa Milk, 143
Gold Milk, 144
Choco Maca Elixir, 145
Sesame Hemp Revitalizer, 145
Tropical Smoothie, 146
Berry Green Smoothie, 147
TEMPLATE: Green Smoothie, 147
Maca Horchata, 147
High-Protein Vanilla Almond Shake, 148

11. Savory Snacks and Appetizers   150

Smokey Salsa, 151
Glorious Guacamole, 151
Avocado Mousse–Stuffed Tomatoes, 152
Lemon Garlic Steamed Artichokes, 153
Curried Crispy Chickpeas, 154
Broiled Artichoke Fritters, 155
White Bean Artichoke Dip with Arugula,
   155
Sun-Dried Tomato Tapenade, 156
Kalamata Rosemary Hummus, 157
TEMPLATE: Hummus, a.k.a. Bean Puree,
   159
Truffled Cashew Cheeze, 159
TEMPLATE: Soft Plant-Based Cheeses, 160
Veggie Lettuce Boats, 160
Gold Bar Squash Chutney, 161
Okra Bruschetta, 162
Buffalo Cauliflower, 163
Curried Garbanzo Cakes with Poppy Seeds,
   164
Kentucky Baked Portobello Nuggets, 165
Grilled Plantain Kebabs, 166
Black Bean Tostones, 167
Quinoa Amaranth Cakes, 168
Pecan Veggie Pâté, 169

TEMPLATE: Raw Pâté, 170
Creamy Herb Polenta, 170

12. Salads and Sides   172

Super Sprout Salad, 173
TEMPLATE: Ultimate Salad, 174
Simple Chop Salad, 174
Asian Cucumber Salad, 175
Green Papaya Salad, 175
Simple Sauerkraut, 176
Quick Kimchi, 178
Watercress with Pistachios and Currants, 179
Waldorf Salad, 180
Caesar Salad, 181
Pickled Okra, 181
TEMPLATE: Pickled Veggies, 182
Provençal Salad, 183
Tomato Avocado Salad, 183
TEMPLATE: Kale Salad, 184
Curry Kale Salad, 184
Ranch Kale Salad, 185
Sesame Kale Salad, 186
Walnut Taco Salad, 187
Raw Walnut Crumble, 188
TEMPLATE: Legume and Vegetable Salad, 188
Black Bean and Corn Salad, 189
Ginger Rainbow Chard, 189
TEMPLATE: Simple Green Sauté, 190
Garlicky Greens, 191
Roasted Zucchini and Corn, 192
Chili Lime Grilled Asparagus with Mushrooms and Bell Pepper, 193
Broasted Brussels Sprouts, 194
Broiled Cauliflower with Sun-Dried Tomatoes, 194
Steamed Italian Baby Bok Choy, 196
Three Greens with Tomato Sauce, 197
Edamame Arame Salad, 198

Parsnip Fries, 198
Cauliflower Steaks with Ethiopian-Spiced Almonds, 200
Cream of Kale, 201
Smashed Roasted Cauliflower and Parsnip, 202
Israeli Couscous Tabouli, 203
Green Quinoa, 203
Golden Rice, 204
Unfried Rice, 205
Spicy Pinto Beans, 206
Spaghetti Squash with Broccoli, 207
Date Glazed Sweet Potatoes, 208
Wasabi Garlic Twice-Baked Potatoes, 209
Pearled Barley with Mushrooms and Corn, 210
Quinoa Chickpea Pilaf, 211
Grilled Mediterranean Vegetables and Quinoa, 212
TEMPLATE: Grain Vegetable Dish, 213
Mushroom Kasha, 213
Herb-Roasted Potatoes, 214
Fingerling Potatoes with Pesto, 215
Green Beans with White Bean Fennel Sauce, 217

13. Dressings and Sauces   219

Oil-Free Orange Tarragon Dressing, 220
Oil-Free Asian Umeboshi Dressing, 220
Simple Flax or Hemp Oil Dressing, 221
Cilantro Lime Vinaigrette, 221
Strawberry Vinaigrette, 222
TEMPLATE: Vinaigrette, 223
Golden Turmeric Dressing, 223
Raw Hempseed Ranch Dressing, 224
Caesar Dressing, 225
Horseradish Dijon Dressing, 226
Oil-Free Macadamia Wasabi Dressing, 226
Creamy Pepita Dressing, 227

TEMPLATE: Creamy Dressings, 228
Creamy Lemon Tahini Dressing, 228
Oil-Free Creamy Sweet Potato Dressing, 229
Cilantro Mint Chutney, 229
Raw Tamarind Sauce, 230
Zesty Chimichurri Sauce, 231
Smoky BBQ Sauce, 231
Ancho Chili Sauce, 232
Easy Cheezy Sauce, 233
Almond Dipping Sauce, 233
Creamy Mexican Dipping Sauce, 234
Roasted Red Pepper Sauce, 235
Sweet-and-Sour Sauce, 236
Simple Roasted Squash Sauce, 236
Raw Coconut Curry Sauce, 237
Tahini Oat Sauce, 238
Fire Roasted Tomato Sauce, 239
Oil-Free Mushroom Gravy, 240

14. Soups and Stews   242

Healing Broth, 243
Watermelon Gazpacho, 243
Raw Cucumber Fennel Soup, 244
Raw Carrot Brazil Nut Soup, 245
TEMPLATE: Raw Vegetable Soup, 246
Miso Vegetable Soup, 246
Congee with Fenugreek, 247
Asian Noodle Soup, 249
Creamy Asparagus Soup with Corn, 250
TEMPLATE: Creamy Vegan Soup, 251
Ital Roasted Squash and Sweet Potato
    Soup, 251
Italian Spring Vegetable Soup, 252
Curried Broccoli and Great Northern Bean
    Soup, 253
Smoky Split Pea Soup, 254
Moroccan Chickpea Stew, 255
Mexican Two-Bean Soup, 256
Kitchari, 257

15. Main Dishes   259

Raw Collard Veggie Rolls, 260
Simple Baked Tofu, 260
Maple Baked Tempeh, 262
Baked Falafel, 262
Nori Rolls, 263
Designer Seed and Nut Crust Pizzas, 265
Simple One-Pot Meal, 266
TEMPLATE: One-Pot Meal, a.k.a.
    Monk Bowl, 267
Roasted Veggies and Beans, 267
Raw Coconut Curry Vegetables, 268
Millet Black Bean Veggie Burgers, 269
Magnificent Mushroom Burgers, 270
TEMPLATE: Veggie Burger, 272
Black Bean Grits, 272
Ratatouille, 273
TEMPLATE: Quiche, 274
Broccoli Dill Quiche, 274
Lemon Tempeh with Kale and Rice Noodles,
    276
Mushroom Cauliflower Tacos, 277
BBQ Roasted Tofu with Collards, 278
Tempeh Fajitas, 279
Jamaican Patties, 280
Sloppy Joes, 281
Grilled Eggplant Towers with Cashew
    Ricotta, 282
Millet Squash and Broccoli, 284
Cauliflower Casserole, 285
Corn Casserole, 286
TEMPLATE: Vegan Loaf, 287
Lentil Walnut Loaf, 288
Thai Curry Vegetables, 289
Creamy Lentil Saag, 290
Mexican Seitan-Stuffed Peppers, 291
Broccoli Rabe Penne Pasta with Oil-Free
    Cream Sauce, 292
TEMPLATE: Simple Vegan Cream Sauce, 293

16. Desserts and Sweet Snacks   **294**

Superfood Trail Mix, 295
TEMPLATE: Superfood Trail Mix, 295
Choco-Chia Pudding, 295
Raw Chocolate Pudding, 296
Strawberry Cashew Cream, 297
Banana Mango Ice Cream, 298
Raw Hemp Energy Balls, 298
TEMPLATE: Raw Energy Balls, 299
Crunchy Chocolate Buckwheat Clusters, 299
Raw Apple Crumble, 300
Mixed Fruit Kanten, 301
Fruit-Sweetened Baked Pears, 303
Chocolate Pecan Dipped Fruit, 304
Cranberry Walnut Power Krispy Bars, 305
Sweet and Spicy Baked Plantains, 306
Pumpkin Pudding, 307
Apricot Oat Bar, 308
Raw Carrot Ginger Cake, 309
TEMPLATE: Simple Cookie Recipe, 310
Almond Butter Chocolate Chip Cookies, 310
Fruit-Sweetened Pistachio Peach Cobbler, 311
TEMPLATE: Fruit Cobbler, 312
Fruit-Sweetened Black Bean Brownies, 312

Vegan Fusion   314
Metric Conversion Chart   318
Comprehensive Nutrient Reference Guide   319
Notes   339
Clinical Wellness Programs Utilizing a Whole Food Plant-Based Diet   341
Additional Resources   344
Acknowledgments   351
About the Experts   352
About the Contributors   354
Vegan Fusion Culinary Immersions   356
Index   357
About the Author   377

Foreword

In the over forty years in which I have been in medical practice, the causes of the major diseases that devastate Western societies—clogged arteries, high blood pressure, obesity, diabetes, and a host of inflammatory diseases involving the joints, intestinal tract, skin, and various other organs—have become apparent.

The force that is causing Westerners to become grossly obese, clogged up, diabetic, inflamed, toxic, and cancerous is not some genetic mutation, exotic virus, or mysterious toxin—and the cure is not in some new pill, potion, or procedure. The cause and cure of all these dreaded diseases can all be summed up in three words: "It's the food!"

Instead of eating whole foods in their natural forms, as people have done for millennia, today many Americans and others in Western nations pour too many flesh-based, dairy-laden, overly processed, devitalized, hypersugared, and stealthily salted foods into their system—hour after hour, day after day, year after year.

Eating this way is analogous to pouring diesel fuel into the gas tank of your car's V6 engine. Diesel fuel is basically kerosene. This oily fuel would clog the fuel lines and foul the sparkplugs, similar to the way saturated animal fats, cholesterol, and vegetable oils stiffen, inflame, and eventually clog the arteries and foul the insulin receptors, manifesting in high blood pressure, diabetes, heart attacks, strokes, cancers, and various inflammatory diseases.

For the past three decades, my medical practice has largely evolved into nutritional counseling, with the goal of keeping people out of hospitals and off operating tables through wiser food choices and a healthier lifestyle. Daily, I see the power of a whole food, plant-based diet to prevent diseases that I was told in medical school were "relentlessly progressive"—atherosclerosis, diabetes, colitis, rheumatoid arthritis, and obesity; what's more, I've seen the power of food to actually reverse these conditions, to the amazement of both the patient and myself. As the nutrients from a life-enhancing food stream of colorful salads, hearty vegetable soups, a generous helping of green and yellow vegetables, and succulent fruits pours through the body, these chronic conditions can melt away.

Simply put, a whole food, plant-based diet is, by far, the most powerful healing modality I know. And it is the affordable, life-sustaining, hunger-fighting, planet-saving antidote for what ails us as individuals and a society.

The foods presented in *Healing the Vegan Way* have qualities that naturally help reverse disease:

- Lower in sodium and high in potassium, which makes them the cornerstone for lowering high blood pressure

- Rich in soluble and insoluble fiber that creates digestive regularity, the basis for healing colitis and other inflammatory bowel diseases
- High in phytonutrients that reduce the risk of breast, prostate, and other cancers—and, sometimes, can help to actually reverse them
- Free of cholesterol, low in saturated fats, high in plant sterols—so atherosclerotic blockages in the arteries begin to melt away with the very first meal
- More favorably balanced with omega-3 fats and other anti-inflammatory lipids and plant constituents—so they help reduce inflammation throughout the body
- Lower in caloric density, so people can eat lots of sumptuous soups, salads, vegetables, stews, potatoes, quinoa and other whole grains, and fruits and still become lean and healthy

These foods, prepared with the delightful flavorings and cooking techniques of world cuisines, are the best-tasting medicines ever. Speaking as a physician, what's not to like?

As a passionate environmentalist, I know that all the major environmental disasters that loom before us—deforestation, soil erosion, water depletion, water pollution, global warming—are primarily driven by the industrial production and consumption of animal flesh. If one cares about the planet, the future, and the children and grandchildren who will come after us, it is time to realize that the single most effective thing we can do to improve our own health and the health of life on this planet, is to reduce—or better yet, eliminate—our consumption of animal products.

At long last, the truth of the underlying cause of our health crisis and impending environmental disruption is gradually being recognized. Changing human understanding—and far more challenging, human eating habits—is another matter.

Our consumption of salt, sugar, and oil-laden fast foods and convenience foods is addictive, and we're eating more of these foods every year. The industrial-scale production and consumption of these foods spawn and sustain giant industries, and government subsidies and policies protect these businesses and perpetuate unhealthy habits. And in our culture, eating meat is the glorified norm and is growing in popularity. All of this makes a societal transition to a plant-based diet seem like a David-and-Goliath challenge.

Our species prides itself on its intelligence, but despite knowing that a whole food, plant-based lifestyle is the key to salvaging the health and lives of millions of individuals, we have been reluctant to give up our flesh-eating habits so far. If we are to make this future-saving transition in time and on the societal scale that is required, we need some magic.

Fortunately, plenty of magic is around these days. People everywhere are opening to new ways of seeing and nourishing themselves, and this openness will catalyze the great societal sea change toward plant-based foods. By creating great tasting, easy-to-prepare vegan food, chefs, culinary teachers, and home cooks like you will provide major magic to help this miracle come to pass.

When a delicious piece of meat-free lasagne or lentil pâté melts in the mouth of a skeptical omnivore who then says, "Oh, if that is vegan food, I could eat that!" you are hearing that magic at work. This is how vital progress is made—bite by bite, bowl by bowl.

No one I know can make that magic happen better than Mark Reinfeld. Mark is an experienced and talented vegan chef who not only loves his craft of making plant-based ingredients taste surpassingly good, but he loves food itself as a manifestation of the energy of life. He also obviously loves people, the animals, and the Earth, as his warm, open heart shows in all his writings and recipes.

In *Healing the Vegan Way,* Mark presents both basic and advanced principles for creating a delicious menu of vegan foods that will help heal all the tissues and organs of the body—while also bringing delight to the tongue and palate. Now, there's one tasty prescription!

So, put yourself in "Dr. Mark's" capable culinary hands and you will enjoy the world's most delicious therapy that will bring healing to you, to your loved ones, and to our planet. Here's healing medicine to be savored, celebrated, and shared! Bon appétit!

—Michael Klaper, MD

Bite by Bite, Bowl by Bowl:
A Recipe for Healing

For as long as I can remember, I have been interested in exploring the healing qualities of food—discovering the impact that our food choices have upon our health. *Healing the Vegan Way* is the culmination of over twenty years' work in the vegan and raw food culinary world, and I'm excited to have this work be a part of your journey to wellness.

Several leading medical doctors and registered dietitians collaborated with me to demonstrate that many of the major health challenges facing our society today can be addressed by adopting a well-balanced, whole food, plant-based diet. To further support you on your healing path, I offer recipes that provide both the nutrients we need to thrive, as well as the delectable flavors to keep you yearning for more!

May you experience the joy and abundant health that the plant kingdom has to offer!

With thanks and aloha,
Mark

If you have specific and serious health concerns, you should consult with a qualified health-care professional before making substantial changes to your diet.

How to Use This Book

Part 1 shares the many benefits of plant-based cuisine, highlighting some of the nutritional powerhouses of the plant kingdom and examining other lifestyle factors that will support you in creating a healthy, well-balanced life.

This section also provides a 14-day menu plan that follows the guidelines of the Complete Health Improvement Program (CHIP) developed by Dr. Hans Diehl (see page 19). It concludes with a Comprehensive Nutrient Reference Chart on page 319, where you can learn about the essential nutrients the body needs and their food sources.

Part 2 will help you set up your kitchen and master some basic techniques in vegan natural food preparation before diving into more than two hundred delectable recipes. The recipes in each chapter are listed roughly in order from lightest to heaviest.

Be sure to rotate through as many of the recipes in the book as possible. This will provide you with the greatest array of nutrients. Use these recipes as a starting point for creating your own versions and specialties based on your preferences and whatever ingredients are on hand. Once you have understood the simple concept of a Template Recipe (page 93), you will discover how easy it is to create hundreds of variations to suit your individual taste.

Sidebars and Symbols

Throughout the pages you will see the following sidebars and symbols:

Template Recipe: Follow these guidelines to create hundreds of variations of the featured recipe, see page 93 for more about the Template Recipe.

Chef's Tips and Tricks: We share the secrets that make your life in the kitchen easier and more enjoyable.

Quicker and Easier: Super simple recipe ideas for those on the go.

Recipes for Health

While so many different nutritional theories are out there that it makes the head spin, I kept certain guiding principles in mind as I developed these recipes. First, I wanted to include recipes that incorporated those foods with the highest nutrient density (foods with the greatest amount of vitamins and minerals relative to calories; see Chapter 3). Second, although the recipes were not designed with any particular health challenge in mind, I wanted to create delicious recipes that were lower in salt, processed oil, and concentrated sugars than many alternatives:

Sodium-restricted dishes. Most of the recipes containing salt do so "to taste." If you wish to reduce your sodium intake even further, please eliminate the added salt or soy sauce indicated in the recipe, and add small amounts to taste, if necessary. You can use a low-sodium soy sauce, or replace the sea salt with the Salt-Free Seasoning (page 108). Remember that not all salts are created equal. These recipes were developed using a mineral-rich sea salt. Some sea salts are higher in sodium than others, and the coarseness of the salt will also determine the amount of sodium in a measured amount. (One teaspoon of coarsely ground salt contains less sodium than does 1 teaspoon of finely ground salt.)

Processed oil-free dishes. There is a growing movement in the plant-based nutrition world to avoid processed oils in our diet and to get whatever fat we need from the whole foods directly, instead of from its processed oils. Every recipe in the book is either oil-free or can be easily adapted to oil-free. To limit oils, follow the oil-free versions of recipes, indicated by ◗, and use the water sauté method discussed on page 101.

Soy-free dishes. You can use chopped portobello mushrooms whenever tofu or tempeh is called for in the recipe. You can eliminate the soy sauce, or replace the soy sauce called for in the recipes with coconut aminos, a coconut-based sauce available at your local natural foods store. Please see page 42 for a discussion of the "soy controversy."

Low- or no-sugar dishes. You'll want to steer clear of those recipes higher in sugar, even if that sugar comes from fruit. Please see the sweetener chart on page 89 for some healthful alternatives to white sugar

and visit your local natural foods store to discover the various natural sweeteners on the market. You can make your own date syrup by following the recipe on page 88.

Gluten-free. Virtually all the recipes in this book are gluten-free or can be made gluten-free. Gluten, a protein found in wheat and other cereal grains, is responsible for the grain's elasticity. More and more people are being diagnosed with celiac disease (extreme gluten intolerance)—or are simply cutting gluten out of their diet, for overall health reasons. Some recipes that do contain gluten can be easily adapted to become gluten-free. I have noted on the recipes that do include a gluten product, what to use as a gluten-free replacement.

I have used spelt flour in the recipes that do call for flour. Spelt is an ancient variety of wheat that does contain gluten, though in a form that many with wheat allergies can tolerate. Those with celiac disease are unable to tolerate gluten in any form and should therefore avoid spelt. For a gluten-free flour mix, please see page 105. For the gluten intolerant, please remember to use gluten-free tamari as the soy sauce, and to purchase a gluten-free variety of nutritional yeast—two common ingredients used in the book.

Whenever possible, I recommend using organic ingredients. Organic food is grown without the use of chemical fertilizers and pesticides, most of which have not been fully tested for their long-term effects on humans. For maximum food safety, go organic. Please see page 60 for more information on organics.

I also recommend using a minimum of processed and packaged ingredients. This is much better for your health and is the environmentally sustainable way to go. Also, eating locally grown foods whenever possible ensures optimal flavor and freshness and conserves resources. Growing foods in your own garden or participating in community-supported agriculture programs (CSAs) are the best way to go if you have the opportunity. It's quite fulfilling to see something grow from seed to plant. Farmers' markets, where you can meet the people growing your food, are the next best choice. Ask the vendors how the food was grown, if not labeled "certified organic." Stock up on what is fresh and in season. Using a Template Recipe format (page 93), many of the recipes in *Healing the Vegan Way* can be adapted to include whatever ingredients are available.

For most people, simply gravitating toward a plant-based diet will bring healing to their body and mind that they never imagined possible.

Precepts of a Healthy Life

In addition to our making wise food choices, other aspects of our life require our mindfulness and attention for optimal functioning, stability, wholeness, and happiness. I like to view these other aspects as spokes on the wheel, pillars of the temple, or slices of the pie of our life.

1. Healthy Plant-Based Diet

A healthy diet is essential and complementary for sustainably thriving physically, mentally, and emotionally. Balance and moderation are also key. As you make the shift from an unhealthy, processed, animal product–heavy diet, you may be surprised at the results. Many people who transition from a less healthy diet to one with more plant-based, unprocessed foods report their taste buds and cravings change— the taste buds become more pleased with new and different foods, and the cravings morph from the more standard greasy burger-type food over to leafy greens, grains, and legumes. It is often simply a matter of time and evolution.

Often the transition is challenging, because food culture is so ingrained from an early age, and is tied to our family traditions.

Make a gentle and gradual transition toward healthier, plant-based foods. Slow and steady change is usually the longest lasting. Using the recipes in this book, your transition will be a delicious one—without any feelings of deprivation.

2. Moderate Exercise

Exercising regularly, even in moderate amounts, is a huge slice of the healthy-life pie. Innumerable studies have shown that thirty minutes a day of walking or other body movement vastly decreases the risk of chronic disease and diseases of affluence, and increases mental positivity, attitude, and outlook, as well as increasing life span. Bones and muscles are strengthened and your heart rate is given a refreshing boost. Weight control, endorphin release, increased strength and endurance, better sleep, social connection, and lots of fun are all benefits you can get from a regular exercise regimen.

If you're thinking that sometimes you just don't have the energy for movement, remember that expending energy during exercise actually yields increased energy for the rest of the day, when balanced. Start modestly and work your way up in increments. To remove any dreaded exercise stigma, finding forms of exercise that are fun is a way to feed two birds with one scone. Walking a dog, salsa dancing, playing with kids in a park, using a bike, or walking as transport, rebounding, sports that you enjoy playing with others, yoga, even going to the gym can become activities that you look forward to.

3. Positive Attitude

Optimism or pessimism can extend from thinking patterns to health patterns. Studies show increasingly that positive thinking is absolutely key to stress management, which in turn can extend to vibrant health. A positive attitude can increase the quality and length of life span, dissuade the possibility of onset of depression or distress, provide greater resistance to chronic disease, and improve coping mechanisms in the event of more challenging episodes.

Even the Mayo clinic emphasizes this idea on their website, listing the many health benefits of positive thinking, including increased life span, better resistance to seasonal colds, and lower rates of heart disease and depression.[1]

A friend shared an amazing story on the importance of a positive attitude. His friend won a world-class handball tournament. "When I made a good shot, I said, 'Good shot.' When I missed a shot, I said, 'Nice try!'" He did not beat himself up when he missed the shot, but kept the positive attitude and kept moving forward.

Observing our own self-talk—and changing the negative to positive—can take a lot of patience and persistence. But the results are so worth it! A positive outlook toward the events in our life, and our interpretation of them, can do worlds of good for mental and physical health.

The idea that our thoughts can affect our health has been studied widely in recent years. Bruce Lipton has been a pioneer in looking at the importance of epigenetics, what factors in an individual cause genes to turn on and off, in his book *The Biology of Belief*. Other notable books on this subject include *The Anatomy of Hope*, by Jerome Groopman, MD, *The Instinct to Heal*, by David Servan-Schreiber, MD, PhD, and *Love, Medicine, and Miracles*, by Bernie Siegel, MD, all written by medical doctors who have witnessed the power of the mind both personally and in practice. They all cite numerous studies on this topic.

There is an entire field of study called psychoneuroimmunology (PNI), also referred to as psychoendoneuroimmunology (PENI), which focuses on the interaction between psychological processes and the nervous and immune systems of the human body.

4. Adequate Rest and Meditation

Are you someone who always feels tired, getting to bed after midnight, only to have to rise at six a.m.? You're not alone. In this go-go-go culture, many of us simply do not take enough time in the day to get the proper amount of sleep—which differs for everybody regardless of the recommended average for adults of eight to nine hours per night. Brains often are in a near-constant state of processing. Calming them to stillness now and then will do wonders for mental and physical health.

Sleep is paramount to our ability to learn and process memories. Not only that, sleep restores expended energy, gives muscles the chance to repair, and influences hormone release for vital body function. Sleep quality is a major factor for rest—at least two hours per night of deep or REM sleep is optimal.

Adequate rest also correlates with optimal nutrient absorption. Because sleep disorders can result in digestive difficulties, compromised liver detoxification, and suboptimal immunity, quality sleep is absolutely required for these functions to happen. To help with proper rest, it is recommended to finish eating earlier in the evening rather than later, and allow for proper winding-down time—the stomach should spend the night resting, not digesting!

In addition to rest, some form of practice to calm our restless mind, and manage stress and stressful thoughts, can be a wonderful way to increase your well-being. There are numerous forms of meditation and spiritual practices (try yoga for both mind and body benefits!). Even five minutes a day of powering down and finding inner calm can be a good practice. Find and explore one that resonates with you, and you may be amazed at the difference it makes.

5. Periodic Cleansing

Even with a healthy diet and wellness practice, environmental toxicity from air and water pollution to chemicals and building cleaners—and stress can cause toxins to accumulate in the body. Some common environmental toxins include phthalates and BPA used to make plastics; VOCs (volatile organic compounds) found in drinking water, carpet, paints, deodorants, cleaning products, and air fresheners; heavy metals, such as arsenic, mercury, lead, aluminum, and cadmium, found in drinking water, fish, vaccines, pesticides, preserved wood, antiperspirant, building materials, and dental amalgams; and triclosan, found in antibacterial soaps, some deodorants, toothpastes, cosmetics, kitchenware, and children's toys. These are all known to cause potential immune and endocrine system dysfunction. The lungs, liver, kidneys, and skin do a diligent job of removing toxins daily, but cleanses help the body along with this considerable task.

Cleanses can help escort out impurities, persistent parasites, germs, and abnormal cells. With any cleanse, digestion function is of utmost importance. A wide variety of options exist for digestive cleanses, including a vegan cleanse, whole foods cleanse, juice cleanse, colon cleanse, raw foods cleanse, and others. The idea behind all of these is to give the digestive system a rest, with some sustaining nutrients (as in a juice, smoothie, or broth regimen), or just lightening the digestive load by avoiding processed foods. (Page 68 provides information on a sample raw foods cleanse.)

An effective cleanse can be anywhere from one to three days a week to a few days a month, or even longer depending on individual needs. Always consult with a qualified health-care practitioner before embarking upon any cleansing regimen.

6. Engaging Community and Social Life

In 1943, famed psychologist Abraham Maslow published his hierarchy of human needs, and demonstrated that being loved and belonging are as important as food and shelter to find personal fulfillment.

Many people avoid scheduling social time into their hectic life. Even if brief, those moments spent with a good friend or family member, helping a neighbor with a project, working in the community garden, or even playing with kids at the park are activities that feed and nourish us as well. Volunteering, getting involved in organizations or meetups, attending fun community events, and doing group exercise are all good ways to expand on this piece of the pie.

Community can also support healthy lifestyle practices. Find a group cooking immersion like the ones we offer through Vegan Fusion (see page 357), or a local chapter of the Community Complete Health Improvement Program (CHIP; see page 341); the group's encouragement and shared sense of purpose is a powerful aspect of these programs' success. In fact, more health and medicine practitioners are moving toward the group model of care because of how effective group support can be.

As you work to incorporate these practices into your daily life, you will notice how a deeper sense of wholeness and satisfaction naturally arises.

part one

THE HEALING

CHAPTER 1

Preventable Health Challenges

When diet is wrong, medicine is of no use.
When diet is correct, medicine is of no need.
—AYURVEDIC PROVERB

Research continues to mount that many of the major health challenges facing society can be prevented and reversed through adopting a plant-based diet. The evidence indicates that the overconsumption of the saturated fat and cholesterol in animal products leads to serious health problems, such as obesity, heart disease, diabetes, hypertension, gout, kidney stones, and certain forms of cancer.

According to statistics from the World Health Organization (WHO), noncommunicable diseases (NCDs), such as cancer, heart disease, lung disease, and diabetes, are responsible for 63 percent of deaths worldwide—double the number of deaths from infectious diseases (including HIV/AIDS, tuberculosis, and malaria), maternal and perinatal conditions, and nutritional deficiencies combined. The principal known causes of premature death from NCDs are tobacco use, poor diet, physical inactivity, and harmful alcohol consumption. NCDs can be prevented.

They affect not only high-income countries, but middle- and low-income countries as well. By 2020, NCDs are expected to account for seven of every ten deaths in the world; however, in the United States, they already do. These projections suggest that NCDs and the death, illness, and disability they cause will soon dominate health-care costs and are causing public health officials, governments, and multinational institutions to rethink how they approach this growing global challenge.

The WHO recommends that health practitioners, policymakers, community members, and industry leaders must work together in a multilateral fashion to create comprehensive solutions to this growing challenge. The real change must come through education and expansion of access to whole plant foods so that individuals may choose to gain control of their own health.

According to the International Data Corporation's 2014 paper on chronic disease burden, "Health behavior is one of the most important determinants of health, and at the same time it is the one that people can influence. It has been suggested that healthy lifestyle practices, such as healthy diet, regular exercise, control of weight, smoking, sleep and stress management, and moderate use of alcohol, would prevent 90% of type 2 diabetes, 80% of coronary heart disease, and 70% of stroke."

Stated otherwise: Much of the current "health-care crisis" can actually be easily addressed by making a shift toward a vegan diet. And the solution affects not just our health but the worldwide economy, as well. You may not realize the connection between the pothole on your street and what people are eating for dinner. But when you contemplate all of the financial resources that are directed toward treating preventable diseases, and consider the impact that redirecting those resources toward social services, education, infrastructure, and so forth—would have on society, you will see that the connection is not so farfetched.

When exploring the following list, please keep in mind the cost of treating these challenges, both in terms of human suffering, as well as the social cost of preventable medical bills.

Heart Disease

Heart disease, or cardiovascular disease, refers to a variety of health ailments that include coronary artery disease, arrhythmias, infections of the heart, abnormalities with the heart muscle, and congenital heart defects. With heart disease, heart attacks, strokes, and/or chest pains can ensue.

Historically, populations that consume a whole food, plant-based diet have a significantly lower proportion of people suffering from heart disease. At one time, only kings and queens suffered from heart disease, gout, and other diseases of dietary excess. Today, that privilege of dying from heart disease has spread to everyone eating the standard American diet (SAD). It has increased since 1985—and simultaneously the standard American diet tends even further toward high fat, high salt, high sugar, and high levels of MSG and aspartame.

According to the Centers for Disease Control (CDC):

- Heart disease is the leading cause of death in the United States for both men and women. People of all ages and backgrounds can get the condition.
- About 610,000 people die of heart disease in the United States every year—that's 1 in every 4 deaths.
- Coronary heart disease is the most common type of heart disease, killing over 370,000 people annually.
- Every year about 735,000 Americans have a heart attack. Of these, 525,000 are a first heart attack and 210,000 happen in people who have already had a heart attack.
- High blood pressure, high LDL cholesterol, and smoking are key risk factors for heart disease. About half of Americans (49%) have at least one of these three risk factors.

The CDC diet recommendation is: Eat a healthy diet that is low in salt; low in total fat, saturated fat, and cholesterol; and rich in fresh fruits and vegetables.

It is becoming increasingly clear that lifestyle changes can prevent or reverse many instances of heart disease. Regular blood pressure checks are important to monitor for hypertension, as well as diabetes and cholesterol checks.

Dr. Caldwell Esselstyn Jr. from the Cleveland Clinic, who wrote the book *Prevent and Reverse Heart Disease: The Revolutionary, Scientifically Proven, Nutrition-Based Cure,* has had immense success treating heart disease with diet and lifestyle changes. His early research showed that certain cultures in the world do not suffer from heart troubles, and thereby he studies those diets: of rural Chinese, of Papua New Guinea highlanders, of central Africans, and of Indians from Mexico.

He believes that prevention and reversal of heart disease lies in the consumption of a whole food, plant-based diet devoid of any processed oils whatsoever. Dr. Esselstyn is well known for saying that such a diet is not in any way "extreme" when compared to the procedure of cutting open the body so as to work on the heart. He says that by following this diet, the consumer will be "heart attack proof," and cites never having to count calories again as one of the benefits of the regimen.

His patients have seen wide rates of success: sharp drops in cholesterol as well as widening of the arteries and thereby recovery from heart disease. He believes heart disease is fully preventable and purely a result of the standard American diet (see page 25).

Dr. Dean Ornish, another pioneer in the cardiological medical world, undertook clinical research that proved even severe heart disease could be reversed not with drugs or surgery but with lifestyle changes, such as diet, exercise, and wellness habits. Dr. Ornish posits that emotional stress, depression, anxiety, low levels of exercise, and eating a diet with too many stimulants and too much saturated fat and cholesterol gang up on the heart in harmful ways.

Following his Spectrum program has resulted in numerous reductions and reversals of heart disease. This holistic lifestyle and wellness program rounds out a diet low in fat and high in unprocessed plant-based foods, regular exercise, stress management, and peer support. The name "Spectrum" refers to the individual choice of how involved the lifestyle changes need to be, personalizing one's needs, preferences, and genetics.

HEALING STORIES

I was diagnosed with nonischemic cardiomyopathy in 2008. I was told that due to my inability to tolerate the drug regimen that I was probably looking at a heart transplant. My heart was three times its normal size and my ability to pump blood was down from a normal 61% to 9%. I was immediately implanted with a pacemaker to await the transplant.

With the pacemaker, I could now tolerate the drugs, all 8 of them. I was constantly fatigued. I still could not walk more than a block. In addition, I went from 117 pounds to 130 in less than six months. I knew I couldn't keep going this way. My doctors were not offering me any other options. Consequently, after reading Dr. Joel Fuhrman's *Eat to Live* I decided that a vegan diet was the way to go.

I changed my diet and my life at the same time. It took me two years to get off all my medications, the transplant was completely off the table, I lost fifteen pounds, and I now dance three times a week with no fatigue. I am also 63 years old. My doctors just couldn't believe the change. They had never seen such a turnaround for a heart condition as severe as mine. I now teach vegan cooking classes and coach whenever possible.

−R.C, Seattle, Washington

Diabetes

A person with diabetes has excessive glucose in the blood. To convert glucose into energy in the cells, the body uses insulin made in the pancreas and released into the bloodstream. In the case of a diabetic, the glucose or blood sugar overpowers the amount of insulin. Symptoms include excessive thirst and urination, fatigue, blurred vision, high blood pressure, infections, and the presence of ketones in the urine, a result of there not being enough insulin in the blood.

According to the Centers for Disease Control:

- Almost 30 million children and adults in the United States have diabetes.
- 86 million Americans have prediabetes.
- 1.7 million Americans are diagnosed with diabetes every year.

It has been shown that a low-fat, plant-based diet improves insulin presence, reduces blood sugar, and helps with weight loss. Weight loss is very effective in preventing the onset of diabetes, as the relationship between overweight and type 2 diabetes is direct. Besides diet, physical activity in the form of regular exercise is a good diabetes counter. Additionally, consuming more plants and plant-based foods may give you more energy and a feeling of lightness—which can help motivate you for physical fitness.

Dr. Gabriel Cousens is an award-winning author of several books and a pioneer in the plant-based medical community. His book *There Is a Cure for Diabetes: The Tree of Life 21-Day + Program,* details the success of this three-week program at the Tree of Life Center in Arizona. In the program, which relies on green juice fasting and a 100 percent organic, nutrient-dense, vegan, low-glycemic, low-insulin-scoring diet—"a cuisine that is sustainable for the duration of one's life, and prepared and eaten with love," he writes in his book. Dr. Cousens has released diabetes patients from medications and insulin shots within four days, and rendered the patient to a nondiabetic state by two weeks.

In a study of 110 participants who participated in this program:

- 28% of IDDM type 2 diabetics reversed their diabetes after 3 weeks with no insulin and a fasting blood sugar (FBS) of less than 100.
- 60% of the NIDDM type 2 diabetics were off all oral medications after 3 weeks with an FBS of less than 100.

• 100% of prediabetics healed.

Dr. Neal Barnard is a physician and clinical researcher with the George Washington School of Medicine, who led the groundbreaking research on treating diabetes naturally that has been published in many leading journals. In Dr. Neal Barnard's *Program for Reversing Diabetes: The Scientifically Proven System for Reversing Diabetes Without Drugs,* he demonstrates that a low-fat vegan diet improves glycemic control and cardiovascular risk factors in randomized clinical trials in individuals with type 2 diabetes. The studies also show that by adopting this diet—free of all animal products and added vegetable oils—individuals can lower their cholesterol, reduce their blood pressure, and lose weight without deprivation.

The book explains how the diet actually alters what goes on in an individual's cells. Rather than just compensating for malfunctioning insulin, like other treatment plans, Dr. Barnard's program helps repair how the body uses insulin. The Physicians Committee for Responsible Medicine reports that his program was found to be three times more effective than the American Diabetes Association's dietary guidelines at controlling blood sugar.

🐾 I am a 66-year-old retired firefighter. Three years ago, in a routine annual checkup with my family doctor, the diabetes test showed that I had a result of 11.6—certified diabetes. My doctor insisted I go on diabetes medication immediately. I was shocked to receive this news as I was in excellent physical condition and not overweight. I was leaving for a trip and needed to take some time to process this news. A close friend gave me a copy of T. Colin Campbell's book *The China Study.* [Note: For more on *The China Study,* see pages 12–13] It was perfect timing.

I now understood why I had become diabetic and I immediately adopted a whole food, plant-based diet. When I returned to Canada three months later I went back to my doctor, who was pleased to tell me that the medication must have worked because my blood test was now 5.6. I told him I never took the pills and had not even picked up the prescription. Instead I had been strictly following a whole food, plant-based diet. He simply could not believe it. I am so happy I read *The China Study* and took this optimal road to health.

—G.T., Toronto, Canada

THE EXPERTS SPEAK
*The Plant-Powered Dietitian,
Sharon Palmer, RDN*

Since I published my first book, *The Plant-Powered Diet,* I have heard from so many people about their successes related to taking on a plant-based diet. One of my most favorite, inspiring stories came from Randy in Oklahoma, which I shared in my book. Here's his story in his own words:

🐾 At the age of 55, I was changing my granddaughter's diaper and I thought, "If I remain diabetic I'm going to lose ten or twelve years of my grandbaby's life." Being from Oklahoma, deciding to become a vegan was a stretch. I imagine I doubled that demographic. It's remarkable: After thirteen days my type 2 diabetes reversed—my doctor was astounded. I started with losing weight, then my doctor took me off all diabetes, cholesterol, and blood pressure meds and my energy skyrocketed. I started hiking six miles—I felt like it, because it didn't hurt anymore due to all the anti-inflammatory foods I was eating. I lost 41 pounds in 14 weeks—I went from a size 40 waist to 28 or 30. Before I had never eaten cauliflower, cabbage or kale. My vegetables were limited to beans, corn and fried potatoes. Now the list of vegetables I eat is lengthy. I use lots of spices to flavor them. Moving to a plant-based diet has been the most intelligent and healthy thing I have ever done. I am planning to walk all the way across the U. S. as a testament to my new lifestyle.

High Cholesterol

Cholesterol helps the body build healthy cells and make hormones. It has a purpose in the body, yet it is not needed in the diet at all; the body, in a healthy metabolic state, is able to make all of the cholesterol it needs.

There are different types of cholesterol. The most well known are LDL, which is artery-clogging, and HDL, which helps remove fats from the bloodstream by escorting them to the liver for removal. A routine blood test will show your total cholesterol number, currently recommended to be under 200, and LDL recommended to be under 130, though some health professionals would agree that having these numbers even lower is actually healthier. The recommended ratio of total to HDL is 3.5 to

1. The different types of cholesterol each have specific biochemical functions that balance each other out when they exist in proper proportions. Since there is no essential need for exogenous cholesterol, the excess amounts taken into the body by eating certain foods can tip the body's cholesterol balance into the disorder known as hyperlipidemia, or high cholesterol. The resulting fatty deposits can become inflamed and clog arteries, keeping adequate blood from flowing to the heart, which can increase heart attack and stroke risk. One danger is that high cholesterol is symptomless.

The American College of Cardiology and the American Heart Association released new assessment guidelines for cardiac risk in 2013, which look at lifestyle risk factors as well; however, the first-line treatment protocol remains statin drugs.

- 73.5 million adults (31.7%) in the United States have high low-density lipoprotein (LDL).
- Fewer than 1 out of every 3 adults (29.5%) with high LDL cholesterol has the condition under control.
- Less than half (48.1%) of adults with high LDL cholesterol are getting treatment to lower their levels.
- People with high total cholesterol have approximately twice the risk for heart disease as people with ideal levels.
- Nearly 31 million adult Americans have a total cholesterol level greater than 240 mg/dL.

High cholesterol is sometimes linked to genetics, but also is largely preventable and/or treatable through diet and exercise, with or without medication. A common correlation is often found between high cholesterol and an unhealthy and inactive lifestyle, and mainly the result of a diet overstocked with animal products. Trans fats, commonly found in many packaged snacks, can play a role in the cholesterol picture, and should be avoided. A shift to a whole food, plant-based diet can bring about large and swift cholesterol point drops, given that plant foods have little to no cholesterol. Cholesterol has continued to be a very prominent topic in nutrition. There is a lot of confusing information out there. The popularity of statin drugs as well as paleo and other diet trends that promote animal fats as a healthy source of nutrients are major contributors to all this confusion.

The oxidation of LDL cholesterol leads to plaque formation that damages blood vessels. This oxidation can be prevented by naturally occurring antioxidants found in high concentrations in plant foods. Plant foods are also high in soluble fiber and healthy polyunsaturated fats, which help to lower cholesterol by allowing the body to properly metabolize cholesterol for use instead of storing it where it can cause damage. So, a plant-based diet has many well-known powerful benefits to cholesterol regulation, along with exercise and an overall wellness plan. Many people experience a dramatic reduction in their LDL cholesterol levels within several weeks of adopting a plant-based diet. This is particularly profound when you consider that cholesterol-lowering medication is one of the most highly prescribed medications!

My journey toward eating plant-based began by accident. It was a simple routine annual visit with my doctor that shook me to my core. The results showed my cholesterol was nearing 200. Which for a woman of color is basically a glaring neon sign for a death sentence. My doctor ordered another test with a visit from me in two weeks, which also included me going to see a cardiologist. This was serious and I was scared. Really scared.

By the end of the week, I'd learned that my body would be best served by following a vegan diet. Yet, I delayed the complete change for a few weeks to learn the basics. Once I felt comfortable, I changed my diet to vegan and my cholesterol went down within a month or two to 150. My body naturally regulated my weight, even though I was not overweight. I did a little yoga, Zumba, and mostly walked.

As time went on, I eagerly dove into the vegan lifestyle without looking back. I did not feel limited in any way. There are a multitude of vegetables, legumes, grains, nuts, seeds, mushrooms, and fruits that heal the body naturally from within. It has been almost 12 years now. I deeply believe that food is medicine in balance.

—J.W., Orlando, FL

Cancer

Cancer is defined as uncontrolled growth of abnormal cells in the body. This faulty response develops when the body's normal control mechanism stops working. Old cells do not die and instead grow out of control, forming new, abnormal cells. The extra cells may form a mass of tissue,

THE EXPERTS SPEAK
Michael Greger, MD

A plant-based diet may also help in averting and/or slowing certain cancers (such as breast cancer, prostate cancer, cervical cancer, and colon cancer). This is in part because plant foods contain antiaging, anticancer antioxidants (on average 64 times more than animal foods), fiber, and phytochemicals, which in some cases can even help repair DNA damage. Even two weeks on a plant-based diet appears to dramatically improve cancer defenses.

The blood of those on plant-based diets is more effective at killing cancer cells than those who eat a standard diet even if they exercise strenuously. But WHY? What secret weapons do plants possess against cancer? There are several ways plants help us prevent and fight cancer. Angiogenesis inhibitors (natural chemicals that starve tumors) in plant foods may help prevent cancerous tumors from connecting to a blood supply. Additionally, restriction of a certain amino acid, called methionine, is best achieved through a plant-based diet, as it starves human tumors of the amino acid necessary for their growth—all while potentially extending our life span.

Another explanation about why cancer rates are lower among those eating plant-based diets may be because of lower levels of IGF-1 (insulin-Like growth factor-1), a cancer-promoting growth hormone, and increased levels of the IGF-1 binding protein due to a reduction of animal protein intake. Your pituitary gland naturally elevates IGF-1 levels when you're a kid so you grow, and then those levels come back down as a young adult. Should your levels stay a bit too high as an adult, though, there's this constant message to your cells to grow, grow, grow, divide, don't die, keep going, keep growing. And so not surprisingly, the more IGF-1 you have in your bloodstream, the higher your risk for cancer. More IGF-1, more prostate cancer; more IGF-1, more breast cancer.[1]

Of course it's not the original tumor that tends to kill you, it's the metastases. IGF-1 is a growth factor—it helps things grow—so, it helps cancer cells break off from the main tumor, migrate into surrounding tissues, and invade the bloodstream. What do you think helps breast cancer get into the bone? IGF-1. And the liver? IGF-1. Lung, brain, lymph nodes? IGF-1. It helps transform normal cells into cancer cells in the first place, then helps them survive, proliferate, self-renew, grow, migrate, invade, stabilize into new tumors, and even helps hook up the blood supply to the new tumor. IGF-1 is a growth hormone that makes things grow—that's what it does. But too much growth when we're all grown up can mean cancer.

How do we avoid excess levels of IGF-1? If you measure the blood levels of IGF-1 before and after eleven days on a plant-based diet with exercise, IGF-1 levels significantly drop. And IGF-1 binding protein levels significantly rise. That's one way our body tries to protect itself from cancer—from excessive growth—by releasing a binding protein into our bloodstream to tie up IGF-1. It's like our body's emergency brake. Yeah, sure, in as little as eleven days a healthy diet can reprogram your body to slow down IGF-1 production, but you still have all that IGF-1 circulating in your bloodstream from the bacon and eggs you had the week before. So, your liver releases a snatch squad of binding proteins to take it out of circulation pronto. Exercise alone can drop IGF-1 levels, but you need the plant-based diet to get those kind of snatch squad levels. 🌿

called a tumor. Some cancers, such as leukemia, a cancer of the blood and bone marrow, don't form tumors.

According to the Centers for Disease Control:

- Cancer is the second-leading cause of death in the United States, exceeded only by heart disease, and accounts for nearly 1 of every 4 deaths.
- Nearly 14.5 million Americans with a history of cancer were alive on January 1, 2014.

Once diagnosis occurs, most people immediately begin a combination of treatments, such as surgery with chemotherapy and/or radiation therapy. Other treatments offered are immunotherapy, targeted therapy, or hormone therapy. Unfortunately, diet and lifestyle are not usually addressed in conventional treatment, despite the fact that a clear connection has been observed between the prevention and reversal of certain types of cancers and diet.

Put simply, research shows that some animal-based foods seem to stimulate growth of abnormal cells in the promotion stage of cancer; and plant-based foods, especially antioxidants, are proven to halt or reverse cancerous cells in the promotion stage. In fact, the National Institutes of Health evidence guide to nursing practices advises that "appropriate dietary guidance is an important component of self-care. Evidence well supports the consumption of plant-based, low saturated fat diets to promote overall health and survival. Oncology nurses should share this information with patients and encourage

the importance of weight management, and the consumption of diets that parallel guidelines set forth in the American Cancer Society guide."

Research has shown that a plant-based diet has reduced or reversed a variety of cancers, including mouth, esophageal, larynx, stomach, lung, prostate, and pancreas. Conversely, research identifies animal products, especially red meat and processed meats, as increasing chances of cancer, especially colorectal.

Meat consists of multiple components, such as heme iron. Meat can also contain chemicals that form during meat processing or cooking. In 2015, the World Health Organization classified processed meat—meaning meat that has been salted, cured, fermented, smoked, or otherwise enhanced for flavor and preservation—as an IARC Group 1, carcinogenic to humans.

As classified by the International Agency for Research on Cancer (IARC), Group 1 is the same category as well-known causes of cancer, such as tobacco smoking and asbestos. The IARC Working Group concluded that eating processed meat causes colorectal cancer. The risk generally increases with the amount of meat consumed. An analysis of data from ten studies estimated that every 50-gram portion of processed meat eaten daily increases the risk of colorectal cancer by about 18 percent. The IARC Working Group also saw an association with stomach cancer, but the evidence is not conclusive. Red meat was classified as Group 2A, probably carcinogenic to humans. Evidence is strongest for an association with eating red meat and colorectal cancer, but there is also evidence of links with pancreatic cancer and prostate cancer.

According to the most recent estimates by the Global Burden of Disease Project, an independent academic research organization, about thirty-four thousand cancer deaths per year worldwide can be attributed to diets high in processed meat. Eating red meat has not yet been established as a cause of cancer, but if the reported associations were proven to be causal, the Global Burden of Disease Project has estimated that diets high in red meat could be responsible for fifty thousand cancer deaths per year worldwide.

There has been no conclusion about whether a safe level of meat consumption exists. In addition to carcinogens, another important topic of study is the influence of certain hormones on cancers, namely insulin-like growth factor (IGF-1). IGF-1 is a natural human growth hormone instrumental in normal growth during childhood, but in adulthood it can promote abnormal growth—the proliferation, spread (metastasis), and invasion of cancer. IGF-1's natural function is to help things grow, so it helps cancer cells break off from the main tumor, migrate into surrounding tissues, and invade the bloodstream.

It seems that animal proteins, because they resemble our own proteins, raise IGF-1 levels, whereas plant proteins seem to lower them.

In a Pritikin study referenced by Dr. Michael Greger, those eating exclusively vegan had significantly lower IGF-1 levels and higher IGF binding proteins than those just eating vegetarian, suggesting that the more plant-based one's diet becomes, the lower one's risk of fueling growth hormone dependent cancer growth. When added to a petri dish with prostate cancer cells, a drop of blood from a person eating a vegan diet showed about eight times' better efficiency at slowing down the rate of growth than did the blood of those on the standard American diet. After a year on a plant-based diet, participants' blood eliminated the cancer.

This study was duplicated at Pritikin with women using three different types of breast cancer cells, and in just two weeks of eating a plant-based diet, their blood significantly slowed down and stopped the growth of cancer cells at a much higher rate than before the two weeks. Further study shows a lasting effect. When people adopt a plant-based diet, their IGF-1 levels go down very quickly, and if they stay on a plant-based diet, their levels continue to drop even further.

The results of these studies were published in several professional journals, including the *American Journal of Clinical Nutrition* and *Nutrition and Cancer*, and concluded that the blood of those on a vegan diet was dramatically less hospitable to cancer.

The China Study, written by researcher T. Colin Campbell and his son, Thomas M. Campbell, documents the results of one of the most comprehensive nutritional studies ever conducted. Its research is based on a twenty-year study of dietary and disease patterns in rural China. The study found that there is a strong correlation between a whole food, plant-based diet and the avoidance or reduction in certain diseases, including cancers. Genes were not shown to be as much of a factor in disease prevalence as diet; instead the researchers surmised that it is the antioxidants in plants that protect the body from free radicals and counteract cancer growth. Furthermore, researchers showed they could turn on and off the growth of cancer cells by the administering and removal of casein, a protein found in cow's milk products.

Ideally this newer understanding of how diet directly affects hormone stimulated cell growth will lead to a more holistic approach in cancer treatment. In the meantime, individuals can improve their body's cancer-fighting abilities by the choices they make every day. Including as many colorful foods in the diet is a good way of absorbing a variety of cancer-fighting nutrients. Red contains lycopene, orange provides beta-carotene, yellow-orange mostly delivers vitamin C, green contains folate, green-white provides lutein, white contains allicins, blue gives anthocyanins, red-purple provides resveratrol, and browns donate fiber, said to be especially effective in countering colorectal cancer.

Obesity

Obesity is commonly defined as an excess of body fat, usually 20 percent and up from a person's ideal body weight, which is derived from a person's BMI (body mass index). Bariatrics is the study and treatment of obesity, and is becoming a more common practice as obesity emerges as a growing health problem.

An obese person is subject to more disorders and debilitations than a person of normal weight, such as heart disease, stroke, diabetes, hypertension, osteoarthritis, and such cancers as endometrial, colon, and breast. Additionally breathing difficulty and sleep apnea, increased risk of bone fracturing, and psychological and social challenges are obesity risks.

- More than one-third (34.9% or 78.6 million) of US adults are obese.
- In 2008 the estimated annual medical cost of obesity in the United States was 147 billion US dollars; this is $1,429 higher per person than the cost of those of normal weight.
- It is estimated that at current trend levels, by 2030, 86.3% adults will be overweight or obese and 51.1% will be obese.

Childhood obesity is a serious problem in the United States. Approximately 17 percent (or 12.7 million) of children and adolescents 2 to 19 years of age are obese. There is some good news: according to a study in the *Journal of American Medical Association* listed on the Centers for Disease Control website, the prevalence of obesity among children aged 2 to 5 years decreased significantly from 13.9 percent in 2003–2004 to 8.4 percent in 2011–2012 compared with 17.7 percent of 6- to 11-year-olds and 20.5 percent of 12- to 19-year-olds. This positive progress is linked to participation in federal nutrition programs as well as more awareness about the dangers of consuming sugar-sweetened beverages.

Most people can understand that with a personal commitment to a healthy lifestyle that includes moderate exercise, being

THE EXPERTS SPEAK
Joel Kahn, MD

Turn the clock back to 1990. It was in July and I was in Ann Arbor, Michigan, just a week into my first job as a hot-shot cardiologist trained to fix any blockage with a balloon catheter. I had just completed four years of cardiology training working side by side with Dr. Geoffrey Hartzler, the world-famous pioneer who developed aggressive angioplasty heart therapy. I knew the answer to heart disease was to put a balloon any and everywhere.

It was during that month that in my mail at home was the prestigious journal *The Lancet*. I was reading the table of contents and saw something that caught my eye: a randomized trial of intensive cardiac lifestyle change that compared a plant-based, low-fat diet to conventional therapy. This study was published by Dr. Dean Ornish, an internist focused on healing heart disease in San Francisco and just a few years older than I was. The study, called the Lifestyle Heart Trial, demonstrated that long-standing heart disease was reversible with intelligent use of the fork, the feet, and a focus on community and stress management. Lifestyle changes combined with group support and hugs could melt plaque away without using my hallowed catheters and balloons. The audacity!

I was fertile ground for Dr. Ornish's groundbreaking contribution to heart disease care. I had been a vegetarian since my undergraduate days. A few years later, after reading *A Diet for a New America* by John Robbins, I moved closer and closer to an entirely plant-based diet due to my concerns about health, the environment,

and animal kindness. Ironically, given what we know today about meat, never did I suspect that the choices I made in my kitchen would turn out to be a therapy to reduce angina chest pain, lower hospital admission rates, and reduce cardiac events.

More reading led me to the work of Caldwell Esselstyn Jr., MD, at the Cleveland Clinic; Nathan Pritikin in Miami; Neal Barnard in Washington, DC; Hans Diehl, PhD, in Loma Linda; John McDougall, MD, in Santa Rosa; and so many more people across the country, all studying the effects of plant-based diets on cardiac disease, diabetes, dementia, obesity, hypertension, and other chronic illnesses.

I began asking every patient I saw to become a student of this lifestyle and appreciate the impact it could have on the length of their days and their life. I started giving them a list of resources to review between visits, written on an Rx pad. Ultimately, I created a website (www.drjoelkahn.com) with these and additional resources, including blogs that I myself began to write on heart disease prevention and reversal.

The science of plant-based eating has grown considerably and I lecture on the topic frequently. Dr. Ornish followed up his Lifestyle Heart Trial with results at five years showing even better reversal of heart blockages with his program. He then went on to track thousands of study participants and showed that this program saved dollars compared to conventional care. This was enough to get Medicare to approve his intensive cardiac rehabilitation program for payment in the last few years.

Dr. Ornish then has gone on to study prostate cancer patients assigned to watchful waiting and randomized them to his program or conventional care. In a year, those following his lifestyle regimen had a reduction in their PSA blood test while the other group had it go up, a worrisome trend for the conventional eaters. He also showed that the blood of his lifestyle group actually killed prostate cancer cells eight times more readily than the usual care group, as if you can make your blood into chemotherapy by eating lots of fruits and vegetables. That is a wild and wonderful thought. Finally, he worked with Nobel Prize–winning researcher Elizabeth Blackburn, PhD, to show that his program activated an enzyme called telomerase and caused gene telomeres to lengthen, all suggesting that his plan was a true antiaging therapy.

Around the same time as Dr. Ornish was publishing his heart disease reversal data, Dr. Caldwell Esselstyn Jr. of the Cleveland Clinic began publishing results he was observing in patients with advanced heart disease that he was treating with a completely plant-based diet without added oils. He presented cases showing dramatic reversal of long-standing blocked heart arteries, relief of chest pain, improved sexual function, and reduced needs for hospitalizations and procedures. He updated his data in 2014 to nearly two hundred patients, showing the same results were sustained.

In further support of the power of a plant-based lifestyle on health have been a flurry of publications from the Adventist Health Study. Loma Linda, California, has the longest life span of any community in the United States and one of the top five in the world, attributed to the residents' plant-rich diet. Beginning in 1958, the habits and health outcomes of the Seventh Day Adventists have been tracked until this day. In 2014 they published their most recent data showing reduced death rates in follow-up of vegan members of the church versus the omnivores. They also showed reduced problems with diabetes, hypertension, high cholesterol, obesity, and many cancers. Not a bad outcome for filling your plate with fruits and vegetables.

Every step of the way, this journey has rewarded me, especially as I see the movement I first read about all those years ago grow and resonate. For instance, a volunteer support group I helped create in Detroit (www.pbnsg.org) for persons who want to prevent or reverse chronic diseases with nutrition drew not the fifty or so members I'd anticipated, but over one thousand—a number I'm sure I never would have predicted in 1990.

The future can be so bright if medical school administrators, hospital executives, chiefs of cardiology, and individual practitioners can appreciate that preventive cardiology using plant-based diets is science-based, good for business, good for education, and the right thing to do. While I still practice interventional cardiology (I don't want to retire those Hartzler-trained hands), what excites me more is the prevention side. I am confident that as many as 80 percent of heart attacks and the majority of heart procedures and events can be eliminated, along with their pain, suffering, and expense, by teaching the next generation the power of their fork, their feet, and their fingers. 🌱

overweight and obese are preventable and reversible states. But confusion about what constitutes a healthy diet can sometimes be the biggest barrier.

It is important to recognize that losing weight is not just a matter of deciding to eat less. Restrictive dieting often leads to deprivation and a yoyo cycle of loss and gain, not to mention guilt and shame when the weight comes back. Scientists are finding that even though we are an obese society, we are also nutrient deficient—we're eating more and nourishing ourselves less! It turns out that the diet of convenience that has developed over the last several decades simply cannot support the needs of our physiology.

The time has come for us to see beyond the temptations of the food industry and listen to our body's true needs. Replacing sugars, fats, and salt-laden processed foods with whole plant foods, especially fruits and vegetables, is the only path out of this epidemic. A foundation of healthy nutrition from plants is what provides the energy, motivation, and clarity of mind to then make further lifestyle improvements.

According to Dr. Joel Fuhrman, "The key to optimizing your health and achieving your ideal body weight is to eat predominantly those foods that have a relatively high proportion of nutrients (noncaloric food factors) to calories (carbohydrates, fats, and proteins)."

The more nutrient-dense food you consume, the more you will be satisfied with fewer calories and the less you'll crave low-nutrient, empty-calorie foods. (For more on nutrient density, see Chapter 4.)

Mental and Emotional Health Imbalances

Generalized fatigue, mood swings, and episodes of depression or anxiety, even at subclinical levels, are things most people have experienced at some time. All of these complaints can have a multitude of causes and a wide range of specific details, depending on the individual.

There are several ways that plant nutrients can help support us during times when energy is low, stress is high, or emotional stability becomes a challenge to maintain. A plant-heavy diet can help us avoid foods that may exacerbate energy and mood fluctuations during times of stress, when the first impulse is to grab something sugary, fried, or salty to satisfy an emotional need. When our cells are receiving positive support through proper macro and micronutrients, we are much better equipped to adapt to outside stressors that use up nutrient reserves. Proper nutrition also helps to maintain the integrity of our immune system.

Some examples to keep in mind are:

- Phytonutrients. A variety of colorful foods, such as beets, red bell peppers, berries, sweet potatoes, and others, provide an array of protective and restorative phytonutrients, including plenty of antioxidants, which reduce inflammation in the body and brain.
- Trace minerals, found in foods grown in healthy soil, provide cofactors necessary for the formation of certain hormones that stabilize mood and support clear thought patterns.
- Fiber, found naturally in fruits and veggies, improves digestion, helps alleviate sluggishness and clears wastes and toxins from the body, leading to a lighter, more energized state.
- Whole grains help release tryptophan, an amino acid that supports the release of serotonin in the brain. Choose low-glycemic options, such as brown rice, or ancient grains, such as quinoa, amaranth or millet.
- Legumes, such as beans, green peas, and edamame, provide magnesium, a mineral needed by every organ in the body. Magnesium promotes many things from a healthy heart to muscle relaxation to strong bones. It also plays a role in the development of serotonin, a neurotransmitter that regulates mood.
- Green vegetables offer a healthful dose of vitamins B6 and B9 (folate). B vitamins are critical for brain health, reducing the risk for both memory loss and depression, and also play important roles in neurological health and energy production.
- Healthy fats. Omega-3 fatty acids found in walnuts, hemp/flax/pumpkin seeds, and avocados improve circulation in the brain, leading to improved mood and memory function. Healthy fats improve nerve cell communication and transport of mood-stabilizing chemicals through cell membranes. Researchers from the National Institutes of Health report that omega-3 fatty acids are as effective as commonly prescribed antidepressant drugs at treating major depressive illness.

A study published in the March-April 2015 *American Journal of Health Promotion* reported impressive results of diet change.[2] Close to one hundred GEICO employees, who were either overweight or diagnosed with type 2 diabetes, adopted a low-fat, high-fiber vegan diet. After eighteen weeks, the study participants lost an average of 10 pounds, lowered LDL cholesterol by 13 points, and improved blood sugar control if they had type 2 diabetes. Another exciting result was that they also boosted productivity while alleviating symptoms of depression, anxiety, and fatigue.

Hope Is on Our Plate

It is well known that plants have the power to heal and transform our lives. Science is just at the infancy stage of understanding the interplay between food and health.

A comprehensive meta-analysis research study published in 2014 in the *British Medical Journal* found that after looking at several databases of cohort studies from various populations ranging from the 1950s up to 2013, they concluded that intake of fruit and vegetables is the most common factor associated with a reduced risk of mortality from all causes, including cardiovascular disease. They noticed a close dependent relationship where risk of all causes of mortality was decreased by 5 percent for each additional serving a day of fruit and vegetables, by 6 percent

Eating seven or more portions of fruit and vegetables a day reduces your risk of death at any point in time by 42% compared to eating less than one portion, reports a UCL study published in the *Journal of Epidemiology & Community Health* in 2014. Researchers used the Health Survey for England to study the eating habits of 65,226 people representative of the English population between 2001 and 2013, and found that the more fruit and vegetables they ate, the less likely they were to die at any age.

- Eating seven or more portions reduces the specific risks of death by cancer and heart disease by 25% and 31% respectively.
- Compared to eating less than one portion of fruit and vegetables, the risk of death by any cause is reduced by 14% by eating one to three portions, 29% for three to five portions, 36% for five to seven portions and 42% for seven or more.

for fruit consumption, and by 5 percent for vegetable consumption.

These are just a small sampling of major health challenges that can and have been improved by adopting a plant-based diet. More are being discovered all of the time. Change can begin today, with you.

The Limitations of Modern Medicine

The accomplishments of modern medicine have been prodigious. We have seen the development of proton accelerators that can zap cancers, surgical robots that can be employed in performing coronary bypass surgeries, and advances in molecular biology and genetics that can open doors to amazing new worlds. And yet these advances in high-tech medicine to take care of acute and episodic diseases have not altered the advances of our modern killer diseases.

Rarely found some one hundred years ago, cardiovascular disease (coronary heart disease and stroke) and cancers of the breast, prostate, colon, and lungs are now claiming every third and fourth American life, respectively.[3] Disturbingly, the chance of becoming a diabetic in America for a newborn baby is now one in three.[4] And we have no medical cure.[5] These are chronic diseases. And often, the best we can do with chronic diseases is to manage them symptomatically. But the medical cure for most of them is elusive. Concurrently, we have seen an enormous rise in the prevalence of excess weight where now two out of three American adults are overweight or obese.[6] As a result, manufacturers have to supersize everything from shirts to pants and from gurneys to coffins.

And yet, many of these chronic diseases, currently consuming more than 80 percent of our national health care budget, are largely preventable and even reversible.[7] Modern epidemiology has unraveled the mystery: most of our modern killer diseases are lifestyle related. They relate to the use of tobacco, sedentary living, and, preeminently, to our rich diet. The answer, then, is not a mechanical or pharma-cological approach, but a lifestyle-based approach to attack the causes of these diseases.

Connecting the GDP and Modern Killer Diseases

Examining the global distribution of these chronic diseases, a strong economic gradient emerges: the higher the national income (GDP [gross domestic product]), the greater the prevalence of these diseases. The massive China Study, masterminded by T. Colin Campbell, PhD, of Cornell University, for instance, clearly showed two clusters of diseases in China: "diseases of affluence" (coronary artery disease, stroke, hypertension, diabetes, osteoporosis, and cancer of the breast, prostate, lung and blood) and "diseases of poverty" (pneumonia and tuberculosis, digestive diseases, cancer of the stomach and liver, and infectious and parasitic diseases).[8] While the diseases of affluence correlated closely with the level of economic development and the abundance of processed food and animal products high in fat and protein, the diseases of poverty were predominantly intertwined with poor sanitation, nutritional deficiencies, and poor food quality because of a lack of refrigeration.

Changes in the Diet Composition

Developing countries in the past had to rely predominantly on "foods-as-grown." They relied basically on corn and beans, potatoes and yams, wheat and rice, and plenty of fruits and vegetables. These inexpensive yet nutritionally and fiber-rich plant foods were naturally very low in fat, salt and sugar. They provided more than enough protein, even though the intake of animal protein was usually quite low and with

continues

continued from previous page

that also the consumption of cholesterol and saturated fat. Most of the calories consumed then came from unrefined complex carbohydrates, the body's preferred and clean-burning fuel to meet its energy requirements.

As the GDP increased, however, dietary energy sources changed drastically. The largely unrefined complex carbohydrate foods, high in starch, which used to make up the majority of the total calories consumed, became refined white flour products, such as pies, pastries, pastas, and pizzas. Potatoes turned into Pringles. Corn turned into Doritos. Wheat turned into Zingers. And beans and grains turned into hamburgers and sirloin steaks.

With food technology being able to create new taste sensations on one hand, and with advertising being able to create a mass market on the other, the diet composition underwent a major overhaul, where the largely unrefined complex carbohydrates became a minority player. In their stead, calorie-dense, processed foods, usually high in sugar, salt, and fat, as well as meats, sausages, eggs, and cheese high in fat, calories, salt, and cholesterol, became the dominant energy carriers.

The Food Revolution

Even in our country, food just isn't the same as it was some hundred years ago. Back then, the American diet consisted largely of "foods-as-grown" coming mostly from local gardens and nearby farms. Those foods were supplemented with a few staples from the general store and some meat from range-fed cattle and "home-grown" chickens. At the time of our great-grandparents, in this country they didn't slaughter 1 million animals an hour. And they didn't have forty thousand slickly packaged, cleverly promoted products waiting at the local supermarket. And they didn't have over 100,000 fast-food outlets spending billions of dollars advertising take-out service. Families in those days sat at their own tables, and they ate their own freshly cooked food and home-baked bread.

But times and serving sizes have changed. Many of us spend more than 65 percent of our food dollars "eating out." Our livestock is fattened in feedlots where a lack of exercise, antibiotics, and "growth enhancers" produce bigger cattle faster and juicier meat with about twice as much fat as range-fed cattle. And 150,000 chickens are now raised in factory farms under one roof, never seeing the sun in their lifetime. And hogs have now been reduced to breeding machines and cows to mere milk producers. Today's farm produce is almost exclusively processed, refined, concentrated, sugared, salted, and chemically engineered to produce taste sensations that are rich in calories and poor in nutritional value. Advertising, marketing, taste, "mouthfeel," and culinary "bliss points" have created a demand that addicts and produces big profits and big bodies.[9]

Plant-based whole foods, on the other hand, are nutritionally balanced. They don't need nutrition labels. Refinement, however, strips these foods of most of their fiber and nutrients. Processing adds calories, subtracts nutrition, and contributes myriads of chemical additives, including an amount of salt that exceeds ten times the body's minimum requirement. Today, close to 50 percent of the calories eaten are now empty calories almost totally devoid of any significant nutritional value. No wonder so many people are overfed and undernourished.

The least nutritious foods with the most sugar are the most widely advertised. Enormous resources of advertising go far toward the destruction of more sensible eating habits. And large governmental subsidies support the meat and dairy industries. And remember: meat is the single largest source of fat in the American diet, and its excess protein may contribute to kidney disease, gout, osteoporosis, and cancer.[10] But even more serious is the heavy load of saturated fat that most animal protein foods carry, and the trans fats found in crackers, cakes, pies, and foods sold in crinkly bags. These fats are prominently involved in increasing the rates of cholesterol synthesis by the liver, thus creating excessive cholesterol production that is reflected in the typically high blood cholesterol levels, which prominently drive our circulation-related disease epidemic. This includes, among others, coronary heart disease and stroke, Alzheimer's, memory loss and senility, hearing and visual acuity loss, erectile dysfunction, renal disease, peripheral vascular disease, and type 2 diabetes.[11]

Making the Change—and Getting Results

Today, more than ever, we have become victims of our own lifestyle. The contribution of the medical care system to the health status of Western nations is marginal, since it can do little more than to serve as a catchment net for those who have become victimized by their culture or who have become victims of their own choices.

Large sophisticated studies have shown that 63 to 80 percent of all major coronary events before the age of sixty-five could be prevented, if Americans simplified their diet to lower their blood cholesterol levels to less than 180 mg/dL, their systolic blood pressure to <125, and quit smoking.[12]

Dean Ornish, MD, convincingly argued that a plant-based, whole food diet coupled with exercise and stress management could reverse not only atherosclerotic plaques in coronary patients but also indolent prostate cancer.[13] Caldwell Esselstyn Jr., MD, at the Cleveland Clinic, showed that of the "walking dead" cardiac patients, 74 percent were still alive after twenty years by adopting a simple plant-based, whole food program that reversed atheroscle-

rotic plaques.[14] Of his diabetic patients, 71% percent were off their oral medications within four weeks and with normal blood sugar levels. Neal Barnard, MD, demonstrated the effectiveness of a plant-based, whole food program in reversing type 2 diabetes.[15] Of his diabetic patients, 71 percent were off their oral medications within four weeks and with normal blood sugar levels.

Intensive therapeutic lifestyle change (ITLC) programs, such as CHIP (Complete Health Improvement Program) offered by the Lifestyle Medicine Institute (with over 70,000 graduates from its community-based educational intervention program), have seen their patients reverse their chronic conditions within weeks by markedly improving their dietary and lifestyle habits.[16] Centered around on a lifestyle improvement intervention that aims for a plant-based, whole foods diet, the clinical results have been published in more than 30 thirty peer-reviewed articles.[17] (For more on these programs, see pages 341–343.)

Outlook and Doing It!

As they begin to understand the cause-and-effect relationship between their diet and their diseases and their level of health and healing, many people will give up the excesses of the "good life." Instead they will opt for the "best life" with its elegant simplicity, as you find so powerfully presented in Chef Reinfeld's people-tested recipes.

Moving towards a vegan diet is a responsible choice. Many people who have done so have learned and experienced that moving towards a plant-based, whole food diet will do more to heal their chronic diseases than all the pills and procedures.[18] They have learned that while health may not be everything, without health, everything is nothing. 🌱

CHAPTER 2

A Cornucopia of Nutritional Theories— Which Is Right for You?

The reverse side also has a reverse side.
—JAPANESE PROVERB

There are many nutritional theories, and each one has many advocates with vast bodies of evidence supporting its approach as the correct one, even as the only correct one. I personally believe that a plant-based diet that includes a great variety of colorful, whole food ingredients is the healthiest choice for humanity, both for our body and our planet. Once you take the other factors into consideration (the environmental impact of a plant-based diet compared to a meat-based one, including water usage, land usage, pollution, carbon emissions, etc.), you will see that the evidence is staggering in favor of a plant-based diet as the most sustainable and humane form of feeding ourselves (see page 314 for more information). But for the moment, the important thing to understand is that a plant-based diet is *at least as healthy* as any other dietary option out there.

There's a lot of misinformation about plant-based diets, and many people have questioned whether going without animal foods can give you adequate nutrition. So, can we meet all of the body's nutritional needs on a plant-based diet? The answer is a resounding YES.

More than twenty years ago, the US Department of Agriculture (USDA) and the US Department of Health and Human Services affirmed that all the body's nutritional needs can be met through a well-planned, plant-based diet.

More recently, the American Dietetic Association, now called the Academy of Nutrition and Dietetics, the largest group of food and nutrition professionals, restated its position that "well-planned vegan and other types of vegetarian diets are appropriate for all stages of the life cycle, including during pregnancy, lactation, infancy, childhood, and adolescence." It is the association's official opinion as well as that of the Dietitians of Canada that "appropriately planned vegetarian diets, including total vegetarian or vegan diets, are healthful, nutritionally adequate, and may provide health benefits in the prevention and treatment of certain diseases."

The association goes on to say, "The results of an evidence-based review showed that a vegetarian diet is associated with a lower risk of death from ischemic heart disease. Vegetarians also appear to have lower low-density lipoprotein (LDL) cholesterol levels, lower blood pressure, and lower rates of hypertension and type 2 diabetes than non-vegetarians. Furthermore, vegetarians tend to have a lower body mass index and lower overall cancer rates. Features of a vegetarian diet that may reduce risk of chronic disease include lower intakes of saturated fat and cholesterol and higher intakes of fruits, vegetables, whole grains, nuts, soy products, fiber, and phytochemicals."

May this forever dispel the myth that a vegan diet is inherently lacking in nutrients. While it is true that many individuals will benefit from supplementation at certain times in their life, a well-varied, whole food, plant-based diet does provide all the

THE EXPERTS SPEAK
Michael Greger, MD

While a plant-based diet has been shown to be the healthiest diet, please keep in mind the following: two vitamins are not available in plants: vitamins D and B_{12}. There is a serious risk of B_{12} deficiency if no supplements or B_{12}-fortified foods are consumed, a particular danger for pregnant and breastfeeding mothers and their infants. It can lead to vegetarian's myelopathy (degeneration of the spinal cord), paralysis, a variety of other problems, and thickened arteries, and can shorten one's life span. Two other nutrients to keep an eye on are iodine—which is harmful in too great or too small amounts (it is especially important during pregnancy, and can be found in sea vegetables) and zinc.

The convergence of evidence suggests that an affordable plant-based diet can help prevent and even reverse many of the top killers in the Western world. This could save Medicare billions of dollars, but medical training continues to underemphasize nutrition education, in part, perhaps, because lifestyle interventions go against the prevailing conventional wisdom. The USDA, in formulating its dietary guidelines, has been accused of both acting with bias and ignoring relevant research (for further reading, Google the McGovern Report). However, the most recent guidelines take a step in the right direction by recommending a shift to a plant-based diet, which Kaiser Permanente, the largest US managed-care organization, supports.

Lifestyle medicine attempts to find, prevent, and treat the causes of disease. The power of plants is exemplified by the fact that in modern medicine plant compounds form the basis of many critical medications, but it's better to prevent disease in the first place. 🌱

protein, calcium, iron, and all other vital nutrients needed for us to thrive.

The Round Table

Imagine a group of people sitting at a round table. If I place a bowl of fruit in the center of the table and ask everyone, "Is this healthy?" many people would answer yes immediately. But the answer depends who is sitting at the table. If for instance, at the table there is a raw foodist, a fruitarian, a macrobiotic person, a paleo diet advocate, an Ayurvedic doctor, a low-carb person, a low-fat person, and a sugar-free person, everyone is going to give a different opinion on whether or not it is healthy. Imagine how complex it can get when each person details his or her carefully thought-out version of optimal diet components as well as the best sources and amount of proteins, fats, grains, sugars, and other nutrients.

If I were sitting at the table, my response would be that there is a plant-based solution to every health challenge we face. Yet, even within the framework of a plant-based diet, the opinions vary widely on these topics. What is the best ratio of fats to proteins to carbohydrates? What percentage of raw foods is optimal in our diet? Are complex carbohydrates okay? What about concentrated sweeteners?

But Is It Healthy?

Consider this metaphor: our health and physical constitution is like a pane of glass. Some people are gifted with a very thick pane of glass; they have a strong constitution and seem to defy all known rules of nutrition. (These are the 90-year-old cigar aficionados who can eat whatever they want.) Other people, for whatever reason, have a thinner pane of glass, perhaps when their immune system or health is challenged.

All of our dietary habits and lifestyle choices are like tossing a pebble at the pane of glass. Some pebbles are bigger than others. Occasionally having some heated oil in your diet, or some refined sugar every now and then, for most of us, is like having a small pebble tossed against the window. Doing hard drugs would be like tossing a giant boulder into the pane of glass. No matter how thick the pane of glass, this habit will cause serious damage.

With this perspective on nutrition, instead of looking at some food or lifestyle choice as being healthy or unhealthy in itself, it becomes more about the interplay between our current physical health and how frequently we engage in various food and lifestyle choices. For instance, someone with blood sugar issues would not want to toss even one pebble of a concentrated sweetener at that pane, and those with cardiac issues would avoid sprinkling it with processed oils.

We are all biophysically unique and what works for one person may not work for someone else. Also, what may be right for you at one time in your life and in a particular season or climate may not be right in other times and places. It is up to each of us to conduct an ongoing experiment to see what works best for us. And your doctor or nutritionist can always help you determine the right approach for you.

The Standard American Diet (SAD)

The standard American diet is the name for the way many in Western society choose to eat; this habit usually consists of lots of processed carbs (cereals, breads, pasta, cookies, cakes, etc.), processed meat products, and a few fruits and veggies. It is full of hydrogenated oil, high-fructose corn syrup, sodium nitrate, and monosodium glutamate (MSG), and lacking in basic essentials, such as vitamins and minerals. The standard American diet is all about convenience, where fast and packaged foods have become a way of life. The fast pace of our lives has made "quick" and "cheap" characteristics that often override any real conscious choices.

However, the consequences of this lifestyle are not so convenient or easy to digest. Most packaged and fast foods have virtually no nutritional value. They are pretty packages housing plenty of calories in the form of now known addictive and inflammatory substances: processed salt, sugar, and fat. If these items are part of your daily intake, then you may well be on the fast track to being overfed and undernourished, and in time heading down the path of disease. The SAD contains foods that are directly related to many degenerative diseases.

Any step you can take away from the standard American diet is a step in the right direction.

Diets A to Z

The poor state of health that we have found ourselves in interestingly coincides with society's simultaneous obsession with how to become more beautiful, thin, fit, and sexy. The demand for quick and easy fixes still predominates making any true fundamental change, so the search for the "perfect" diet can seem never-ending when you don't see results. The following list is by no means comprehensive, but is intended to highlight the vast differences in popular nutritional theories so that you can make an informed decision about your health.

Alkaline diet

Also known as the alkaline acid diet, the alkaline diet is based on the fact that the body is slightly alkaline. A standard diet consists of many acid-producing foods, which use up the body's energy resources to excrete. Some believe that lack of energy, nasal troubles, anxiety, cysts, and too frequent colds, headache, and flu are results of an acidic diet. To bring the body into balance, the alkaline diet highlights fruits, vegetables, nuts, and legumes.

It celebrates a return to the diet of long-ago ancestors, who were eating before modern farming techniques and crops were born. It is thereby minimally processed and excludes processed grains, dairy, salt, grain-fed meat, and sugar as being the main culprits in acid release. The first person to talk about the benefits of an alkaline diet was the New York physician William Howard Hay, who discussed his theories in the books *Health Via Food* and *Weight Control* in the 1920s and '30s. While there are many proponents of this diet, it has not been subject to many rigorous studies.

Anti-inflammatory Diet

The anti-inflammatory diet is also sometimes referred to as the wellness diet. It makes the connection between persistent inflammation in the body and serious ailments, such as heart disease, cancers, obesity, and Alzheimer's. It is also reputed to reduce triglycerides and hypertension, and ease stiff joints or arthritis. Inflammation as we know it is the cornerstone of the body's healing response, bringing more nourishment and more immune activity to a site of injury or infection. But when inflammation persists beyond its purpose, it damages the body and causes illness. Stress, lack of exercise, genetic predisposition, and exposure to toxins (such as secondhand tobacco smoke) can all contribute to this uncontrolled chronic inflammation. Dietary choices play a major role as well, as foods can be a type of environmental trigger. Therefore the diet instructs on what foods cause inflammation and are to be avoided and what foods help to alleviate already-present inflammation.

Since the importance of addressing inflammation is widespread in wellness practices and even conventional medicine, there are many different versions of this diet.

Ayurvedic Diet

Ayurveda, meaning "science of life," is a five-thousand-year-old traditional science originating in India. Ayurvedic diet adherents eat according to their constitution to maintain the ultimate balance between three doshas (mind-body types), which represent how the five basic elements combine to form energy in the body. They are: Vata dosha (space and air), Pitta dosha (fire and water), Kapha dosha (water and earth). Each individual is born with a unique constitution, called the prakriti, and it can be influenced positively or negatively by how that person digests food and eliminate waste.

Ayurvedic eating, being all about balance, encourages the consumption of six tastes—salty, sweet, sour, pungent, bitter, and astringent—preferably in each meal. Lunch is the biggest meal of the day because Ayurveda teaches that the digestive fire is strongest at midday. The diet excludes caffeine, high amounts of sugar, alcohol, most animal products except for ghee (clarified butter), and most processed foods. Ayurveda places high importance on digestion, so herbal and plant remedies are often used to support digestion.

Ayurvedic diets can be highly individualized since each person has a different constitution, so consulting an experienced practitioner for evaluation can be beneficial.

Anti-Candida Diet

Several diets are focused on normalizing out-of-balance intestinal flora. *Candida albicans,* a yeast fungus, is normally present in the microbiome of all bodies, but can cause health disturbances to arise when it grows in excess. A *Candida* cleanse diet eliminates anything that may contribute to its proliferation, to eliminate what is referred to as yeast syndrome—an array of symptoms affecting all body systems and including headaches, severe PMS, yeast infections, brain fog, fatigue, depression, and other disorders of the immune, endocrine, and nervous systems.

Removed from the diet: yeast, cheese, white flour, sugar/artificial sweeteners, caffeine and alcohol, fruit/juice, most dairy (except for ghee, butter, kefir, and probiotic yogurt), beans, root vegetables, some mushrooms, meat except for salmon and sardines, grains and glutens, additives, vinegars, and some nuts.

Often blamed for excess *Candida* in the system are antibiotics, which kill both good and bad bacteria, allowing room for the fungal growth to take over. Routine use of antibiotics could lead to compromised gut health over time, and a gradual increase in symptoms that can evolve over several years. The aim of the diet is to reduce any excess of *Candida* in the system, restore the immune system, and regulate yeast production in the body.

The idea of regulating *Candida* production gained some traction after Dr. C. Orian Truss proposed in a research journal that *Candida albicans*, a yeast growing on the warm interior membranes of the body, could play an important role in problems throughout the body.[1] He decided to put some of his own chronically ill patients on a sugar-free diet and the antifungal drug nystatin, and do his own research. These patients' health dramatically improved. Despite Truss's research and several other books about the topic, the diet continues to be controversial in conventional medicine.

GAPS (Gut and Psychology Syndrome) Diet

The phrase "Gut and Psychology Syndrome," coined by Dr. Natasha Campbell McBride, highlights the connection between digestive function and the brain; the main idea behind the diet is that toxins escape from the GI tract because of damaged gut lining, or "leaky gut," leading to a host of digestive problems, food allergies, and psychological issues.

The GAPS diet was derived from the specific carbohydrate diet (SCD) created by Dr. Sidney Valentine Haas to naturally treat chronic inflammatory conditions in the digestive tract. Through her own research, Dr. McBride took the SCD protocol and adapted it specifically for those with learning disabilities, psychiatric and psychological disorders, and problems with the immune system and digestion. The GAPS diet removes foods that are thought to be difficult to digest and damaging to gut flora (no dairy or sugar; low fruit and grain) and replaces them with nutrient-dense foods (bone broth, probiotic foods) to restore gut health.

For SIBO (small intestinal bacterial overgrowth), the established treatment diets are GAPS (see page 27), the low FODMAP diet (LFD; see page 31), or a combination of these diets. There is little scientific evidence to back up this diet, however.

Gluten-Free Diet

A gluten-free diet is indicated for those with a diagnosis of celiac disease, where even a small trace of the protein gluten is harmful, and for those with gluten intolerance, in which small or large amounts of gluten cause digestive discomfort. Other symptoms can include lethargy, musculoskeletal and neurological pain, skin reactions, and a foggy mind. This diet has become increasingly common, even among those who don't have celiac disease or gluten intolerance, with the huge popularity of books such as *Wheat Belly*, by cardiologist Dr. William Davis, and *Grain Brain*, by neurologist Dr. David Perlmutter, which connect the intake of all processed grains to almost any current health complaint. Many people have found relief from chronic struggles, such as migraines, fatigue, or irritable bowel syndrome (IBS), and have recovered from autoimmune conditions, such as rheumatoid arthritis and Crohn's, by eliminating gluten from their diet. Some theories as to why this intolerance is so prevalent are being looked at from the inside out, but as of this writing, research on gluten's effect on the body is still inconclusive.

Excluded from the diet are any form of barley, rye, wheat, kamut, triticale, and spelt. Oats and other grains that do not have gluten in them may become contaminated if processed in a shared facility, or even grown in fields close to grains containing gluten, and therefore can theoretically cause a reaction as well, unless certified as gluten-free. Ingredients to watch out for are hydrolyzed protein, textured vegetable protein, and all derivatives of wheat, oats, rye, and barley (including barley malt, modified starch, most soy sauces, and natural flavorings).

A product can only be labeled "gluten-free" if it has been processed in a separate facility from anything containing gluten. The increase in prevalence of this diet has raised awareness in the food industry, and now many markets and restaurants are savvy about offering truly gluten-free options.

Glycemic-Index Diet

The glycemic-index diet is essentially a ranking of foods based on the amount of carbohydrates they contain into three categories:

- High-GI foods (70 or higher): white rice, white bread, pretzels, white bagels, white baked potatoes, crackers, sugar-sweetened beverages.
- Medium-GI foods (56–69): bananas, grapes, spaghetti, ice cream, raisins, corn on the cob.
- Low-GI foods (55 and under): oatmeal, peanuts, peas, carrots, kidney beans, hummus, skim milk, most fruits (except those listed above and watermelon).

The glycemic load (GL) gives a fuller picture of a carbohydrate's effect on blood sugar than glycemic index alone. It looks at how much of that carbohydrate is in a serving of a particular food. The carbohydrate in watermelon, for example, has a high GI. But there isn't a lot of it, so watermelon's glycemic load is relatively low. A GL of 20 or more is high, a GL of 11 to 19 inclusive is medium, and a GL of 10 or less is low.

One unit of glycemic load approximates the effect of consuming 1 gram of glucose. Glycemic load is calculated by multiplying the grams of available carbohydrate in the food times the food's GI and then dividing by 100. For example, a cup of white rice has a high glycemic load, a large banana has a medium glycemic load, and 2 cups of popcorn has a low glycemic load.

Participants on the glycemic-index diet will eat primarily from the low-GI category, eating some medium-GI foods but only dabbling in the high-GI foods. One challenge of this diet is that only foods containing carbs get ranked, so it is important to remember to incorporate other macronutrients into a plan for an overall balanced diet, more like the approach recommended by Jennie Brand-Miller in her development of this diet.

The concept was developed by Dr. David J. Jenkins and colleagues in 1980–1981 at the University of Toronto in their research to find out which foods were best for people with diabetes. The American Diabetes Association recognizes this index as a valuable resource.

Ketogenic Diet

The ketogenic diet is a high-fat, adequate-protein, low-carbohydrate diet that forces the body to burn fats rather than carbohydrates. Normally, the carbohydrates contained in food are converted into glucose, which is then transported around the body and is particularly important in fueling brain function.

However, if there is very little carbohydrate in the diet, the liver converts fat into fatty acids and ketone bodies. The ketone bodies pass into the brain and replace glucose as an energy source. The diet is used in medicine primarily to treat refractory epilepsy in children. An elevated level of ketone bodies in the blood, a state known as ketosis, leads to a reduction in the frequency of epileptic seizures.

Now popularized as a quick way to lose weight, this "diet" works in the same way as any of the low-carb/high-protein and -fat diets, such as Atkins and South Beach, by utilizing a state of ketosis to mobilize stored fat. Although appealing to those trying to slim down quickly, extreme use of ketogenesis is not meant to be done long term and should be used only under medical supervision to avoid potentially dangerous metabolic problems.

Low-Carb Diets:
Atkins, South Beach, and Zone

Several controversial diets have centered on reducing carbohydrate intake. The most popular include the Atkins Diet, the South Beach Diet, and the Zone Diet.

Atkins Diet

The Atkins diet rates high for quick weight loss, but lower for nutritional completeness and sustainability. The key diet theory is that when you eliminate carbs from your diet, the body burns fat cells for its energy needs, and thereby you lose weight. The premise is the same as the ketogenic diet, as well as other higher-protein and lower-carb diets that have caught the attention of the weight-loss market. Without the immediate source of glucose, you burn the stored fat, and ketones are released that supply the body's energy needs.

Dr. Robert C. Atkins developed the diet after reading a 1958 research paper, "Weight Reduction," by Alfred W. Pennington in the *Journal of the American Medical Association*. Atkins used the study to resolve his own overweight condition and wrote the first best-selling book about the diet in 1972. The Atkins Nutritional Approach, as he dubbed the diet, gained widespread popularity in 2003 and 2004. At the height of its popularity, one in eleven North American adults was on the diet. In reports of those following the Atkins diet, long-term weight loss is less

common than short term. Trouble with diabetes and heart health have emerged for some on the diet.

South Beach Diet

Dr. Arthur Agatston, a cardiologist based in south Florida, initially developed this diet for his chronically overweight heart patients. While the traditional low-fat diets being recommended to his heart patients were not working for weight loss, cholesterol, or blood sugar levels, Agatston noted that his patients on the Atkins diet were experiencing weight loss. He was reluctant to recommend the trending low-carb Atkins diet because of the saturated fats and limitation of carbohydrates containing fiber and other nutrients. So, he used other medical research to build an eating plan that categorized fats and carbohydrates as good or bad and emphasized lean protein and fiber. The plan also limits excess sugars, as they can disrupt hormonal balances and promote cycles of hunger and weight gain.

Dr. Agatston's diet is similar to Atkins but differs in its definition of "bad" carbs vs. "good" carbs as well as favorable fats. Agatston's goal was to emphasize healthy food choices, rather than getting caught up in choosing either low-fat or low-carb.

Zone Diet

The Zone diet is considered to be in the low-carbohydrate diet school, yet is meant to provide more of a balanced intake of nutrients so as to ensure satiety. Its name comes from the zone where carbohydrates, fat, and protein are properly balanced in a place where weight loss, wellness, and peak performance is achieved without much effort. Like other less strict low-carb diets, it uses the glycemic index to recommend the best carbohydrate food choices.

It seems to promote taking food in dosages similar to the way medication is taken. This diet proposes that the precise ratio between proteins and carbohydrates is essential to "reduce the insulin to glucagon ratio, which purportedly affects eicosanoid (fatty acid) metabolism and ultimately produces a cascade of biological events leading to a reduction in chronic disease risk, enhanced immunity, maximal physical and mental performance, increased longevity and permanent weight loss."[2] Weight is lost almost exclusively from fat and not from muscle or water weight. In addition to weight loss, drops in cholesterol have been reported, although, as with other low fat diets, the research has been inconclusive.

The Zone diet was created by Barry Sears, a biochemist, and promoted in his 1995 book *The Zone: A Dietary Road Map*. He says he was motivated to do this because of his own desire to avoid dying of a heart attack, a fate of which all other men in his family had been early victims.

Low FODMAP Diet

The low FODMAP diet is not a weight-loss plan but a treatment for IBS. FODMAP (fermentable oligosaccharides, disaccharides, monosaccharides and polyols) is a term for short-chain carbohydrates, combinations of which are found in many common foods:

Apples
Apricots
Asparagus
Artichokes
Blackberries
Cauliflower
Cherries
Garlic
Honey
Legumes
Mangoes
Milk and yogurt
Mushrooms
Nectarines
Onion
Peaches
Pears
Persimmons
Plums
Rye and rye bread
Snow peas
Soft cheeses (cottage cheese, cream cheese, ricotta)
Sugar snap peas
Sugar substitutes, including inulin, sorbitol, mannitol, xylitol, and isomalt
Watermelon
Wheat

These foods can be problematic for people with IBS, because FODMAP is poorly absorbed in the small intestine and rapidly fermented by bacteria in the gut, causing gas, bloating, and abdominal pain. The idea is to reduce the amount of FODMAP consumed and gradually reintroduce foods so as to identify which may be causing your particular symptoms. Following the low FODMAP diet can be a difficult prospect, and since the diet is intended to help people with IBS pinpoint food intolerances, it requires the guidance of an expert dietitian who has been trained in the area. If you experience IBS or often have abdominal symptoms, your doctor may recommend this diet, but while many foods are restricted at first, the goal is to get you back to the widest variety of foods that your system can tolerate.

Low-Sodium Diet

The body needs about only a quarter-teaspoon of salt per day, but generally people often consume more than five teaspoons a day.

A low-sodium diet, by definition, reduces your intake of sodium to a bare minimum, which is recommended to be between 1,500 and 2,000 milligrams per day, and 140 milligrams per serving. A low-sodium diet is indicated for those with heart disease, hypertension, fluid retention and swelling, and is recommended as general practice for middle-aged and older adults. Being aware of sodium intake is a good idea for everyone, especially since it, like sugar, is often snuck into packaged foods you may not expect, including those claiming to be healthy or natural. Regular consumption of these products can cause cravings for more salt than we really need, and actually limit our ability to taste the true flavors of our food.

It is also important to realize that sodium does have very important functions in the body. It only becomes a problem when it is out of balance with other minerals, such as potassium, magnesium, and calcium, which we know collectively as electrolytes. Sea salts and other pure mineral salts are better choices than regular table salt for this reason.

The DASH (dietary approaches to stop hypertension) diet is a low-sodium regimen promoted by the US-based National Heart, Lung, and Blood Institute to prevent and control hypertension. It is also recommended by the United States Department of Agriculture (USDA) as one of its ideal eating plans for all Americans.

The DASH diet is based on National Institutes of Health (NIH) studies that examined three dietary plans and their results. None of the plans were vegetarian, but the DASH plan incorporated more fruits and vegetables, low-fat or nonfat dairy, beans, and nuts than the others studied.

One of the key suggestions for lowering sodium in a diet is reading food nutrition labels very carefully, as well as lowering intake of processed items by instead using whole foods and refraining from adding salt. Good flavor substitutes in place of salt are lemon, spices, herbs, garlic, ginger, vinegar, and pepper.

Macrobiotic Diet

Macrobiotic, meaning "great life," is an unrefined, natural foods–only diet. It is a lifestyle emphasizing the understanding of the rhythms of life for optimum wellness and happiness, using a food = happiness equation. Christoph Wilhelm Hufeland, an eighteenth-century German physician, first used the word *macrobiotics* in the context of food and health in his book *The Art of Prolonging Human Life* (1797). George Oshawa is credited with developing and popularizing the diet in Japan in the 1930s, and his student Michio Kushi went on to introduce modern macrobiotics to the United States in the early 1950s, essentially creating the natural foods movement in the '60s with his popular Erewhon Market.

Macrobiotic diets have a predominance of grains, often 50 to 60 percent, considered the best food to eat. The rest of your daily food intake is rounded out with 20 to 30 percent from land vegetables, 5 to 10 percent from sea vegetables, and 5 percent from soups. Sodium and potassium are the primary elements in food that define its yin/yang qualities that affect our well-being. Fat is avoided in the diet, but fish and some animal products are sometimes included.

The diet prescribes eating locally grown and in-season products, theorizing that these items are more in tune with our rhythm than those flown in or eaten out of season. In summer, the diet calls for fewer foods and in winter, cooked food is used as a source of heat. Food is meant to be chewed completely, until it is liquid, before swallowing, and meals should end when one is 80 percent full.

Mediterranean Diet

The Mediterranean diet is a very common and well-accepted nutritional recommendation originally inspired by the traditional dietary patterns of Greece, southern Italy, and Spain that gained widespread recognition in the 1990s.

It's generally accepted that the folks in the countries bordering the Mediterranean Sea live longer and suffer less than most Americans from cancer and cardiovascular ailments. The not-so-surprising secret is an active lifestyle, weight control, and a diet low in red meat, sugar, and saturated fat and high in produce, nuts, and other healthful foods.

The Mediterranean diet has been associated with a decreased risk for heart disease, and it's also been shown to reduce blood pressure and "bad" LDL cholesterol. This makes sense if your Mediterranean approach largely shuns saturated fat and includes healthier mono- and polyunsaturated fats in moderation.

The latest evolution of the Mediterranean diet has been elucidated in Julieanna Hever's book *The Vegiterranean Diet*. In her words, "The Mediterranean diet has been the gold standard dietary regimen for decades, and with good reason: it has been linked to lowered risks of chronic conditions such as heart disease and diabetes. By focusing on whole-plant foods that promote long-term wellness and ideal weight management, we can reap the benefits of the most researched and beloved diet, made even healthier."

Oil-Free Diet

Excluding all oils is the cornerstone of the oil-free diet. This diet subscribes to the theory that no oil is good for the body's health and wellness, not even so-called healthy oils, such as olive or coconut. The main health critique of oil is that it damages blood vessels by stripping them of important disease-fighting cells.

Oils are a processed food and are very calorie dense. Processing oil strips the plant of its nutrients, leaving a highly concentrated substance with a lot of saturated fat and calories. Additionally, it takes many more ears of corn, for example, to make a tablespoon of oil, than a person would normally consume, resulting in an overabundance of concentrated richness.

The oil-free diet suggests replacing oil with water for frying or dry frying with nothing but a pan on low heat. Simply leaving oil out of recipes is another technique, or subbing in avocado, nut, or seed butters.

This diet is advocated by several health advocates, including Dr. Caldwell Esselstyn Jr., author of *Prevent and Reverse Heart Disease* (see page 344), as the optimal diet for heart health.

Paleo Diet

The paleo diet has other names, the caveman or Stone Age diet, coming from its premise that a return to what is supposed to have been eaten in prehistoric times is the most natural diet for the modern day body. The diet holds that weight loss and avoidance of modern-day disease such as diabetes, heart disease, and cancer are all results of cavemanlike eating, since many health concerns today are attributed to carb and processed-heavy eating.

A focus on hunting and gathering frames the eating guidelines for paleo eating. Meat that is lean and optimally fresh is plentiful on the diet, as is poultry and fish. Lots of fruits and vegetables and fats, including eggs, nuts and seeds, and "good" oils, are included as well. Excluded is everything that originates from more modern-day farming, such as dairy, wheat, potatoes, refined sugars or oils, salt, beans and grains, or anything processed.

Some nutritional deficiencies can materialize for paleo dieters, since so many nu-

THE EXPERTS SPEAK
Michael Greger, MD

Eating low on the food chain reduces our exposure to dietary antibiotics and industrial toxins that concentrate in animal fat (a problem multiplied by the feeding of slaughterhouse byproducts to farm animals) that may contribute to multiple diseases. Plant-based diets reduce our exposure to mercury and other toxic heavy metals, advanced glycation end-products (AGEs), and cadmium, as well as xenoestrogens in fish, which may interfere with male fertility, and estrogenic meat carcinogens in cooked meat that stimulate breast cancer cells and may affect fetal development. Luckily, eating plants not only reduces our exposure to these toxins, but also may protect us against subsequent damage. A cooked meat carcinogen (abbreviated PhIP) found in fried bacon, fish, and chicken may not only trigger cancer and promote tumor growth, but also increase cancer's metastatic potential by increasing its invasiveness.

Contrary to popular myth, people eating plant-based diets have healthy bones and higher blood protein levels than omnivores do. Plant-eaters get more than enough protein. Plant-eaters average fewer nutrient deficiencies than do average omnivores, while maintaining a lower body weight without necessarily losing muscle mass. Those eating plant-based diets may experience enhanced athletic recovery. 🐢

trients from beans and grains are missed. It is also possible that the emphasis on meat may result in an excessive daily consumption of animal proteins and fats. Another drawback is the lack of solid evidence about what exactly and in what proportion cavemen were eating. Insects, for instance, are known to be a part of the Paleolithic diet. If you find a paleo cookbook that includes a chapter on insects, please let me know.

Raw or Living Foods Diet

A raw food diet is based on the principle that food is best eaten in its most natural state, that is, uncooked or low-heat cooked, and unprocessed, or minimally so. A raw diet consists chiefly of plant foods, although some will consume raw eggs, raw milk, or cheese made from raw or unpasteurized milk, and in some cases, raw meat. Purists will eat exclusively raw foods, while other raw dieters aim for 75 percent or more raw (called a High Raw Diet). Alcohol, caffeinated products, and refined sugars are generally left out of a raw diet.

Preparing meals involves chopping, blending, soaking, sprouting, juicing, and dehydrating, to create dishes without traditional cooking methods. If heating or dehydrating, raw foodists do not turn the heat up beyond 115° to 118°F. Advocates explain that raw or living foods have natural enzymes, which are critical in building proteins and rebuilding the body, and that heating these foods destroys the natural enzymes needed for the digestion process, may alter the vitamin content of a food, and can leave toxic materials behind.

Benefits claimed from a proper raw food diet include its abundance of fiber, the variety and high nutritional density from consistent consumption of fruits, vegetables, nuts, and seeds, a trim physique, clearer and brighter skin, and high levels of energy. See Chapter 4 for more on the benefits of raw foods.

SOS (No Salt, Oil, Sugar) Diet

The SOS diet eliminates all added salt, oil, and sugar.

Eating a whole foods, unprocessed diet provides the body with adequate salt, oil, and sugar content, which is less than some of us believe. The body's salt need is less than ¼ teaspoon; oils needn't be more than 10 percent of caloric intake per day, and are plentiful in nuts, seeds, avocados, and the like. Naturally occurring sugars from fruits, vegetables, and complex carbohydrates give plentiful energy to the body.

New discoveries in science prove that industrial, processed, sugar-, fat-, and salt-laden food—food that is made in a plant, rather than grown on a plant, as Michael Pollan would say—is biologically addictive. We are all subject to more and more of them if partaking of the standard American diet.

Dr. David Kessler, a Harvard-trained doctor and former head of the US Food and Drug Administration, wrote the best-selling book *The End of Overeating*. He describes how the food industry and restaurant chains engineer foods to be just as addictive as cigarettes by triggering the reward system in the brain to get us hooked on sugar, fat, and salt. The food industry uses science to engineer the perfect taste, color, texture, look and smell, creating the "bliss point," a common industry term for the resulting neurochemical addiction.

For example, a bag of potato chips doesn't just satisfy hunger and deliver calories. The salt, sugar, and fat combine to make it perfectly addictive. The starch in the chips causes glucose levels to rise, which results in a craving for more. This also stimulates the brain to release dopamine, the feel-good chemical, when we eat them, leading to a craving that is actually more for the dopamine. Giving up these substances can be an extreme challenge, but when the brain and the taste buds begin to adapt, successful SOS-free dieters become more sensitive to them and find it easy to adjust to a new lifestyle of freedom from them.

Great ways to begin to reduce SOS in the diet are: creating meal rituals at home, thus eating out less; going to restaurants that you know will accommodate requests; consuming fewer packaged, processed, or premade items; crowding SOS out with satisfying whole food substitutes; and simply removing all SOS from the kitchen.

This way of eating is advocated by both Dr. Esselstyn and Dr. Campbell as the ideal formula for maintaining optimal health.

Starch Solution Diet

The Starch Solution, by Dr. John McDougall, states that there is a specific diet that best supports the health of every animal. According to him, the ideal diet for humans is based on starches. Recent research has shown that we produce up to eight times more starch-digesting enzymes in our saliva than do other primates. According to Dr. McDougall, starch-based diets date as far back as the Neanderthals (later than the Paleolithic period); with evidence showing its existence throughout even the Aztec

and Mayan civilizations. The one thing each of these civilizations held in common is that they were all lean, fit, and healthy—the polar opposite of the typical individual in the modern-day Western world.

Dr. McDougall developed his own diet program after working with his mentor, Dr. Roy Swank, and observing his work with multiple sclerosis (MS) patients benefiting from the very low-fat Swank diet. Dr. Swank later gave his approval for using the high starch diet in MS, and this led to a 2009 study on MS and the McDougall diet through Oregon Health and Science University (OHSU).

The diet recommended in the McDougall program consists of 70 percent starch (rice, potatoes, beans, etc.—he considers these to be low-fat, high nutrient, and satisfying comfort foods). The remaining foods would consist of 10 percent fruit and 20 percent vegetables. You center the food on your plate on starches with the addition of nonstarchy vegetables and fruit to add color and flavor. You can also add fat-free seasonings for variety and to make your meals more interesting.

The diet avoids all meat, fish, dairy, eggs, animal fats (such as lard and butter), vegetable oils (including olive oil), and processed and packaged foods. Avocado, dried fruit, fruit juice, nuts, seeds, and simple sugars, such as maple syrup, are best consumed in small quantities as part of a starch-based meal. If you want to accelerate weight loss or are recovering from a chronic disease you are advised to avoid these foods altogether.

Numerous individuals that have adopted the starch-based diet under the

For millennia, food has been the necessary fuel that nourishes our physical bodies. Our relationship to food and its consumption, however, is interwoven with shifting cultural attitudes that have a profound effect on our mind and soul. Over the centuries, the shared experience of eating food has held different meanings for millions of individuals. It is the most powerful and easily attainable drug, one that uses all five senses to directly connect to our emotions. It can nourish, it can comfort, and it can calm. But it can also bring on a guilt that inflicts pain and wreaks havoc on both our physical body and our soul.

Our relationship to food can become unhealthy, and the term we most commonly recognize for this is eating disorder. The truth is, specific patterns of behavior that encompass our relationship to food do not always exist in well defined, compartmentalized categories, such as anorexia or bulimia; disordered eating affects us all. Disordered eating as a set of behaviors does not only describe those individuals that restrict or binge on food, but represents an entire continuum of behaviors. Food restriction, overeating, physical purging, purging through excessive exercising, or taking part in compulsive obsessive food rituals are just some examples of disordered eating.

These behaviors are the product of powerful thought patterns that start to distort reality, induce cognitive distortion, and lead to detrimental physical effects on various organ systems in the body. With time, many people succumb to a poor quality of health and life. Too often they come to the attention of mental health professionals and physicians only when concerned loved ones intervene or when the individual can no longer bear to suffer with the intensity of his/her thought patterns and uncontrollable compensatory behaviors.

The vast majority of Americans have some type of disordered eating and most are unaware that it exists. Fast food's conveniences come with the cost carried by all food that is processed: the inclusion of additives and addicting chemicals that fuel the modern paradox of an overfed and undernourished nation. We crave foods that inflame our body, contributing to weight gain and chronic illnesses such as diabetes and hypertension. Illnesses that spring from these sources often require the chronic intake of pharmaceutical medication and ongoing medical care.

To add to the confusion of food choices is the multibillion-dollar diet industry and its pursuit of the next blockbuster fad.

What if we were to take a moment to think: what drives my food choices? How do these choices affect my energy, concentration, and sense of well-being from meal to meal? Visualize food as fuel and ask yourself: is the fuel I am ingesting helping me feel well and content with life? If the answer is no, fear not. You can change. The power your food has over you can be altered, and starting new wholesome patterns today can affect your health outcomes for years to come. Choosing the right building blocks in eating whole vegetables, fruits, and grains is the foundation of the road leading to a healthier relationship with food.

In my practice I have seen firsthand the life-altering changes that take place when incorporating a healthy relationship to food with nutrition and lifestyle. Choosing to have your food come from the earth, eating a rainbow of colored vegetables and fruits, and limiting the amount of packaged and processed foods will give you all the vitamins and minerals you need and produce dramatic changes in how you feel and move through life. Ultimately, what we say about all relationships is most true with food: we truly are the food we keep. 🌱

leadership of Dr. McDougall have reported relief from symptoms of arthritis, heart disease, diabetes, cancer, and obesity.

Sugar-Free Diet

Awareness of the damage sugar can cause as well as its extreme prominence in daily life has become a major hot topic in the diet world. However, sugar is still a major ingredient in the most common foods consumed on a daily basis. We now understand that weight gain is less often a matter of overeating and more connected to the effect that sugar has on metabolism.

Sugar both drives fat storage and makes the brain think it is hungry, setting up a "vicious cycle," according to Dr. Robert Lustig. The main problem with sugar, and processed fructose in particular, is the fact that the body has a very limited capacity to metabolize it. According to Dr. Lustig, you can safely metabolize about 6 teaspoons of added sugar per day. But the average American consumes 22 teaspoons of added sugar a day. All that excess sugar is metabolized into body fat, and leads to all the chronic metabolic diseases we see people struggle with.

Since sugar appears in so many unsuspected items, avoiding it completely can be a major challenge. Some on a sugar-free diet avoid white refined sugar, while others go all the way to keep even natural fruit sugar out of the diet, consuming exclusively savory items.

Those living with diabetes are familiar with the importance of glucose regulation, and "sugar-free" foods as well as sugar substitutes have long been marketed as health products.

From a whole food, plant-based perspective, it is important to avoid all artificial sweeteners. Although some researchers insist that they are safe in reasonable amounts unless there is a metabolic intolerance, perhaps staying as close to nature as possible is the best approach in navigating the endless controversial topics around food. Stevia or luo han, from a leaf and a fruit, respectively, can be used instead of sugar and/or artificial sweeteners; fresh fruit in lieu of canned fruit or in recipes calling for a bit of sweetness; and spices instead of sugar can add flavor to your meal.

The easiest way to dramatically cut down on your sugar and fructose consumption is to switch to a diet of whole, unprocessed foods, as most of the added sugar consumed comes from processed fare.

80/10/10 Diet

The 80/10/10 diet is also known as a low-fat raw vegan diet and claims to be optimal for athletic performance and general wellness. The name comes from the recommendation that 80 percent of food calories come from simple carbohydrates, 10 percent from protein, and 10 percent from fat. To achieve this ratio, 90 to 95 percent of calories should be from sweet fruit, 2 to 6 percent from leafy greens, and 0 to 8 percent from nuts and seeds. The prescription is for two or three fruit meals in the earlier part of the day, and a large vegetable salad in the later part of the day, almost all in an uncooked form.

This diet was developed by Dr. Doug Graham, a lifetime athlete who has been eating a raw food diet for almost thirty years, after an observation that many raw fooders eat too much fat. Although the diet is the foundation of the program, Graham emphasizes the importance of addressing other lifestyle factors, which include exercise, sunlight, adequate sleep, and emotional balance.

Theorizing that in nature, no animal cooks food and cooking alters its natural state, everything is eaten in its raw form. Additionally, the diet holds that any more than 10 percent protein calories in the body is toxic, and the same goes for fats, especially oils, which are not in their whole food state and thereby harmful. Grains are not included in the diet since they need to be cooked, and nutritionally have less potency than live fruits and vegetables.

Dr. Graham says that other low-fat vegan diets rely too much on cooked starches, such as rice, bread, and potatoes, as the main source of calories; and because they taste bland, we usually add sugar, salt, and fats, which compromises their potential health value. Huge amounts of fruits and vegetables can be consumed to obtain adequate calories, which is necessary to thrive on this diet. For example, 4 pounds of watermelon may make up a meal, and dieters are advised to consume approximately a pound of leafy greens, such as lettuce, spinach, and celery, each day.

The List Goes On

The list of the various diets could fill the pages of the entire book.

There are cleansing and fasting diets such as the fast diet, where you can eat whatever you like for five days and reduce your calories on the remaining two days. There is also the eat-right-for-your-blood-type diet, which makes dietary recommendations based upon a person's blood type. (I do attribute my positive attitude to my blood type [B-positive], with no offense to those with B-negative.)

As you can see, many of these diets make recommendations that are diametrically opposed to one another. (The raw food diet conflicts with the macrobiotic diet. The low carb diets conflict with the Starch Solution, and so on.) In my opinion as soon as we bring mindfulness into our food choices, and step away from the highly processed Standard American Diet, most people will experience beneficial results. The question is, how long-lasting are these results? Everyone wants the magic bullet that will make us all healthy and thin with no real effort. And that just doesn't exist—though looking to nature through a whole food, plant-based diet sure is a step in the right direction.

During the past decade of educating people on the topic of nutrition, I have encountered many predominant myths regarding our ability to meet all of our nutritional needs on a plant-based diet. Here are some of the bigger myths, plus the easy debunk.

Myth #1: Protein and carbohydrate are "food groups."

Truth: Protein and carbs are two of the three macronutrients (the third being fats) that are contained in many foods, which are then categorized into food groups. Carbohydrates, proteins, and fats are called macronutrients because the body requires them in relatively large amounts for normal functioning. No food is purely protein or purely carbohydrate, and therefore cannot be truly categorized into one group. The truth is that all foods have some combination of these three macronutrients, along with other micronutrients.

Myth #2: It is impossible to get enough protein eating only plants.

Truth: Most intact foods contain at least a little protein, so by eating a diet with variety, vegetarians and vegans can eat all the protein they need without special supplements. Even rice and veggies can do the trick. Not to mention the higher plant-based protein foods, such as legumes, nuts, and seeds. Simple as that.

Proteins in the body are constantly broken down and resynthesized and we require essential amino acids from our diet to replenish our reserve. The Recommended Dietary Allowance (RDA) for protein for adults is approximately 0.8 g/kg of body weight, which ends up being around 10 percent of our total daily calories. Because of their rapid growth, infants (similar to certain athletes) have the highest RDA for protein, at 1.5 g/kg of body weight. Protein demands increase during pregnancy and lactation to a level of 1.1 g/kg. The RDA for an adult weighing 140 pounds (63.6 kg) is a mere 51 grams of protein, an amount easily consumed in a day.

While we really only need around 5 to 6 percent of our total calories from protein to replace what is excreted, the average American is taking in 15 to 16 percent, and those on trendy high-protein diets are eating upward of 20 to 30 percent.

Myth #3: We need to avoid carbohydrates.

Every few years, carbohydrates are vilified as public enemy number one and are accused of being the root of obesity, diabetes, heart disease, and more.

Truth: Whole plant foods containing carbohydrates (along with other nutrients) are a foundation of good health. The fact is that approximately 97 percent of Americans are not getting the minimum recommended daily intake of fiber. Remember that plants contain carbohydrates. If we severely restrict carbohydrates, we also restrict important sources of fiber as well as phytochemicals, the two most important nutrient groups for preventing and healing disease.

Fiber is a type of carbohydrate and is only found in plant foods. The recommended minimum intake for fiber is approximately 38 grams per day for men and 25 grams per day for women. This is a case where even more is likely better. The usual fiber intake among Americans, however, is woefully lacking at only 15 grams daily.

Individuals with high fiber intake tend to have lower risks of coronary heart disease, stroke, hypertension, diabetes, and obesity.

Fiber-rich foods are protective against colorectal cancer, and increasing fiber intakes improves gastroesophageal reflux disease (GERD) and hemorrhoids. Some fibers also lower blood cholesterol and glucose levels. Additionally, fibers feed the healthy bacteria that reside in your gut and provide nutrients and other health benefits.

Carbohydrates are critical sources of energy for several body systems. Nourish your body and help shield yourself from chronic disease by getting plenty of carbohydrates from fruits, whole grains, and legumes. This way of vibrant eating will naturally dampen the appeal of heavily processed grains and sugars.

Myth # 4: Exclusively vegan diets are lacking in nutrients.

Truth: The Academy of Nutrition and Dietetics agrees that a diet that concentrates on a variety of whole plant foods is the most nutrient dense way to eat. The large database of nutrition science consistently concludes that the healthiest type of food pattern includes a high intake of fiber, phytochemicals, and antioxidants, as well as a minimization or elimination of saturated fats and processed foods—all of which you get with a plant-based diet.

The nutrients most commonly recommended in supplementation, such as vitamins B_{12} and D, DHA/EPA omega-3 fatty acids, and certain minerals, are for all people interested in optimal health, not only those who eat exclusively plants. Nutritional research is still speculating on reasons that we may need to supplement in this day and age. Loss of nutrients through processing of foods, transportation of foods long distances, changes in soil composition due to agricultural practices, food sterilization practices, decreases in intake of sea vegetables, as well as less time spent outdoors in nature, may all contribute to some loss of nutrients.

With the same amount of protein, most plants also contain fiber, significantly more beta-carotene and other phytochemicals, folate, vitamins C and E, magnesium, calcium, and iron. Plants have zero cholesterol and a more health-promoting fatty acid profile.

Vitamin K has been another topic of discussion. Phylloquinone (K1) is found primarily in plant foods, such as green leafy vegetables. Because another form of it, menaquinone (K2), is not found in plant foods, some have suggested you need to eat animal products to have adequate vitamin K status. According to Jack Norris, RD, of veganhealth.org, "The scientific consensus has been that either of the two types of vitamin K are adequate, especially regarding vitamin K's blood-clotting activity."[3]

Myth # 5: Saturated fat is now good for us and should be eaten without restriction.

Truth: There is a clear association between saturated fat and heart disease. A recent article in *Time* magazine, titled "Eat Butter," caused mass confusion.

The article cited an analysis of recent studies that concluded research does not clearly support that a reduction of saturated fat can reduce heart disease. Some major problems with the studies were pointed out; for example: they adjusted for high blood cholesterol levels and even the lowest intakes of saturated fats were above recommended levels.

Walter Willett, a physician and researcher from Harvard, asked for the study to be pulled because of its potential danger to the mainstream audience. The problem is that the message was misinterpreted to mean that now animal fats are healthy foods.

Saturated fats—found primarily in animal foods—have been determined to increase risk for cardiovascular disease and other chronic conditions over decades of research. Thus, the American Heart Association has most recently

continues

continued from previous page

recommended a maximum of 5 to 6 percent of our total calories come from them and it is therefore best to follow these guidelines.

Changing the general public understanding of differences in types of fats is important in addressing this epidemic. Healthy essential fats are necessary to our physiology. Whole foods, such as nuts, seeds, and avocado, provide a variety of important nutrients; enhance absorption of fat-soluble nutrients; and contribute to satiety. After analyzing the preponderance of data on fats, it is pretty clear that the type of fat far outweighs the overall quantity consumed in terms of optimal nutrient consumption.

Myth # 6: Soy is dangerous.

Talk about a bad rap! Manboobs, cancer, infertility, hypothyroid . . . the list of accusations against this powerful bean seems endless, yet any search for a definitive biochemical truth behind them will be a challenge to find. This one food has a history of about thirteen thousand years of cultivation and over five thousand research studies.

Truth: Soybeans have a higher amount of digestible protein than any other legume. They are a great source of phytonutrients, omega-3 fatty acids, and fiber, as well as iron, potassium, folate, and magnesium. Isoflavones in soybeans have been associated with a decreased LDL cholesterol and a protective action from breast cancer incidence and reoccurrence by blocking excess estrogen uptake.

As with any foods, it is optimal to choose organic or non-GMO, when possible, and to aim for a whole source rather than a highly processed version, which can have fewer nutrients. However, organic soybeans lightly processed into miso, tofu, and tempeh are absolutely wonderful and can add a terrifically satisfying flavor and texture to many whole food plant meals.

Myth #7: Dairy is important for bone health; milk does a body good.

Truth: Cow's milk is an excellent food source for calves, which typically gain approximately eight times their weight by the time they are weaned. Human mother's milk is excellent nourishment for human babies, and its composition is very different from cow's milk. Of course, milk is best known for providing calcium—but it is far from being the only source of calcium available, or even the best one.

The calcium in kale is absorbed much better than that in milk. There is 96 mg absorbable calcium in a serving of dairy milk, which is comparable to 1/2 cup of Chinese cabbage, 1 1/2 cups of kale, 5.4 ounces of calcium-set tofu, or 1 1/3 cups of plant-based milk.

Bone health is complex and multifactorial, incorporating genetics, gender, age, and lifestyle factors, such as exercise and overall dietary intake. A plethora of nutrients play powerful roles and work synergistically to keep bone mineralization functioning in a healthy way. In addition to calcium and vitamin D, other crucial characters include protein, potassium, phosphorus, magnesium, zinc, copper, manganese, soy isoflavones, and vitamins B_{12}, C, and K.

As it turns out, the nutrients found in plants can more than meet your daily requirements. Also, a person's level and type of exercise as well as hormone balance are very important factors in bone health.

Myth #8: Iron deficiency is an expected challenge in plant-based diets.

Truth: While iron deficiency is the most common nutrient deficiency in the world, the prevalence is the same in vegan vs. meat-eating groups.

Because nonheme iron found in plants is not absorbed as easily as heme iron found in animal products, it is recommended that vegans aim to eat more iron-rich foods than nonvegetarians.

Eating a variety of plants will easily provide more than enough of this important nutrient. More compelling is the fact that higher intakes of iron (that is, from animal products) appear to be health-damaging due to its high oxidative effects, which supports the benefits of sourcing iron from plants.

Considerations: Phytates (antioxidants found in certain nuts and seeds, legumes, and whole grains) and tannins (bitter polyphenols found naturally in seeds, fruit skins, and leaves) can inhibit the absorption of iron from foods. Adding vitamin C–rich foods and organic acids with iron sources, soaking and sprouting nuts and seeds, having coffee and tea away from meals, and rotating greens to change up oxalate intake (kale, broccoli, bok choy, and napa cabbage are all low in oxalate) will help attenuate this effect. Also, using a cast-iron skillet, taking small amounts of blackstrap molasses, and snacking on dried apricots can help keep iron levels optimal.

These are just some of the many myths surrounding a wholesome, healthful plant-based diet. I end by reiterating the position of the Academy of Nutrition and Dietetics in the fact that a well-planned vegan diet is appropriate for all stages of the life cycle. 🍎

CHAPTER 3

The Pillars of the Plant Kingdom—Nutrient-Dense Foods for Optimal Health

The doctor of the future will no longer treat the human frame with drugs,
but rather will cure and prevent disease with nutrition.
—THOMAS EDISON

On some levels, all plants may be considered superfoods, in that they provide us with the nutrients we need to thrive. Some foods stand out in terms of their nutrient content. *Nutrient density* is generally accepted to be the vitamin and mineral content of a food per weight of food or unit of energy. Whole foods tend to have the highest nutrients compared to the calories they give.

Nutrient profiling is not new, but it's not an exact science or well defined, either. A few groups have been taking on the task of trying to rank vegetables, greens, fruits, and superfoods in order of nutrient density, and sometimes the opinions and methodology differ. It is based on either nutrient-to-nutrient ratios, nutrient-to-calorie index, or calorie-to-nutrient scores. Generally, density can depend on the percentage of the Recommended Dietary Allowance

(RDA) of each nutrient provided. Superfoods that are high in phytochemicals, such as berries, are often left off the lists because there is not any standardized recommended intake amount of phytochemicals.

For a definition of the macro and micro nutrients that follow, please see the Nutrient Reference Guide on page 319.

Here is a short selection of some of the heavy-hitting, nutrient-dense foods. But don't limit yourself to these foods! Take time in your local natural foods store or farmers' market and explore the incredible variety of the plant kingdom.

Vegetables and Greens

Beets
Beets have the most natural sugar of any vegetable, and their most common

use, in fact, is as a source of manufacturing beet sugar. Just out of the ground, their earthy flavor is a big draw, as are their naturally occurring nitrates. A good source of folate, beets also feature niacin, pantothenic acid, vitamin B_6, iron, manganese, magnesium, and copper. They are one of the only vegetables to feature glycine betaine, which protects cells and enzymes from external stressors. Beets are considered to be a blood-building and a liver-loving food.

Beet Greens

Resist any autopilot instinct to toss your beet greens into the compost pile—give them a second chance as a go-to dark leafy! Although they may be a bit more bitter than their leafy green counterparts, the bitterness increases enzymes to help with digestion. Beet greens are well worth your while, as known by the Romans, who used to eat the greens and save the beets for medicines.

Beet greens not only have a higher nutritional profile than the beets themselves, but they have more iron than spinach. You can also find high protein, zinc, phosphorus, fiber, and antioxidants, especially vitamin A.

Bok Choy

Bok choy is a member of the cabbage family and often used in Asian dishes. It contains excellent quantities of vitamin A, B_6, C, and K. It is very low in calories, yet has ample fiber. The lutein and zeaxanthin in bok choy contribute their eye health and antiaging properties. Magnesium, potassium, and phosphorus as well as calcium and folate are also present. The sulfur-containing compounds found in bok choy have been shown to reduce the risk of certain types of cancers, such as breast, prostate, and lung.

Broccoli

A cruciferous vegetable best known for its large quantities of vitamin C and fiber, broccoli also packs in vitamin A, B complex, iron, zinc, and phytonutrients. It is reputed to lower the risk of a common cold, keep digestion smooth, lower cholesterol, and protect against diabetes, heart disease, as well as some cancers. Its phytonutrients act as anti-inflammatories and can lower the effects of some common allergens while concurrently boosting the immune system.

Cabbage (Green and Red)

From the Brassica family, cruciferous cabbage ranks extremely high in terms of its delivery of some of the most powerful antioxidants, such as glucosinolates, which encourage detoxifying enzymes to do their work in the body. The humble and inexpensive green cabbage boasts a lot of vitamins C and K, as well as dietary fiber: one of the best sources out there.

Red cabbage has some slight advantages over green: ten times more vitamin A, more vitamin C, and double the iron, with all the dietary fiber and antioxidants and a beautiful dark red/purplish color.

Chard

Swiss chard, or simply chard, is the green that comes in varieties of colors imprinted in the stem. Find it with swatches of yellow, red, or purple, white, and orange in the stems, veins, and leaves, which explains its other name, rainbow chard.

Consuming one cup provides way more than your daily requirement for vitamins A and K. Nitrate content means chard may be helpful in lowering blood pressure and supplying energy for premier athletic performance. Its antioxidant, alpha-lipoic acid, may lower glucose levels for diabetes management. It also has an impressive chlorophyll content. If you are concerned about or sensitive to the oxalic acid content of chard (oxalic acid may inhibit thyroid function), boiling the leaves for three minutes will disperse the acid.

Collard/Mustard/Turnip Greens

These greens are some of the most nutrient dense in the plant kingdom, alongside kale. They are purportedly most nutritious when consumed raw or lightly steamed. As with kale, their richness in vitamins, minerals, carotenoids, antioxidants, and fiber are said to prevent cancers, protect against the damaging effects of free radicals, and bolster the immune system. Collard, mustard, and turnip greens are most renowned for their vitamin A, C, and K, calcium, folate, and antioxidant chlorophyll content. Turnip greens contain significant potassium quantities.

Green Beans

Green beans, or string beans, are not a bean in the classical sense of the word, which usually refers to legumes, such as black beans, kidney beans, and lentils. Green beans are more similar to other pod vegetables, such as okra and sugar snap peas. They provide benefits that include chlorophyll, fiber, folate, riboflavin, potassium, iron, and magnesium, not to mention vitamins A, C, and K. As such, green bean consumption contributes to enabling the immune system to maximize performance and eliminating harmful free radicals in the body.

Kale

Kale is a low-fat, no-cholesterol leafy green renowned for its extraordinary nutrient density and healthy antioxidant properties. Its concentrated nutrients, high fiber, and sulfur-containing phytonutrients strengthen the immune system, and are said to protect against heart disease and certain types of cancer, such as prostate and colon, detox the liver, and lower blood cholesterol levels.

Kale contains plant-based omega-3 fatty acid alpha-linolenic acid, and is high in vitamins A, B_6, C, and especially K (a reputed Alzheimer's preventative). Its minerals include copper, calcium, potassium, manganese, and phosphorus, and also naturally occurring carotenoids lutein and zeaxanthin, which provide eye health. Consuming kale allows for high iron and calcium absorption, while protecting from vitamin A deficiency, osteoporosis, anemia, and cardiovascular disease.

Mushrooms

Although they come in many different varieties, most mushrooms deliver good quantities of protein (almost twice the amount of other common vegetables), vitamins, unsaturated fatty acids, and cholesterol-lowering and heart-healthy dietary fibers. Selenium, potassium, riboflavin, and niacin are prolific in mushrooms. Additionally, mushrooms are low in calories and sodium, and can be very filling, resulting in some cases in weight loss.

Onions

The onion is esteemed for its antiseptic, anti-inflammatory, and antibacterial properties, and its high fiber and low calories. It has been shown to reduce blood glucose level, blood pressure, and cholesterol, decreasing risk of coronary artery disease, stroke, and type 2 diabetes. It also can reduce chest congestion and decrease chances of catching a cold. Onions contain B-complex vitamins, vitamin C, and the minerals potassium, phosphorus, and magnesium. Quantities of sulfur, beneficial for liver detox, are present in onions. Onion flavonoids act as antioxidants against tumors and bolster the immune system. Quercetin is found in high amounts in the outer skin, so saving a little skin to add to your soup can be beneficial.

Peppers (Red)

Peppers are classified as fruits but commonly thought of as in the vegetable category. They are high in phytochemicals, with antioxidant qualities that help neutralize cell damage. Differently colored peppers have different nutrients, and red peppers specifically contain fiber, folate, manganese, and vitamins A, B_6, C, and K. The reputed anticancer agents beta-carotene and lycopene are found in red peppers. Hot red peppers get their fire from capsaicin, which also give a pepper more of an antioxidant effect and releases endorphins.

Radishes

A root vegetable with a 90 percent water content, radishes are low in saturated fat and cholesterol while also antifungal and antibacterial. Providing plenty of roughage, radishes are filling, which can help with weight loss. Radishes have been used successfully to treat jaundice because they increase the supply of fresh oxygen to the blood, purifying and detoxifying. They also relieve symptoms of piles, since they aid digestion and the excretory system. Their high water content acts as a diuretic and thereby aids urinary disorders by increasing urine content.

The flavonoids that color radishes may reduce heart disease, cancer, and inflammation, and their potassium can help lower blood pressure.

Spinach

Spinach, believed to be of Persian origin long, long ago, hasn't gone out of style despite the upsurge in more popular-of-late greens, such as kale, and that's because it is a powerful superfood with lots of nutrients in every leaf and stem and a mild flavor that hides easily in many smoothies. Some say that the nutrients in spinach are more available when it is lightly cooked instead of consumed raw.

Most of its very few calories come from protein, and it is likewise loaded with non-heme iron, calcium, and magnesium, and has more potassium cup for cup than banana. As if that weren't enough, spinach also packs in the vitamin K, fiber, phosphorus, and thiamine.

Pairing spinach with another ingredient that offers vitamin C is helpful in making spinach's valuable iron more absorbable for strength and energy.

Sprouts

Sprouts are lauded for their high enzyme content, which acts as a catalyst for many body functions. Beans, nuts, seeds, or grains can be sprouted by a function of soaking and humidifying them over the course of some days, and the result is an increase in the quality of the protein. Fiber, essential fatty acids, and vitamin content is also increased with sprouting, specifically vitamins A, B complex, C, and E. Additionally, such minerals as calcium and magnesium attach to the sprouts' protein, making them more bioavailable. Sprouts have the triple bonus of being nutritional powerhouses, locally sourced, and quite inexpensive—you can even grow them at home (for more on sprouting and soaking, see pages 67, 105).

Squash

Squash as a term is somewhat broad, as it is inclusive of pumpkins, gourds, and zucchini as well, with a pretty long list of varieties, and an even longer history of cultivation. Excellent quantities of vitamin A, alongside B_6, C, E, thiamine, niacin, and folate, can be found in most varieties of squash, as well as the minerals magnesium, manganese, copper, calcium, potassium, and iron. Because they are a good source of carotenoids, we get to experience many of their glorious colors and patterns. Rounding out this list of benefits of squash are essential antioxidants and anti-inflammatory compounds.

Sweet potatoes

Sweet potatoes are a reliable source of vitamin A in the form of beta-carotene, with 400 percent of your daily needs met in one medium-size potato. Fiber and potassium are the other heavy hitters in these satisfying carbs, which can be sweet as candy and filling as can be. They also come in colors: some are orange; others are shades of yellow and purple. Sweet potatoes also deliver vitamins B_6, C, D, and iron and magnesium. Their skin alone provides potassium, fiber, and quercetin, an immunity booster.

Do you stay up late at night wondering what the difference is between a sweet potato and a yam? Sweet potatoes and yams are actually two different species of root vegetable, grown in different areas of the world. The USDA labels the orange-fleshed sweet potatoes "yams" to distinguish them from the variety with creamy white flesh. Actual yams, native to Africa and Asia, have an almost black, barklike skin and white, purple, or reddish flesh.

Tomatoes

Tomatoes are a win-win-win, since they provide ample nutrients alongside low calories and are free of fat. Besides all this, they are a stellar flavor enhancer. Tomatoes are said to be good for digestion and for maintenance of healthy liver function. Their vitamin A is essential for vision maintenance; the antioxidant lycopene is likely to lower heart disease and cancer risks; and vitamin C, potassium, and iron help to regulate the health of our blood. Tomatoes are dense in phytonutrients, some of which are shown to prevent clumping of platelet cells.

A Cornell University study showed that cooking actually enhances the nutritional value of tomatoes by increasing the lycopene content that can be absorbed by the body, as well as the total antioxidant activity. So, while fresh grown tomatoes are a terrific vitamin C-rich snack, tomato sauce is a great way to enjoy even more antioxidant benefit. It has been shown that most nutrients are retained when used whole, less so with skins removed.

Watercress

Watercress, as the name indicates, is a water plant with bountiful nutritional benefits, and has a peppery, somewhat bitter flavor. It has anti-aging properties, such as lutein, which helps preserve eye health into older age. It is also known for natural iodine content. Watercress is said to have anticancer properties as well, providing both antioxidants and oxygenation to cells aided by its high chlorophyll content. Along with vitamin E (an antioxidant that helps protect and repair your skin), watercress also contains vitamins A and C, beta-carotene, calcium, iron, and zeaxanthin.

Fruits

Apples

Apples are high in antioxidants, including quercetin, which promotes the body's endurance. Heart healthy, apples can help with a great fiber content and help lower cholesterol. Because they have many phytonutrients and antioxidants, apples may protect against effects of free radicals and reduce risk of developing cancer, high blood pressure, and heart disease. The vitamins C and B complex, and the minerals calcium, potassium, and phosphorus are all present. Apples are a great digestion improving food, due to their high insoluble fiber and ample water content. See the box on page 302 for a list of some of the more popular varieties.

Berries

Berries are a low-calorie treat that is high in fiber and antioxidants. There is a wide variety of berries available, including blueberries, blackberries, strawberries, cranberries, raspberries, lingonberries, and gooseberries. The phytonutrients and flavonoids inherent in berries are theorized to prevent the growth of certain types of cancer. Some berries contain lutein, important for maintaining good vision. Blueberries are good for stabilizing and strengthening blood vessels. Cranberries in their whole, unsugared form are well reputed for helping ease bladder infections. And all berries are helpful choices for blood sugar regulation.

Citrus Fruits

Citrus fruits are most famous for delivering a strong dose of vitamin C, without fat or cholesterol. Citrus fruits contain calcium, potassium, folate, and vitamin A. They also have many beneficial phytochemicals, which may reduce risk of chronic diseases, such as cardiovascular disease, cancer, and the risks that accompany skin damage. Citrus fruits are known for fighting weight gain, protecting against type 2 diabetes, lowering risk of stroke, possibly stalling cancer development and tumor growth, and enhancing eyesight.

Papayas

Papayas have proven nutritional and digestive qualities. Easy to digest, the fruit has a high quantity of soluble fiber. When ripe, papayas have one of the highest vitamin C contents, more than citrus fruits. Vitamin A, B-complex vitamins, folates, potassium, and calcium are also well represented. More rarely consumed because of their potent peppery flavor are the black seeds, which have strong medicinal properties as an anti-inflammatory, antiparasitic, and pain reliever. Pregnant women are cautioned against consuming large quantities of papapa due to their potential abortive effect and disruption of fetal development.

Plums

Reddish blue and purple, the color pigment in plums, is due to anthocyanins, which provide the benefit of antioxidant richness to disperse free radicals in the body, alongside beta-carotene and chlorogenic acid, the antioxidant in green coffee extract touted for its benefit of lowering blood sugar and blood pressure as well as providing sustained energy. The hefty quantity of potassium in plums helps the body manage hypertension and prevent strokes. Plums are relatively low on the glycemic index and aid in controlling blood sugar, with high carbohydrate content, making them good for energy. They contain ample quantities of vitamins A, C, and K. Due to plums' significant levels of insoluble fiber content, some turn to this fruit, more so in their dried form as prunes, for healthy bowel maintenance.

Seeds

Chia

Chia seeds are full of omega-3s, supplying energy boosts and heart health benefits and lowering blood pressure and cholesterol. They have a high protein content, along with fiber, iron, calcium, and antioxidants. The manganese and phosphorus in chia seeds contribute to strong bone health. The tryptophan and omega-3s in chia seeds can act as a mood enhancer, increasing brain function, and their consumption can reduce hunger.

Flax

Flaxseeds are one of the original foods recommended by Hippocrates. They are most nutritionally beneficial in a just-ground state, are best known for their content of omega-3 fatty acids, with their heart-healthy effects, as well as lignans, with their antioxidant qualities. Additionally, flaxseeds contain both soluble and insoluble fiber. Evidence over the years has shown that flaxseeds may reduce rates of cancer, heart disease, stroke, and diabetes. The lignans can reduce inflammation, easing pain of arthritis, and reduce plaque buildup, which can unclog arteries.

Hemp

Cited as one of the most nutritious seeds in the world, hemp seeds, also known as hemp hearts, truly contain a lot of nutrition in a small seed package. In themselves, they are a complete and easily digestible protein, with all twenty known amino acids. They provide the ideal balance of essential fatty acids: omega-3, omega-6, and gamma-linolenic acid. Very high in vitamin E, they also contain magnesium, which helps counter the ill effects of stress, B vitamins, iron, and zinc. Just a few tablespoons of this superseed sprinkled on salads or blended into smoothies and dressings, can give you all of these nutritional benefits.

Pumpkin

Pumpkin seeds are also known as pepitas, and can be eaten raw, cooked, sprouted, or toasted. They offer a wealth of nutrients including 7 grams of protein per ounce. Pumpkin seeds also contain amino acids, unsaturated fatty acids, and bountiful minerals, such as calcium, potassium, niacin, and phosphorus. They also offer ample amounts of most B vitamins, and vitamins C, D, E, and K, as well as beta-carotene and lutein.

Pumpkin seeds may also be good for prostate health, as the omega-3s, monounsaturated oil, carotenoids, and zinc found in them have shown benefits in counteracting the possibilities of prostate cancer. If that isn't enough, pumpkin seeds are anti-inflammatory and contain the third-highest content of phytosterols after sunflower seeds and pistachios. Phytosterols are known to reduce blood levels of cholesterol, enhance the immune response, and may decrease risk of certain cancers.

Sesame

Sesame seeds are best known for containing an extraordinary amount of calcium and magnesium. They are a great source of protein and fiber as well as amino acids essential for growth. They provide the B-complex vitamin niacin. The seeds also contain minerals, such as manganese, copper, iron, phosphorus, and zinc. They have the highest phytosterols, which help in lowering bad cholesterol, of any nut or seed. They also contain antioxidants that lower free radicals, and folic acid, which is beneficial to pregnant women.

Sunflower

Likely the most nutrient-dense seeds available and best eaten raw, protein-rich sunflower seeds provide good quantities of calcium, copper, iron, magnesium, selenium, and zinc. Vitamins B_6 and E, folic acid, niacin, and thiamine are in sunflower seeds, which are also complete with fiber and natural plant hormones. With a significant oil content, they are a good source of low-cholesterol polyunsaturated oil, which is said to lower the risk of heart attacks and other cardiovascular disease.

Nuts

Almonds

Versatile almonds appear in many forms, including almond milk, and make a tasty and nutritious snack all on their own. They are commonly available raw or roasted. Their high mineral, protein, and fiber content makes them among the healthiest of nuts. They are most bountiful in vitamin E, copper, magnesium, and unsaturated fatty acids. Their phytosterols may help prevent heart disease, lower cholesterol, and reduce risk of cancers.

Almond butter is considered to be a more healthful alternative to the ever-so-popular peanut butter. This is due to the increased incidences of allergic reactions to peanuts, as well as possible contamination from aflatoxin fungus (a mold that is common to peanuts—although improved storage and handling practices have greatly reduced the risk of contamination).

Brazil Nuts

These earthy nuts are best known for their high selenium content. Snacking on just two to four a day will provide enough of the daily need of selenium, an antioxidant that plays a critical role in the liver's normal function and is necessary for the liver to convert T4 into the active T3 form of thyroid hormone, which all the cells in the body need to function properly. Brazil nuts provide ample protein and fat as well as several important nutrients, such as folate, choline, magnesium, calcium, and phosphorus.

Cashews

Snackable cashews are known for their mineral supply: iron, selenium, zinc, copper, and phosphorus, which are all key to regulate good health functioning of the body. You'll profit from the presence of vitamins B_6, E, and K in cashews as well. No-cholesterol nuts with mostly the good kind of fat, cashews also contain proanthocyanidins, which are said to restrict cancer cells from replicating.

Pecans

Pecans are a tasty source of energy, with their high fat content including monoun-

saturated oleic acid. Consuming pecans is said to decrease the level of bad cholesterol (LDL) and increase good cholesterol (HDL). They also contain beta-carotene, ellagic acid (believed to be an anticarcinogen), lutein, zeaxanthin, and exceptional vitamin E. Additionally, pecans have many minerals, such as manganese, potassium, calcium, iron, zinc, and selenium.

Pistachios

Reputed to lower body weight and lower risks of heart difficulties, pistachios are a rich-tasting nut containing protein, fiber, and some unsaturated fat. Per serving, pistachios pack more potassium and vitamin K than all other nuts, while providing plenty of copper, vitamin B_6, thiamine, phosphorus, and magnesium. As inflammation fighters, the L-arginine in pistachios makes the lining of arteries more pliable and thereby less at risk for clots, while vitamin E acts as a plaque preventative. Not only beneficial for heart health, the carotenoid content of lutein and zeaxanthin in pistachios is a potent boost for eye health.

Walnuts

Walnuts are the only nut with a significant amount of alpha-linolenic acid. Unlike some other nuts, their fats are primarily polyunsaturated. Although calorie dense, walnuts contribute to a satiated feeling. The omega-3 fatty acids, phytosterols, and antioxidants in walnuts have potential to reduce cancer rates. They are known as a potent food for the mind, promoting brain health (and they're even shaped a bit like the brain!). Walnuts may prevent heart disease and lower cholesterol. They have a large quantity of vitamin B$_6$ and E, folate, thiamine, and manganese.

Grains

Amaranth G

Exceptionally small in size, amaranth is gaining in notoriety because of its astronomical content of top-quality and digestible nutrient content. It has an enormous quantity of manganese, iron, fiber, and lysine, an important amino acid, as well as primary proteins albumin and globulin. Interestingly, it tops many vegetables in mineral content, such as phosphorus, calcium, and iron, as well as carotenoids. It is also the only known grain to have vitamin C content, which makes its iron more absorbable.

Barley

Versatile barley is most nutritious in its whole form: hulled, brown, unpearled—all of which contain gluten. It is plentiful in soluble and insoluble fiber, potentially reducing risks of colorectal cancer. Appearing in barley are manganese, iron, niacin, and protein, in addition to its impressive fiber content. It also may help control blood sugar levels, increase breast milk supply for lactating women, help with weight control, lower glucose levels on the glycemic index, and also lower blood pressure and cholesterol.

Brown Rice G

The versatility of whole-grain brown rice makes it a favorite accompaniment to many dishes. Its impressive fiber content makes it a great choice as a nutritional powerhouse, possibly promoting cardio-vascular health and protecting against certain types of cancer, all while giving a feeling of satisfied fullness, helping with weight management. Because less processing allows its fiber and essential fats to remain intact, brown rice may help lower the risks of both diabetes and high cholesterol. Brown rice provides strong doses of manganese, selenium, and magnesium, as well as phytonutrients, with their anti-inflammatory and antioxidant properties.

Buckwheat G

The name often causes confusion—buckwheat is a seed and not a wheat or grain, and is in fact gluten free. The hulled seeds of the plant are called groats. Buckwheat is available in raw or toasted form (called kasha). The raw form is used widely in raw food cuisine in such dishes as granola, and as the base of cakes and pizza crusts. You can also sprout the kernel for buckwheat sprouts. Buckwheat contains fiber for healthy digestion plus all nine essential amino acids, including lysine, as well as iron, magnesium and manganese, zinc, and copper. It also has two flavonoids: quercetin, which promotes healing, and rutin, which is known for protecting eye health and reducing high blood pressure.

Couscous

Couscous is one of the few food sources of selenium, a trace mineral that is needed in small quantities to reduce buildup of plaque and bad cholesterol in the blood vessels. It is not a grain itself but is a kind of pasta made from semolina. It is a reliable protein, fiber, B vitamins, and manganese source.

Farro

Dating back to the Etruscans, farro (also known as emmer) got its name from its status as a top-of-the-line wheat, or pharaoh's wheat. Big on protein, fiber, iron, zinc, niacin, and folate, farro is filling and a unique alternative to rice and quinoa, and fabulous as an easier-cooking risotto. Farro comes in pearled and semipearled, and in long, medium, or cracked forms. *Pearled* refers to the outer bran being removed for faster cooking times; therefore whole or semipearled are nutritionally more fiber-rich, though they may require soaking and a longer cooking time.

Millet ⓖ

One of the few grains that has an alkalizing effect on the body system, millet is emerging as a more locally grown and economical alternative to quinoa—its cousin in terms of size and cooking time (which means that they can be mixed together for a multigrain dish). Millet contains serotonin, helpful for mood balancing. It has a high protein content and promotes antioxidant activity. Additionally, you will find high B vitamins and the minerals iron, zinc, magnesium, and calcium in millet.

Quinoa ⓖ

While botanically a seed, quinoa is commonly referred to as the ancient grain of the Incas. Quinoa leads the pack of nutritional grains with the highest nutrient profile of all and twice as much fiber as other grains with easy digestibility. It delivers a high dosage of complete protein, having all nine essential amino acids. Quinoa contains B vitamins, especially B_2 (riboflavin) as well as good content of vitamin E. It is also known as a good source of iron, magnesium, potassium, zinc, and calcium, and the antioxidant manganese. Lysine, used by the body for tissue repair, is found in quinoa. Quinoa is also available ground into a high-protein, low-carb gluten-free baking flour, or made into flakes as a substitute for oats.

Spelt

Spelt is an ancient variety of wheat that contains less gluten than common wheat, but does have some; those with wheat intolerances may find it more digestible because of its high water solubility. Although dense in nutrients, its flour makes baked items light and low on crumbs, with a mild nutty flavor. With a hefty protein content, spelt also delivers niacin, phosphorus, copper, iron, zinc, and magnesium.

Steel-Cut Oats ⓖ

Also called Scotch or Irish oats, steel-cut oats are the whole toasted oat grain (as opposed to the rolled or quick version) and are most nutritious in this unprocessed form. Oats are well known for helping to eliminate fat and cholesterol from the body. Steel-cut oats are associated with a decreased risk of heart disease, diabetes, hypertension, and obesity. They have a wealth of B vitamins, magnesium, protein, calcium, and fiber. Naturally gluten-free, oats can be contaminated with gluten if processed in the same facility (or even grown in an adjacent field) as a gluten-containing grain, so be sure to check the packaging for a product's gluten-free certification if necessary.

Triticale

The name *triticale* comes from the cross of names for wheat and rye, *triticum* and *secale*, fitting because this plant was bred by crossing wheat with rye, with a resulting higher protein content than either wheat or rye, with more of the amino acid lysine. It is usually sold as flour but can also be found in whole-grain form called triticale berries, which must be boiled until soft. Both berries and flour contain handsome protein, fiber, folate, and magnesium quantities.

Legumes

Black Beans

High in fiber and protein, black beans are an extremely nutrient dense food. Iron, calcium, potassium, magnesium, folate, zinc, and phosphorus are all present in black beans. Black beans, available dried and in cans, have more free radical–neutralizing antioxidants than other beans.

Fava Beans

Also known as broad beans or field beans and a member of the pea family, these extra-large beans are extra-packed with nutrition. They come canned, dried, or in a pod. Count on fava beans for folate, manganese, vitamin B_1, iron, phosphorus, magnesium, copper, and potassium, not to mention protein. They are low-calorie and filling, supplying ample fiber for the day.

Garbanzos

Garbanzo beans, or chickpeas, well known as the bulk of hummus, are also well known as a fantastic protein source. Available dried and in cans, as well as ground as a gluten-free flour, they are also known for very impressive content of folate and manganese. Additionally, you'll find copper, phosphorus, iron, and magnesium within. Notable as well are their molybdenum and antioxidant phytonutrients. Similar nutrient content is available canned or cooked from dry beans.

Great Northern Beans

Great northern beans are also known as white beans and are extremely versatile as they take on the flavors of whatever they're mixed with, more so than other beans. Like other beans, they are good sources of protein, iron, fiber, and potassium. Another benefit of great northern beans is the presence of folate, a water-soluble B vitamin that helps with protein metabolism.

Kidney Beans

A good source of both soluble and insoluble fiber, kidney beans are named loosely after their shape. As with many beans, they are protein-packed, especially when combined with rice to form a complete protein. Their iron content is another plus, as is their manganese, both of which contribute to energy boosts. Their calcium and folate content enhances bone health. Kidney beans, available dried and in cans, also contain vitamin K and thiamine.

Lentils

Lentils are high in nutrition, low in calories, and easy and quick to cook compared to other legumes. Varieties include brown, red, black, and green, all of which vary in flavor and texture. Their high quantity of soluble and especially insoluble fiber makes for easy digestion, providing a full feeling. They are a strong protein source, with protein making up 26 percent of their calories. They contain plenty of folate, a B vitamin, as well as magnesium, and are a good iron source. Additionally, lentils provide potassium, calcium, zinc, niacin, and vitamin K, and may reduce the risk of heart disease.

Soybeans

Soybeans can be eaten in many forms including tofu, tempeh, and soy milk. The beans are a tasty snack in themselves (edamame). All forms are extremely important sources of protein and fiber in a super low-cal package with healthy unsaturated fats. Soybeans contain vitamins B_6 and K, riboflavin, and folate, and the minerals manganese, magnesium, phosphorus, and iron.

Split Peas

Big on fiber, split peas are super filling and move cholesterol-containing bile out of the body, lowering levels of bad cholesterol. They also are helpful in stabilizing blood sugar levels, which can help in the prevention and management of diabetes. Peas are considered heart-friendly because they have been shown to help reduce plaque in blood vessels, with their notable content of anti-inflammatory fats and the antioxidant vitamin E. They also conquer the effects of sulfites by detoxifying them with the mineral molybdenum. Split peas contain significant amounts of protein, minerals, B vitamins, and isoflavones, which may reduce the likelihood of breast or prostate cancers.

Cayenne Pepper

Cayenne pepper's heat improves blood circulation and aids digestion, increasing the appetite in some cases. Its active ingredient, capsaicin, is used for treatment of aches and pains of muscles or joints. Additionally, cayenne removes toxins from the body and may prevent growth of cancer cells. It is used as an anti-inflammatory and antifungal. Flavonoids give cayenne its antioxidant properties.

Cinnamon

A spice from tree branches with two varieties, the more common Ceylon cinnamon has been used since ancient times to treat sore throat, arthritis, and coughs. Cinnamon is used in diabetes and hypoglycemic management because it has been shown to improve glucose and lipid levels, and may have use in the inhibition of Alzheimer's disease. It is known to be both lipid lowering and antibacterial, according to many published studies.[1] It also can relieve the pain of arthritis and other ailments with its anti-inflammatory properties. This spice is versatile, as it can work well both in sweet and savory creations. Although usually consumed in small amounts, there are traces of fiber, iron, calcium, and manganese in cinnamon.

Fenugreek

Fenugreek is a strongly flavored spice in powder or seed form, and its leaves and shoots can also be consumed in salads. It is remarkable for its ability to improve muscle performance because of its balance of high protein and sustaining carbohydrates. According to Dr. Greger, a muscle strength study showed that fenugreek produced a "significant impact on both upper- and lower-body strength and body composition in comparison to placebo in a double blind controlled trial."[2]

There are many vitamins and minerals in fenugreek, as well as polysaccharides, which can help lower bad cholesterol levels. Its amino acids are said to lower blood sugar levels in those with diabetes. It has been used historically to treat digestive issues, prevent or treat weight gain from its bulky fiber content, and to improve the secretion of milk from nursing mothers. Fenugreek is believed to have fed the Roman legions as they marched across Europe and the Middle East and is promoted as a booster in high-endurance training.

Garlic

Classified as both a food and a medicinal herb, garlic is a healing powerhouse. It fires up digestive enzymes and boosts the immune system. It has been shown to lower bad cholesterol levels and blood pressure as well as to prevent blood clots, with heart-protective benefits. An antibiotic, antioxidant, and antiviral, garlic is rich in sulfur and reputed cancer-preventing compounds. Consumption may reduce pain in those with arthritis. Garlic is also thought to improve the body's absorption of iron.

Ginger

Extraordinarily medicinal, ginger is showing promising results in many studies to be more effective against some infections than antibiotics and may protect cells against cancer. It is perhaps best known for its anti-inflammatory and immunity-boosting properties, healing the intestinal tract, and counteracting nausea and motion sickness. Studies have also shown prevention and treatment of diabetes, reduced arthritis pain, and improved mobility.

Ginger contains vitamins B_5 and B_6, and such minerals as potassium, manganese, copper, and magnesium. The health-benefiting compound gingerol gives raw ginger its antibacterial properties. Cooking transforms gingerol into zingerone, a chemical that gives ginger its strong distinctive flavor and has been shown to be effective against stomach upset from *E. coli*.

Turmeric

Turmeric, an orange spice whose main component is curcumin, is one of the most potent anti-inflammatories, a natural antiseptic/antibacterial that speeds up wound healing, and is strongly antioxidant. Turmeric's other wide-ranging uses include pain relief, fighting free radicals, aiding with fat metabolism, treating depression, and possibly slowing the onset and development of Alzheimer's disease.

Other Superfoods

Cacao

Cacao is widely appreciated for its theobromine, a mild stimulant that can aid in depression treatment, and anandamide, a lipid with feel-good effects. A sense of alertness comes from cacao's phenylethylamine.

There is also a high content of sulfur, magnesium, iron, and flavonoids, which act as antioxidants. The polyphenols in cacao prevent blood clotting, also lowering bad and increasing good cholesterol. Raw unsweetened cacao offers more nutritional benefits than when the cacao is processed as cocoa or milk/dark chocolate.

Chlorella

Chlorella, a type of algae that grows in fresh water, is available in powdered, tablet, capsule, or liquid form in most natural foods stores. It has natural detoxification properties because it bonds to the accumulated chemicals, pesticides, and heavy metals that the body acquires just by living in today's environment. Chlorella may also counteract side effects of radiation, increasing white blood cell counts, and can increase good bacteria in the digestive tract. It is 50 percent protein and contains all essential amino acids, many B vitamins, vitamins C and K, and folic acid, plus calcium, iron, and potassium.

Cultured Foods

Cultured, or fermented, foods, such as sauerkraut, kimchi, kombucha, and miso, have undergone a process whereby natural bacteria feed on sugars and starches in the food and create lactic acids. This helps preserve the food and its nutrients, and also creates enzymes, probiotics, B vitamins, and fatty acids. Long associated with gut health, fermentation renders foods more digestible, and is recommended for improving digestive conditions. Recent studies have linked the gut with health throughout the body, including immune system functioning and mental health; supporting your gut health with cultured foods may help more than just digestion!

Goji Berries

Goji berries are bright red, chewy berries that have a distinct sweet/tart/slightly bitter flavor. Also known as wolfberries, they originated for medicinal purposes in ancient China to treat the eyes, liver, and kidneys. Unlike other berries, they are most commonly found in a dried form, but like other berries, their antioxidant content is high, with additional benefits for eye health, perhaps due to their taurine content. They are unique among other fruits for their high protein levels, with all the essential amino acids. Goji berries also contain vitamins A and C, iron, calcium, zinc, and selenium.

Maca

With origins in South America, maca root, a relative of the turnip, has been used for two thousand years. There is now renewed interest because of its great variety of health benefits. It is believed to improve resistance to disease and is proven to enhance the effectiveness of the adrenal glands, which are connected to energy levels. It is plentiful in B vitamins as well as vitamins C and E. Calcium, zinc, iron, magnesium, phosphorus, and amino acids are also in maca root. Its glucosinolates may reduce risk of cancers and have antifungal, antiparasitic, and antibacterial effects. Memory and sexual function enhancements are reputed to accompany maca consumption. Maca is usually dried into a powder, which works well in smoothies and raw desserts, as it has a mild flavor, described as malty, which often goes unnoticed. It can also be found encapsulated as a supplement.

Moringa

The moringa tree is native to India, and the leaf, from which a powder is made, is a phenomenal nutrition source, with ninety known nutrients and extraordinary concentration of vitamins and minerals. The leaf's compounds are antibacterial and contain substances that lower blood pressure. Moringa is a natural energy booster that simultaneously detoxifies, as it is known to be used to purify water The leaves are used traditionally in cooking, and can be made into a tea with a pleasant mild and slightly spicy flavor. Add a spoonful of the powder to your smoothies or juices.

Noni

The noni berry grows on a tree called canary wood and comes in powdered, pulp, or juice form. It has been used historically to treat menstrual cramps, urinary tract infections, arthritis, and diabetes. Nowadays, more recent studies have shown that the antioxidants and anti-inflammatory content of the noni fruit may prevent stroke, and that drinking the juice may reduce pain sensations. Cholesterol lowering and antibacterial e. coli fighting properties have also resulted from noni consumption. The juice is high in vitamin C, while the noni pulp also contains vitamin B_3, iron, and potassium.

Sea Vegetables

There are thousands of types of sea vegetables, which are classified into categories by color, known either as brown, red, or green. Each is unique, having a distinct shape, taste, and texture. The most commonly eaten sea vegetables are nori, hijiki, wakame, arame, kombu, and dulse. They are often sold in a dried form and used as is, or simply soaked for five to ten minutes before adding to a dish.

Easy ways to incorporate sea vegetables are by making nori vegetable rolls, or keeping a container of kelp flakes around as a condiment for seasoning foods.

The strength of sea vegetables is sky high and readily bioavailable mineral content, including calcium, selenium, iodine, magnesium, potassium, iron, and zinc, with iodine in some as well. They additionally have compounds that help remove toxins from the body. Sea vegetables have been present for around 2 billion years, and all contain chlorophyll, phytonutrients, and protein. See page 86 for more information about sea vegetables.

Spirulina

Available in powdered, tablet, and capsule form, spirulina is a blue-green algae derivative made up of 62 percent amino acids. Spirulina is a superfood especially high in protein, bioavailable iron, and calcium. The chlorophyll in spirulina enhances the immune system and removes toxins from the blood, while its carotenoids help protect cells from damage. It contains gamma-linolenic acid, an essential fatty acid, which has anti-inflammatory properties. Other nutrients found in spirulina are B-complex vitamins, beta-carotene, vitamin E, manganese, zinc, copper, iron, and selenium.

Organically Grown Foods—
for Your Health and the Health
of the Planet

A few words about organics and GMOs:

I recommend purchasing organic ingredients whenever possible. The Organic Trade Association states, "Organic farming is based on practices that maintain soil fertility, while assisting nature's balance through diversity and recycling of energy and nutrients. This method also strives to avoid or reduce the use of synthetic fertilizers and pest controls. Organic foods are processed, packaged, transported, and stored to retain maximum nutritional value, without the use of artificial preservatives, coloring or other additives, irradiation, or synthetic pesticides."

While there has been some conflicting information published about the nutritional benefits of organically grown food, there is no disputing that many of the chemicals in commercial pesticides and fertilizers have not been tested for their long-term effects on humans. Nonorganic foods substantially increase our exposure to these chemicals, as well as to antibiotic-resistant bacteria. There is also the human rights issue of the tens of thousands of agriculture workers on nonorganic farms, many of whom are diagnosed with pesticide poisoning each year. In my opinion, the risks of using these toxic chemicals far outweigh any potential benefits.

Organically grown foods represent a cycle of sustainability that improves topsoil fertility, enhances nutrition, and ensures food security. Organic farmers employ farming methods that respect the fragile

You'll find a comprehensive nutrition chart on pages 319–338; this chart will help you choose nutrients and foods that provide support for and promote the optimal functioning of specific body systems.

balance of our ecosystem. This results in a fraction of the groundwater pollution and topsoil depletion that's generated by conventional methods.

Purchasing local, seasonal, and organically grown food is also an extremely effective way to reduce your environmental impact. Buying local saves the huge amount of energy it takes to transport food—sometimes across oceans and continents. For more information on organic farming, visit your local farmers' market and talk to the farmers. You can also check out the websites for the organic organizations listed in the appendix.

OMG! GMO Alert

A GMO (genetically engineered and modified organism) is a plant, animal, or microorganism that has had its genetic code altered, typically by introducing genes from another organism. This process gives the GMO food characteristics that are not present in its original form. Many feel this practice goes against nature and poses a profound threat to people, the environment, and our agricultural heritage.

There are even GMO seeds that are referred to as assassin seeds. The plant that grows from these seeds produces seeds that are infertile. This prevents the replication of the genetic bond. This means that

Not all produce is created equal. The Environmental Working Group (EWG) puts together a list of those commercially grown foods with the highest level of pesticides and those with the lowest levels of pesticides. The "Clean 15" were found to contain little to no traces of pesticides. While the list changes each year that the EWG tests the produce, the culprits generally remain the same; you can check online at www.ewg.org for the most up-to-date list.

Those with the highest levels of pesticides are referred to as the "Dirty Dozen," which tested positive for forty-seven to sixty-seven different pesticides.

You can identify organic produce by looking at its PLU, which should begin with a "9." Always purchase the "Dirty Dozen" organically.

"The Clean 15" (little to no traces of pesticides)

- Asparagus
- Avocados
- Cabbage
- Cantaloupe (domestic)
- Cauliflower
- Eggplants
- Grapefruits
- Kiwis
- Mangoes
- Onions
- Papayas
- Pineapples
- Sweet corn
- Sweet peas (frozen)
- Sweet potatoes

The "Dirty Dozen," Plus

This is the current list of produce on the "Dirty Dozen" list:

- Apples
- Celery
- Cherry tomatoes
- Cucumbers
- Grapes
- Nectarines (imported)
- Peaches
- Potatoes
- Snap peas (imported)
- Spinach
- Strawberries
- Sweet bell peppers

Plus these that may contain insecticides:
- Hot peppers
- Blueberries (domestic)

farmers must constantly purchase seeds every year from the companies that manufacture them.

GMO seed manufacturers maintain that this makes the seed more pest resistant, promotes higher yields, or enhances nutrition. But the long-term effects of these seeds on our health, our genetic pool, the environment, and other life forms that make up the complex web of life we all share are still unknown. As with the use of chemical pesticides, it is simply not worth the risk. Eating organic foods eliminates GMO from our food supply.

There is a continuous push in the United States to have genetically modified foods labeled as such. This legislation has been fiercely resisted by the companies that manufacture the GMO products and those that profit from their sale. Over sixty countries around the world, including the entire European Union and even China, insist on labeling. In fact, many communities around the world have succeeded in becoming GMO-free.

Please support this important movement to move our agriculture away from genetic engineering and toward truly sustainable agriculture. For more information, you may visit the Non-GMO Project at www.nongmoproject.org. You can tell whether your produce has been genetically modified by looking at the PLU label. Numbers beginning with "8" indicate a GMO product.

CHAPTER 4

The Extraordinary Health Benefits of Raw Whole Foods

If it came from a plant, eat it; if it was made in a plant, don't.
—MICHAEL POLLAN

As we have seen, there are countless nutritional theories, many of which are in direct contradiction to one another.

With so many conflicting ideas on what foods we should avoid, is there any agreement on what to include? While the recommended percentage varies, most would agree on the importance of including fresh fruits and vegetables in our diet as a way to prevent disease and early death. While you may not follow a completely raw diet, the benefits of including some uncooked raw fruits and vegetables in your daily meals are undeniable. Numerous resources are available for those seeking to embrace more of a raw food lifestyle. For a comprehensive guide to raw foods, you can check out my book *The Complete Idiot's Guide to Eating Raw*.

Raw Food Revolution

Raw foods, also called "living foods," have not been cooked or processed.

Gabriel Cousens, MD, one of the strongest modern-day supporters of live food nutrition, writes, "Living or raw food means it has not been processed in any way, including cooking. Because of this none of the heat sensitive micronutrients have been destroyed. . . . Although there is some variation in research findings, most agree that over 50% of the B-vitamins are destroyed by cooking. Thiamine (B-1) losses have been recorded up to 96%, folic acid loses up to 97%, and biotin losses up to 72%. Vitamin C losses are up to 70–80%." Some raw foods tend to have more bioavailable vitamins, minerals, enzymes, phytochemicals, and disease-fighting flavonoids. Furthermore, cooking alters the ingredient away from its most natural state.

Raw food advocates report more energy and greater health and mental clarity by preserving vital nutrients, many of which are thought to be destroyed in the heating process. For instance, a review by researchers at the University of California, Davis found that vitamin C levels decreased by 15 to 55 percent in home cooking.

Often, when someone mentions being on a raw diet, the question that follows is, "How raw are you?" This is because many people on a raw food diet do include some cooked food in their meals—which means a raw diet does not have to be an all-or-nothing enterprise. In fact, it is very common to be 75/25 raw/cooked (a 'high raw" diet) or indeed, 50/50. In the end, every body needs to experiment with different combinations of percentages and ingredients to include raw or cooked, to find the right fit.

While healthy diets can run the gamut from fully cooked to fully raw, many agree that including a certain percentage of raw, unprocessed foods is a basic tenet for gleaning an optimal nutritional intake. A thoughtful balance of raw foods in the diet can counteract some of the deficiencies in a purely cooked diet, and add nutritional elements that may not exist in the same forms in a cooked food regimen.

HEALING STORIES

Managing Type 2 Diabetes with Vegan, Raw, Whole Foods

🐦 I am a retired registered nurse and took one nutrition class while I was attending nursing school. I come from a Scandinavian family, and their diet is high in eggs and rich dairy products. Type 2 diabetes does not run in my family; however, hypercholesterolemia runs rampant on my mother's side of the family. Almost all of my aunts and uncles are on some sort of statin. As a child, I was quite tall and very slender. I was so slender that I was constantly teased about being skinny. I could eat whatever I wanted, whenever I wanted and would never gain a pound. As an adult, I was too tired to cook whenever I got home from work, so I got into a very bad habit of eating out every night and eating fast food for late night snacks.

On a routine dental cleaning my hygienist told me that my gums were looking and acting "like I was diabetic." I went to my internist and got the bad news that I was a type 2 diabetic. I was getting close to 300 pounds, my blood pressure was 170/100, and my triglycerides were over 800. I was immediately put on metformin and a statin and was told to take the drugs even if they made me sick. I began having diabetic neuropathy in my feet, my vision started blurring, and the diabetes caused a rare form of arthritis called DISH (diffuse idiopathic skeletal hyperostosis).

My rheumatologist told me that he couldn't help me with my arthritis until I got my diabetes under control. He put me on muscle relaxers, pain pills, and an antidepressant. Overmedicated and sleeping 12–14 hours a day, I decided to get out of the denial mode and do something drastic. My internist recommended "a plant-based diet with no egg yolks and no cheese." I didn't know much about diets, so I got on the Internet and started my journey.

I ended up taking a 5-day vegan cooking class. We would cook a dish, stop and eat, and while we were eating would get lessons in nutrition. At first, I was skeptical about taking the class because many vegan dishes are high in carbohydrates, but one of the first things I learned in class was that I could eat carbohydrates; I just had to watch portion control. I learned that eating a small snack over a long period of time can be satiating. After that first class my blood sugar had dropped to 106. This was the lowest that it had ever been after eating a meal. Throughout the entire week my blood sugar levels remained in the 100 range. The hardest part of the class was coming home to central Texas and trying to live a vegan lifestyle in a small town where chicken-fried steak smothered in gravy with barbecue as a side dish is the staple meal. I started spending all of my grocery shopping time in the produce aisle. I have primarily been eating raw since I took the class. I get my sources of protein from beans, raw almonds, almond milk, chia seeds, and flaxseeds. I drink a lot of green smoothies that contain greens, blueberries, apples, raw almonds, chia seeds, flaxseeds, and almond milk. I have learned to buy vegetables that stay fresh in the refrigerator for long periods of time. A few months after the cooking class I had my lab work redone:

- I had lost 60 pounds.
- My blood pressure was 124/80.
- My triglycerides dropped 600 points and are now 224.
- My total cholesterol was 95.
- My HDL was 31.
- My LDL dropped to 19.
- My AIC dropped from 7.1 to 4.4.

All of the lab values that were dangerously high dropped to normal simply because I changed the way I eat, what I eat, and when I eat. It is important to note that I lost all this weight simply from changing what I eat. I couldn't exercise because of the DISH arthritis. I have more energy than I've had in years. I now feel good enough to start exercising! I have had a lifelong battle with depression, and controlling my diabetes has also had a major effect on my depression. I have quit taking the drugs prescribed by the rheumatologist, and I now have more energy, less pain, and my depression is very manageable. I'm slowly weaning myself off of the antidepressants. My internist has now taken me off of the metformin and statin. She wrote in my electronic chart: "diabetes is now controlled by diet." My doctor no longer writes me prescriptions, we trade recipes! Living the vegan lifestyle has turned my life around. I don't like to use the phrase "vegan diet" because being a vegan is about embracing a lifestyle, not a diet.

Enzymes for Health

Dr. Norman Walker, creator of the Norwalk Juicer, and author of the pivotal book *Raw Vegetable Juices: What's Missing in Your Body?* expressing a central idea behind raw food theory, writes, "The basic key to the efficacy of nourishing your body is the life which is present in your food and of those intangible elements known as enzymes." Much of our information about enzymes is based upon the extensive research of Dr. Edward Howell, who spent over fifty years researching the importance of enzymes in human nutrition before writing his book *Enzyme Nutrition*, the unabridged version of which contains over seven hundred references to scientific literature.

Dr. Howell writes, "Enzymes are substances that make life possible. They are needed for every chemical reaction that takes place in the human body. No mineral, vitamin or hormone can do any work without enzymes. Our bodies, all of our organs, tissues and cells are run by enzymes."

According to Dr. Howell, there are three different classes of enzymes—metabolic enzymes, digestive enzymes, and food enzymes. Metabolic enzymes are the catalysts of all reactions within the body; they run the tissues and organs, and convert fats, carbohydrates, and proteins into usable forms of energy. Digestive enzymes exist in the body to digest our food. The three major types are amylase, which digests carbohydrates; lipase, which digests fats; and protease, which digests proteins. The third class of enzymes are food enzymes, which are present in all raw foods and which, according to the raw food theory, begin the digestive process.

Dr. Howell goes on to say, "Where there is life, there are enzymes. Enzymes are sensitive to temperatures above 118 degrees F. Above 120 degrees F enzymes become sluggish . . . at 130 degrees F the life of enzymes is extinct. They are dead."

The Data

To date, scientific literature describing health and nutrition aspects of raw foods or living foods diets is limited, and most studies are of vegetarian diets. A meta-analysis of scientific studies from 1994 to 2004 concluded there to be an inverse correlation between the risk of developing certain types of cancer and eating both raw and cooked vegetables. Consumption of raw vegetables tended to be associated with decreased cancer risks somewhat more often than consumption of cooked vegetables.

Columbia University research in 2008 showed significant improvement in mental and emotional quality of life for participants who enrolled in a program at Hippocrates Health Institute (Florida), consuming a raw vegan institute for one to three weeks. Another American study in 2001 showed fibromyalgia syndrome improved in observational study using a mostly raw vegetarian diet.

It is important to keep in mind that many question the role of enzymes in raw food nutrition. Some nutrients are actually more bioavailable when slightly cooked. Lycopene in tomatoes is said to be released more with cooking, as are the carotenoids in many plant foods, and steaming broccoli helps release their glucosinolates, which have cancer-fighting properties. Others point out that even if the enzymes in raw foods have not been destroyed by heating, once the food enters the acidic nature of the digestive system, these enzymes would be destroyed regardless of whether the food is cooked or raw.

Ways to Get More Raw Foods in Your Diet

Raw food cuisine is not just about munching on raw carrots and celery sticks. The cuisine can be highly refined. Techniques that are used to create raw food dishes include sprouting, culturing, and dehydrating.

Culturing

Culturing, also known as fermentation, is the process of shredding a vegetable, placing it in an airtight container usually with water and salt, and leaving at room temperature for about a week to culture. The vegetable's natural lactobacillus bacteria multiplies, lowering the pH balance and increasing the acidic content. Consuming the result provides a probiotic intestinal aid and brings a bountiful quantity of helpful microorganisms to the system, especially for digestion. Sauerkraut, kombucha, kimchi, miso, and rejuvelac are some of the most common cultured items. See Simple Sauerkraut (page 176) and Quick Kimchi (page 178).

Sprouting

Seeds, beans, and legumes can be sprouted for a fresh raw version. After exposure to water and humidity in the form of rinsing, the seeds, beans, or legumes will germinate and open and a sprout will emerge from them and grow. This includes soaked and germinated nuts and seeds, sprouted grains, and legumes, as well as the sprouted young wheatgrass and other grasses eaten whole or juiced. The process of soaking is used because it activates the proteases, which neutralize the enzyme inhibitors that keep the seed, legumes, and grains from germinating at the wrong time. Germinating and sprouting increases the enzyme content. Starches are broken down into simple sugars, proteins are predigested into easily assimilated free amino acids, and fats are broken down into soluble fatty acids.

Juicing

Fresh juices are an essential part of a raw food lifestyle. Nutrients are released immediately into the cells and bloodstream in a form that's easiest to assimilate. Juices made at home are a convenient and delicious way to get the five to nine recommended daily servings of fruits and vegetables. Enjoy juices on their own or as the base for smoothies, live soups, sauces, and dressings. Chapter 10 provides many recipes for delicious juices, smoothies, and elixirs that will help you to boost your intake of fresh fruit and vegetables.

Healing with Raw Foods and Juices
Steve Prussack, Juice Guru
https://www.juiceguru.com

I'm in my late forties and have more energy than when I was in my twenties. Best of all, I maintain the perfect weight for my body, have the clearest, most focused thinking, and my relationship with my high school sweetheart, Julie, gets better every day. But it wasn't always this way.

When I graduated college, I was overweight and out of shape from (A LOT OF) late-night foods, drinking and smoking . . .

I didn't want to stay that way . . . I mean, who does? So, I hit the gym, changed my diet, and tried to get into better shape.

But no matter what, I couldn't get back to my starting weight. I lacked focus. I couldn't find a sustaining love relationship. I binged on junk food thinking it was healthy (low-fat chicken sandwiches, low-fat cheese pizza, etc. etc. etc.).

And then one day, while looking for a solution, in a used books store, I stumbled upon a book by the '80s icon the "Juiceman" Jay Kordich.

As a young man and a college athlete at the height of fitness, he was diagnosed with a deadly cancer.

Traditional doctors had given Jay a dire prognosis but he wouldn't give up and sought out an alternative.

What he discovered was the power of raw foods and juice made of 100% raw, organic, freshly pressed fruits and vegetables. This is what he credited to saving his life and cleansing his body of cancer.

This happened to Jay in his 20s . . . Jay is now going strong in his 90s, and I am fortunate to have worked with him for years. I started to pay more attention to my food choices. I cut out dairy, meat and processed foods. I started to eat more whole foods. I spent a few years eating nothing but 100% raw vegan. I also wanted to cleanse my toxic past (alcohol, fast food, drugs, you name it) out of my body.

So after a while eating raw vegan, I took the plunge and did a 14-day juice fast.

From then on, I have used juicing regularly as a way to rid my body of stored toxins and excess fat as well as making it a habit to consume more raw foods. I am passionate about the power of juicing and raw foods. I dedicate my life to spreading the message because of the healing I have discovered in my own life. I want to show others an alternative to painful surgeries and medications. It's best said that I am only interested in helping others prevent pain and misery. The healthy, natural way.

Dehydrating

Dehydrating involves heating foods at low temperatures to reduce the water content. This yields foods that are crispy, seem baked, and are easy to store. Dehydrated foods are wonderful for the variety of dishes you can create with them—from snacks to desserts to main dishes. Check out the Raw Apricot Fennel Granola (page 121) and the Designer Seed and Nut Crust Pizzas (page 265) for some dehydrated raw food dishes. You can also create dried fruit, raw crackers, and even raw tacos by using this technique. Dehydrated foods retain most of the nutrients of the original fresh foods. Plus, dehydrated foods are easy to pack and carry when you travel.

Sample Raw Program

Are you looking to include more raw foods in your diet? You can begin simply by increasing the percentage of raw foods at any given meal. If you wish, you can select one or two days per week as your "raw days." These days may feel like a "cleanse" to you since you will be lightening your diet and eating a higher volume of raw veggies and fruits than you ever have done before.

As always, consult with a qualified health-care practitioner if you have any health concerns before or during embarking upon a substantial change in your diet. Remember to drink lots of liquids such as water, and herbal teas.

Here is a suggested 5-day menu plan to help you incorporate more raw foods into your lifestyle. Plan to have Day Three of the program occur on your least busy day, as this will be the day with the lightest food intake.

Day One: Cooked vegan foods
Day Two: Raw vegan foods
Day Three: Fruit, smoothies, and juices
Day Four: Raw vegan foods
Day Five: Cooked vegan foods

Beverages: be sure to drink plenty of water and/or herbal or green tea.

Snacks: Enjoy raw nuts and seeds, fresh and dried fruit, crudités with avocado or raw dips and sauces, apple slices or celery sticks with raw nut butter, and juices and smoothies to keep you satiated during the day.

	Breakfast	Lunch	Dinner
Day One Cooked Vegan	Garden Veggie Scramble (page 128)	Kitchari (page 257) with Super Sprout Salad (page 173)	Simple One-Pot Meal (page 266) with side salad
Day Two Raw Vegan	Simple Breakfast Chia Pudding (page 117) with fruit	Raw Carrot Brazil Nut Soup (page 245) with Simple Chop Salad (page 174)	Walnut Taco Salad (page 187) with Glorious Guacamole (page 151) and Raw Cashew Sour Cream (page 113)
Day Three Smoothies and Juices	Any of the juices, smoothies, teas, and elixirs from Chapter 10	Any of the juices, smoothies, teas, and elixirs from Chapter 10	Any of the juices, smoothies, teas, and elixirs from Chapter 10
Day Four Raw Vegan	Simple Breakfast Chia Pudding (page 117) with fruit	Raw Cucumber Fennel Soup (page 244) with Provençal Salad (pages 183)	Raw Coconut Curry Vegetables (page 268)
Day Five Cooked Vegan	Iron-Rich Morning Glory Steel-Cut Oats (page 127)	Moroccan Chickpea Stew (page 255) and side salad.	Tempeh Fajitas (page 279) and Garlicky Greens (page 191)

CHAPTER 5

Putting It into Practice: Meal Plans

You now know that a whole food, plant-based diet can help you build the foundation for optimal health. If you'd like some guidance on how to get started on a plant-based diet, here is a suggestion for a well-balanced and relatively simple 14-day menu plan.

- Breakfast: Chia Pudding template (page 117), Homemade Granola template (page 126), or Green Smoothie template (page 147)
- Lunch: Ultimate Salad template (page 174), adding legumes to create a more substantial meal
- Dinner: Monk Bowl template (page 267) with side salad
- Snacks: When the craving for snacks hit, do your best to choose the healthiest option. Go for raw or roasted nuts and seeds without the salt. Choose baked chips instead of fried. Consider keeping chopped veggies, such as carrot, cucumber, and celery, on hand for dipping in hummus (page 159) or a seed or nut butter (apple slices in almond butter is one of my go-to snacks).
- Beverages: Drink lots of water, herbal teas, or nonsugary juices.

If you are feeling a bit more ambitious, here is a suggested menu that will leave you satisfied and will give you an experience of many recipes in the book. Feel free to invite a friend of two to join you, so you can share in the preparation of the dishes. You can switch the dinner menu with the lunch menu if you wish to have the larger meal during the day.

The following suggested menu plan was created to meet the requirements of the CHIP program developed by Dr. Hans Diehl (see page 341). To do so, be sure to follow the ⬤ oil-free options of the recipes, and use just a pinch of salt or the Salt-Free Seasoning recipe (page 108) to replace the sea salt and tamari called for in the recipe.

As far as desserts go, you may not want to make a new dessert every day if there are leftovers. If you are pressed for time, and want to create even simpler meals, please use your knowledge of the Template Recipe (see page 93) to create a dish with whatever ingredients you have on hand.

	Breakfast	Lunch	Dinner	Snack/Dessert	Beverage
Day 1	Simple Breakfast Chia Pudding (page 117) topped with fresh fruit and with 2 tsp. ground flax and 2 tbsp. chopped walnuts	Veggie Lettuce Boats (page 159) with Hummus (page 159) and side salad	Creamy Lentil Saag (page 290), Golden Rice (page 204), and side salad	Fruit-Sweetened Baked Pears (page 303)	Galactic Green Juice (page 135)
Day 2	Multigrain Grits (page 126) topped with 2 tsp. ground flax and 2 tbsp. chopped walnuts	Kitchari (page 257) with Curry Kale Salad (page 184)	BBQ Roasted Tofu with Collards (page 278), cooked black-eyed peas (see page 98) quinoa, and side salad	Banana Mango Ice Cream (page 298)	Small glass of Brazil Nut Milk (page 104)
Day 3	Garden Veggie Scramble (page 128) topped with 2 tsp. ground flax and 2 tbsp. chopped walnuts	Raw Carrot Brazil Nut Soup (page 245), cooked pinto beans (see page 98), side salad	Thai Curry Vegetables (page 289), basmati rice, cooked chickpeas (see page 98), Green Papaya Salad (page 175)	Fresh fruit	Gold Milk (page 144)
Day 4	Trifecta Stewed Dried Fruits (page 121) topped with 2 tsp. ground flax and 2 tbsp. chopped walnuts, with gluten-free toast and tahini	Nori Rolls (page 263) with salad, cooked adzuki beans (see page 98)	Tempeh Fajitas (page 279) with Glorious Guacamole (page 151) and side salad	Mixed Fruit Kanten (page 301)	Berry Green Smoothie (page 147)
Day 5	Iron-Rich Morning Glory Steel-Cut Oats (page 127) with 2 tsp. ground flax and 2 tbsp. chopped walnuts	Curried Broccoli and Great Northern Bean Soup (page 253), Basmati Rice (see page 96), and side salad	Monk Bowl with steamed vegetables, quinoa, and roasted tofu cubes (page 267) and side salad	Superfood Trail Mix (page 295)	Basil Rosemary Lemonade (page 141)

	Breakfast	Lunch	Dinner	Snack/Dessert	Beverage
Day 6	Açai Power Bowl (page 120) with 2 tsp. ground flax	Italian Spring Vegetable Soup (page 252) with quinoa, cooked chickpeas, and side salad	Lentil Walnut Loaf (page 288) with Oil-Free Mushroom Gravy (page 240) and side salad	Fresh fruit	Citrus Magic (page 137)
Day 7	Multigrain Grits (page 126) topped with 2 tsp. ground flax and 2 tbsp. chopped walnuts	Monk Bowl with rice, steamed vegetables, and roasted tempeh (page 267), and side salad	Mushroom Cauliflower Tacos (page 277) with Spicy Pinto Beans (page 206) and side salad	Strawberry Cashew Cream (page 297)	Maca Horchata (page 147)
Day 8	Simple Breakfast Chia Pudding (page 117) topped with fresh fruit and 1 tbsp. almond butter	Mexican Two-Bean Soup (page 256), brown rice, and side salad	Nori Rolls (page 263) and Edamame Arame Salad (page 198)	Raw Apple Crumble (page 300)	Sunrise Carrot Juice (page 137)
Day 9	Pepita Pecan Granola (page 124), with rice milk and fresh fruit	Asian Noodle Soup (page 249), cooked kidney beans (see page 98) with Simple Chop Salad (page 174)	Black Bean Grits (page 272), Garlicky Greens (page 191) and Chili Lime Grilled Asparagus with Mushrooms and Bell Pepper (page 193)	Hemp Energy Balls (page 298)	Kale Kolada (page 143)
Day 10	Iron-Rich Morning Glory Steel-Cut Oats (page 127) with 2 tsp. ground flax and 2 tbsp. chopped walnuts	Veggie Lettuce Boats (page 160) with Baked Falafel (page 262), side salad with Creamy Lemon Tahini Dressing (page 228)	Simple One-Pot Meal (page 266), Broasted Brussels Sprouts (page 194), and side salad	Choco-Chia Pudding (page 295)	Açai Spritzer (page 142)

	Breakfast	Lunch	Dinner	Snack/Dessert	Beverage
Day 11	Multigrain Grits (page 126) topped with 2 tsp. ground flax and 2 tbsp. chopped walnuts	Creamy Asparagus Soup with Corn (page 250), Quinoa Chickpea Pilaf (page 211)	Raw Coconut Curry Veggies (page 268), side salad	Cranberry Walnut Power Krispy Bars (page 305)	Tropical Smoothie (page 146)
Day 12	Purple Potato Tempeh Hash (page 130), gluten-free toast with tahini, fresh fruit bowl topped with 2 tsp. ground flax and 2 tbsp. chopped walnuts	Raw Collard Veggie Rolls (page 260), Provençal Salad (page 183), cooked black-eyed peas	Broccoli Rabe Penne Pasta with Oil-Free Cream Sauce (page 292), Super Sprout Salad (page 173)	Fresh fruit	Galactic Green Juice (page 135)
Day 13	Simple Breakfast Chia Pudding (page 117) with fresh fruit and 1 tbsp. tahini	Smoky Split Pea Soup (page 254), brown rice, Ranch Kale Salad (pages 185)	Magnificent Mushroom burgers (page 270), Parsnip Fries (page 199), and side salad	Almond Butter Chocolate Chip Cookies (page 310)	High-Protein Vanilla Almond Shake (page 148)
Day 14	Multigrain Grits (page 126) topped with 2 tsp. ground flax and 1 tbsp. chopped walnuts	Moroccan Chickpea Stew (page 255), with Green Quinoa (page 203), and side salad	Lemon Tempeh with Kale and Rice Noodles (page 276), Super Sprout Salad (page 173)	Raw Chocolate Pudding (page 296)	Rehydrating Watermelon Chiller (page 136)

As a registered dietitian with over 30 years' experience, I am a lover of life, good health, and great food. Fortunately, these are not mutually exclusive, but rather, exceedingly interdependent. It is a miracle of sorts to watch someone reclaim their health by making simple yet profound lifestyle changes. The capacity for the human body to heal from devastating, painful conditions is truly remarkable. The choices we make on a daily basis define our health and longevity—physical activity, social engagement, exposure to fresh air, sunshine and nature, sleep, laughter and joy, avoidance of addictive substances, and, of course, food choices.

Food is the fuel on which our body runs; it provides the structural materials used to build, rebuild, and repair our body tissues, and it supplies the resources needed to manufacture brain cells, muscles, bones, hormones and enzymes. You literally are what you eat, or perhaps more accurately, what you absorb. When we recognize the role food plays in the body, the very notion that what we eat is of little consequence to health utterly defies rationality. Healthy food is, quite simply, critical to achieving and maintaining optimal health.

Plant foods are concentrated sources of dietary components that are consistently linked with favorable health outcomes—antioxidants, phytochemicals, phytosterols, fiber, enzymes, pre- and probiotics, essential fats, unrefined carbohydrates, plant protein, vitamins, and minerals. These compounds work together to turn off disease-promoting genes, reduce inflammation, boost immune function, balance hormones, enhance detoxification enzymes, maintain blood glucose levels, keep blood pressure and blood cholesterol levels in check, and support all body systems.

What are the most important steps a person can take to design a diet that provides the ultimate protection against disease, and the greatest potential for healing? The culinary creations in this book, and the following ten steps, will guide you to a plant-based diet that makes your heart and soul sing, and is essentially bulletproof.

1. Be picky about your macronutrient sources. Your calories come from three macronutrients—carbohydrates, fat and protein. (Some also come from alcohol, but this should not be a significant source of calories for anyone.) The percentage of calories from each of these macronutrients matters far less than where the calories come from. One of the interesting features of the Blue Zone (places where people live the longest, healthiest lives) is that the percent of calories from each macronutrient varies widely within each population. For example, the percentage of calories from fat in various Blue Zones ranges from about 11 to about 38 percent. However, the primary source of macronutrients in all of the Blue Zone populations is whole plant foods—intakes of processed foods are low. Fresh foods from home gardens or local markets are dietary mainstays. The lesson is to stick mainly to whole grains, legumes, vegetables and fruits for carbohydrates. Rely on nuts, seeds, avocados, coconut, olives, and soy foods for fat. Enjoy high-protein plant foods, such as beans, peas, lentils, tofu, tempeh, seeds, and nuts as primary protein sources.

2. Eat the most nutrient-dense diet possible. Nutrient density is a measure of how many nutrients each calorie provides. Some nutrient density charts include not just vitamins and minerals, but fiber, phytochemicals, antioxidants, and essential fatty acids. The more nutrients and other beneficial compounds consumed per calorie, the more protective your diet. The most nutrient-dense foods on the planet are nonstarchy vegetables, with dark leafy greens leading the pack. These foods offer the highest amounts of nutrients per calorie of food. Next come fruit, legumes, starchy vegetables, nuts, and seeds. At the bottom of the charts are fried foods and pure oils, as they provide a lot of calories but very few nutrients.

3. *Think color.* When you select your foods, consider their color. Aim for at least 10 servings of vegetables and fruits each day—preferably at least 3 green, 2 red, 2 orange-yellow, 1 purple-blue, and 1 white-beige. Color is also important for foods in other groups. For example, red, pink, and black beans tend to be more antioxidant and phytochemical rich than white or brown beans. The same goes for rice, quinoa, and other grains—red or black varieties provide some distinct advantages. Use preparation methods that help foods retain their color—for example, do not overcook your vegetables!

4. *Go for variety.* While this might seem like a no-brainer, too often we stick to familiar foods, limiting our exposure to some of the most delicious, nutritious foods on the planet. It is quite a revelation to learn about the differences of foods within the same food group. Each product comes with its own nutritional profile, and its own unique package of protective phytochemicals and antioxidants. For example, within the nut family, almonds are rich sources of calcium and vitamin E, Brazil nuts are loaded with selenium and magnesium, cashews provide zinc and iron, hazelnuts are great sources of manganese, pistachios stand out for their vitamin B_6 and plant sterols, macadamia nuts are one of the few signif-

icant sources of omega-7 fatty acids (a healthy monounsaturated fat), and walnuts are rich sources of omega-6 and omega-3 fatty acids, and antioxidants. We will enjoy the greatest benefits by consuming a delightful selection of foods within each food group.

5. *Support healthy gut flora.* We are just beginning to understand the complexities and consequences of gut flora for human health. A healthy microbiome:

- boosts nutritional status by synthesizing nutrients and enhancing nutrient absorption;
- promotes healthy weight, reducing risk of obesity and chronic disease;
- releases short-chain fatty acids from fiber, providing protection against colon cancer;
- boosts immunity, protects against allergies;
- reduces inflammation, and risk of inflammatory bowel diseases;
- maintains the integrity of the intestinal wall;
- supports and protects brain function.

How do you ensure a healthy microbiome? Begin by consuming plenty of prebiotics from beans, whole grains, onions, asparagus, artichoke hearts, bananas and other whole plant foods. Prebiotics are types of fiber (from plants) that nourish and support beneficial bacteria. Minimize intake of foods that foster the growth of bad bacteria—processed foods, fried foods, refined carbohydrates (starches and sugars), and red or processed meat.

Incorporate food-based probiotics (foods containing friendly bacteria), such as yogurt (there are lots of nondairy choices), fermented vegetables, tempeh, miso, and other fermented or cultured foods. Avoid excessive intakes of

continues

continued from previous page

alcohol. Finally, consider taking probiotics, especially during and following antibiotic therapy.

6. Opt for organic, when possible. Buying or growing organic helps minimize harmful chemicals in your food, and in our environment. Conventional farming practices use pesticides and herbicides that contaminate groundwater, promote erosion, and may be contributing to colony collapse disorder in bees. Persistent organic pollutants and heavy metals move up the food chain, so the plant-based diets provide an advantage in this regard. If you cannot manage 100 percent organic, become familiar with the products that have the highest pesticide content, and if possible, buy these organic. Generally, foods eaten with the skin on (e.g., apples, peaches, pears, berries) pose greater risk than those eaten with peel removed (e.g., pineapple, bananas, kiwi, melon). The Environmental Working Group (EWG) provides a valuable tool on its website rating levels of pesticides in produce. Check out http://www.ewg.org/foodnews/.

7. Eat more raw food. Raw foods minimize the products of high-temperature cooking, such as acrylamide, heterocyclic amines, polycyclic aromatic hydrocarbons, and advanced glycation end-products. They are rich in phytochemicals and antioxidants, and provide enzymes that help us convert phytochemicals into their active forms. Soaking, sprouting, fermenting, blending, and other common raw food preparation techniques boost nutrients, reduce antinutrients, and support favorable changes in gut flora.

8. Meet all your nutritional requirements. Even if you carefully design your diet to include a variety of organic, whole plant foods, it is possible to come up short on some nu-

trients. For people eating completely plant-based, the nutrient of greatest concern is vitamin B_{12}. This is because plants are not reliable sources. It is essential that people eating mostly or exclusively plant foods take a vitamin B_{12} supplement or consume sufficient B_{12}-fortified foods. We also need to think about sources of iron, zinc, calcium, vitamin D, iodine, and omega-3 fatty acids. These nutrients are plentiful in the plant-kingdom, but we do need to be conscious of their sources, and include them in our daily diets. The good news is that it is not difficult to meet all your nutrition needs from plant-based diets—it just takes some nutrition knowhow.

9. Drink water. Liquid calories do not satisfy the appetite control center the way solid foods do. While some beverages provide nutrients, whole foods provide greater satiety, more fiber, and other nutrients, and have more favorable effects on blood glucose. Avoid sugar-sweetened beverages completely, and calorie-free beverages containing artificial sweeteners. Artificial sweeteners appear to confuse your appetite control center, mess with metabolic hormones, and adversely affect gut flora. Water is the best thirst quencher and is calorie-free. Herbal teas are another healthful option. Vegetable juice (especially green juices or tomato juice) or wheatgrass juices are good options for boosting antioxidant status. Nutritious higher-calorie beverages, such as fruit smoothies, and nondairy milks can also have a place in a healthy diet. Smoothies made from nondairy milks, fruit, greens, nut butters, seeds, avocados, and other wholesome foods can make a fast and easy meal replacement.

10. Master the art of mindful eating. Mindful eating is about having a healthy relationship with food. It is about appropriately responding to hunger cues, improving digestion, and fully enjoying and appreciating your food.

It is far more about eating consciously than perfectly. Prepare as much of your own food as possible, and enjoy the process of culinary creativity. Make food preparation a real priority, and give it the time it deserves. Create a relaxing atmosphere for meals, and avoid multitasking while you are eating. Eat at the table, and give your meal your full attention. Make your food look gorgeous and appreciate the smell, color, texture, and taste of each morsel. Chew your food well. Be aware of everyone involved in bringing food to your table, and consume it with a grateful heart. Buy from local farmers and local producers, and avoid foods that support practices that are inconsistent with your values.

part two

THE RECIPES

200 Recipes for Every Season

CHAPTER 6

Preparing Your Kitchen

Great cooking favors the prepared hands.
—JACQUES PÉPIN

In the following chapters, you will embark on a culinary journey that can lead you and your family toward a life of optimal health. Here are some suggestions on how to gear up your kitchen and stock your pantry.

Kitchen Gear

If you are taking an interest in cooking knockout vegan recipes but currently have a bare-bones kitchen, start with these key kitchen items. Having the right tools will make your journey easier, make cooking more appealing, and up your ability to wow your friends with your new plant-based creations. It's exciting and sparks creativity to have a wide selection of tools to work with. Build your kitchen gear over time as your means allow.

Knives: A chef's knife is a multipurpose tool that is designed to suit many kitchen tasks; use it to mince, slice, and chop vegetables and tofu. Other knives to include are a paring knife (for garnishes and peeling) and a serrated knife (handy for slicing bread and tomatoes). You definitely want to work with knives that you are comfortable with, so if you can, go to a kitchen store to see which styles you like best. Some people like heavier large chef's knives. I have gravitated toward the lighter ceramic knives. Ceramic knife blades are lightweight, easy to clean, leave no metallic taste or smell, and are stain- and rust-proof. Check out the Kyocera or Shenzhen brands. The 5 ½-inch santoku style is very popular. For stainless-steel knives, we like Henckels, Wüsthof, and Shun.

Follow the manufacturer's guidelines when it comes to sharpening and storing knives. You will need a special sharpener for ceramic knives, or you can send them back to the manufacturer to be sharpened for a nominal fee.

Bamboo cutting board: A bamboo version of the timeless cutting board resists scarring, looks lovely, cleans easily, and is renewable and earth-friendly, to boot.

Blender: Having a strong blender is super helpful in the kitchen, especially when it comes to raw food preparation and creating creamy soups, sauces, dressings, and plant-based cheeses. A Vitamix is my blender of choice. Visit www.vitamix.com and enter code 06-002510 for free shipping in the continental United States. Hamilton Beach makes an acceptable household brand.

Food processor: It's the tool to use for pâtés and spreads, and for grating larger quantities of carrots, beets, cabbage, and other veggies. There are also mini food processors that come in handy for mincing garlic, chopping small amounts of nuts, or making small portions of spreads so you don't need to get the big one dirty. Cuisinart is a popular brand.

Citrus juicer: Handheld citrus juicers are wonderful for getting the majority of the juice out of the fruits and reducing the need for seed removal.

Finger peeler: This small device slips on to your finger so that you can peel vegetables and fruits without worrying about dropping the peeler.

Zester: Invaluable for zesting citrus and grating ginger, nutmeg, and dark chocolate. Try Microplane brand, which offers various styles to suit your preference.

Garlic press: If chopping and mincing garlic isn't your thing, invest in a good garlic press. Newer models are easy to clean and don't even need clove-peeling.

Sprout bags and nut-milk bags: These handy bags have multiple functions—you can soak nuts and seeds in them, use them as a strainer for raw nut milks or juice, and

go about sprouting large nuts and seeds in them, too.

Toaster oven: It takes less time to heat up, uses less energy, and cooks food faster than a regular oven. Many quick and easy dishes can be prepared on the baking tray.

Juicer: To make the juices in Chapter 10, a juicer is indispensable. Some recommended brands include the Green Star juicer, which is possibly the best juicer in terms of minimal loss of nutrition. It extracts the juice of virtually anything, even wheatgrass, without needing to change parts. It can also process nuts, seeds, and grains. The Tribest Slowstar and the Breville juicers are also popular and highly rated models.

Dehydrator: If you are ready to up your raw food preparation game, it may be time to invest in a dehydrator for making tasty raw snacks, such as kale chips. From preserving excess produce, to making fruit leather, or dehydrated crackers and cookies, a dehydrator can make raw uncooking an adventure. Try the Sedona or Excalibur.

Pots and pans: Cast-iron or stainless-steel pots and pans of various sizes (no aluminum or Teflon). You can start with a 3-quart pot, a 5-quart pot, and a medium-size sauté pan and build from there.

Measuring cups and spoons: Important for accuracy in following recipes, especially for baked goods. I prefer metal to plastic.

Mixing bowls: Use metal or glass. Start with a variety of small, medium-size, and large.

Spatulas: Use wood, strong plastic, or metal. Check out what is available at your local cooking supply store to see which you prefer.

Baking sheets and casserole dishes: Avoid aluminum. You can begin with a medium-size baking sheet and one small and one large casserole dish.

In addition to this list, there are many gadgets and utensils that make cooking fun—and easy.

After you've equipped yourself with the essentials, consider adding the following:

Apron
Bamboo sushi mat, for nori rolls
Basting brush
Colander
Crock pot
Glass containers with lids, for refrigerated food storage
Grater
Griddle/grill: A useful item that straddles two burners and has a griddle on one side and grooves on the other side for grilling
Hand towels
Immersion blender, for making creamy soups without using a full-size blender
Kitchen scissors, for harvesting fresh herbs and opening packages
Mandoline: enables you to slice, julienne, and waffle-cut your favorite vegetables
Mason jars or other glass containers to store grains, nuts, and seeds
Oven mitts and pot holders

Salad spinner
Scoops of various sizes, including a small melon scoop
Spice grinder (a.k.a. coffee grinder) and/or a mortar and pestle, for spices and seeds
Spiralizers: the Saladacco or Spiral Slicer spiralizer turns zucchini, yams, carrots, and any other firm vegetable into angel hair "pasta," wide flat ribbons, or thin slices.
Steamer basket
Strainers
Whisks

The Vegan Pantry

Having a well-stocked pantry will allow you to create a vast array of gourmet vegan cuisine with the least amount of effort. Although most of the ingredients used in *Healing the Vegan Way* can be purchased at your local supermarket, some specialty items may require a trip to the natural foods or ethnic market. Many large supermarkets now have a "natural foods" section. Remember to go for local and organic ingredients whenever possible. Visit ethnic markets to experience the diversity of culinary traditions. You can also check out the Additional Resources section for websites where you can place special orders online.

Please do not be discouraged if you cannot stock up on all of them at once, as there is usually a way to substitute with what you do have on hand. Build your pantry over time. The more variety of foods you have access to, the more motivated you will be to try new dishes.

Consider stocking up on some of these essentials:

Baking and dessert ingredients: To explore the world of desserts, buy baking soda, baking powder, vegan chocolate and carob chips, cocoa powder, pure vanilla extract, and flavorings such as mint, raspberry, orange, almond, coffee, banana, hazelnut, and more. Also consider a few specialty items, such as tapioca flour (or Egg Replacer by Ener-G Foods), shredded coconut, and rose water and other food-grade hydrosols.

Beyond Meat, Field Roast, Tofurky, and other analogue products: Virtually all natural food stores and even many mainstream markets now carry a full section of analogue products—those products that aim to replicate the flavor and texture of the animal products they are aiming to replace. New products are coming out all of the time. There are now plant-based versions of chicken, beef, turkey, pork, chicken, beef, even salmon. These products are typically highly processed, often contain gluten, and may be high in sodium. Most of these I group in the category of transitional foods, along with the transitional condiments (see below). While they may not be part of a whole foods, plant-based diet, I think they are incredible in helping people transition to a plant-based diet. When the craving for animal foods hits, many of these products can satisfy the urge. I liked Beyond Meat in terms of flavor and because, unlike seitan, it is gluten-free. A chicken-style version of Beyond Meat, which I like the best of its products, is available in several flavors. Beyond Meat also produces a ground beef replacement. If Beyond Meat is not available at your local store and you can eat gluten, see if you can find chicken-style seitan. Field Roast and Tofurky also offer products that I enjoy on occasion.

Breads and flour: For breads, experiment with what is available in your local market to discover your favorite. Food for Life has a line of gluten-free breads and English muffins, typically available in the freezer section.

For flours, I like to use white spelt flour to replace whole wheat pastry or white flour. For gluten-free flours, I like Bob's Red Mill multipurpose gluten-free baking mix and also the company's newer 1-to-1 Baking Flour, which can replace the flour called for in the recipes in a one-to-one ratio. For gluten-free baking, you will also want to pick up xanthan gum or guar gum, as a specialty product. These are substances to replace the gluten in other flours that can contribute elasticity to the recipes. I include a recipe for Gluten-Free Flour Mix on page 105. For that recipe you can pick up sorghum flour, brown rice flour, and tapioca flour.

Capers: A peppercorn-size flower bud of a Mediterranean bush, *Capparis spinosa*, native to the Mediterranean and parts of Asia. Capers are usually sun dried and pickled in vinegar brine to bring out their lemonlike flavor. Imparts a tangy, salty flavor to dishes.

Chinese cuisine spices: Five-spice powder, a blend of spices, is common in Chinese and other Asian cuisines. The blend typically contains cinnamon, star anise, cloves, fennel, and Szechuan pepper. Szechuan peppercorns have a slightly lemon flavor and accentuate the heat of other spices, such as chiles, that are used in a dish.

Chipotle chile powder: One of my all-time favorite ingredients. It consists of smoked jalapeño peppers. It imparts a smoky heat to dishes. A little goes a long way.

Coconut milk: Available in most supermarkets; look for the organic canned variety of full-fat coconut milk, for optimal flavor. Low-fat coconut milk is an acceptable alternative for those wishing to cut down on fat. Coconut milk beverages typically are sold in aseptic packages and are less concentrated than the canned coconut milk.

Coconut oil, organic: One of my go-to oils to use for higher-heat sautéing, coconut oil is solid at room temperature and requires no refrigeration.

Dried fruits

Dried herbs and spices: These include allspice, aniseed, basil, bay leaves, black pepper, cardamom, cayenne pepper, chili powder, cinnamon, cloves, coriander, cumin, curry powder, fennel seeds, fenugreek, ginger, mace, marjoram, mustard seeds, nutmeg, oregano, paprika, parsley, rosemary, saffron, and turmeric.

Flaxseeds: either ground or whole.

Fresh herbs: Basil, dill, oregano, ginger, thyme, rosemary, lemongrass, chives, mints, cilantro, mace, marjoram, sage, chervil, turmeric, kaffir lime leaves, tarragon (French and Mexican varieties), Thai basil, and flat-leaf (Italian) parsley.

Fresh fruits and vegetables

Grains and legumes: available in bulk, see page 96–97.

Japanese condiments: Pickled ginger, wasabi powder, and umeboshi plum paste.

Liquid smoke: Purified water that has been infused with smoke. It adds a smoky flavor to dishes. Choose those brands without artificial additives. Use sparingly; a little goes a long way.

Milks, nondairy (soy, rice, hemp, flax, cashew, oat, and almond): An abundance of dairy-free milks are available in the market today, something for everyone's individual taste preferences. The soy milks tend to have the creamiest flavors when added to the recipes. Look for organic, unsweetened, whenever possible. (For homemade, see the Plant-Based Milk Template Recipe, page 104.)

Mirin: A Japanese rice cooking wine with a low alcohol content. It adds a sweet and tangy flavor to dishes.

Miso paste: A salty paste made by fermenting soybeans, grains, and other beans. Purchase unpasteurized, for maximum nutritional benefits. See page 248 for more about miso.

Nut and seed butters: such as almond butter, tahini, cashew butter.

Nuts and seeds: raw, unsalted.

Nutritional yeast: One of my top condiments, it's a vegan source of protein and vitamin B_{12} that adds a cheesy and nutty flavor to dishes. Store nutritional yeast in a cool, dark place in an airtight jar, and use it within a few months. Go for the large flake variety, if possible. I like Red Star brand.

Oils: For maximum freshness, to minimize oxidation and prevent the oil from becoming rancid, be sure your oils are cold pressed and stored in dark jars.

For heating, I like coconut or grapeseed oil. Choose cold-pressed, extra-virgin olive oil. It's from the first pressing and is rich in flavor and nutrients. Other oils to consider include sesame (toasted and light), sunflower, and safflower.

For salads, I like flaxseed oil and hemp oil. These oils have a nutty flavor and are plant-based sources of essential fatty acids. They require refrigeration and are not meant to be heated. You can also try borage and pumpkin seed oils.

Pastas and noodles: Experiment with different styles of gluten-free pasta, such as rice, corn or quinoa. I recommend Tinkyada brand.

Quinoa: Botanically a seed, though commonly referred to as the ancient grain of the Inca, quinoa is high in protein and may be used to replace rice in any of the recipes in the book.

Salts: Go for sea salt over iodized table salt, which is highly refined and contains anticaking agents. Celtic sea salt is a widely acclaimed unprocessed whole salt from France. Himalayan crystal salt is another popular choice. You can also experiment with smoked salts, which add an additional depth of flavor to your dishes.

Those on sodium-restricted diets can use the Salt-Free Seasoning (page 108) instead of salt.

Sea vegetables: These mineral rich foods have been consumed in Japan and around the world since ancient times. They will impart the flavor of the sea to your dishes. They are rich in iodine, essential for proper thyroid function, and are also good sources of folic acid and magnesium, vital for heart health. As always, look for the organic varieties, without added coloring. Varieties to explore include wakame, kombu, nori, kelp, dulse, alaria, laver, hijiki, and sea lettuce. You can also check out raw kelp noodles, available at natural food stores. They are mildly flavored and can be used to create a raw gluten-free "pasta." Toss with your favorite raw sauces.

Smoked paprika: A smoky version of the commonly available paprika. Some varieties are spicier than others, so adjust your quantities accordingly.

Superfood condiments: Culinary superfood supplements that I love to add to smoothies and live desserts include raw cacao powder and nibs, spirulina, hemp seeds, maca powder, and goji berries. Check out the superfood information in Chapter 3 to learn about the amazing benefits of these power foods.

Sweeteners: See the chart on page 89 for a selection of sweeteners to replace white sugar. There are some amazing coconut-based products on the market, including coconut nectar and coconut crystals.

Tamarind paste: The tangy and slightly sweet pulp from the pod of a large tropical tree that is used in several cuisines from around the world, including Asian and South American.

Tempeh: Originally from Indonesia, tempeh consists of soybeans fermented in a rice culture, then cooked. Many different varieties are created by mixing the soybean with grains, such as millet, wheat, or rice, together with sea vegetables and seasonings. Tempeh is high in protein, and has a heavier, coarser texture than tofu. It usually has a mild, slightly fermented flavor. Its color is usually tan with a few dark gray spots. For storage, tempeh may be frozen or refrigerated.

Thai food essentials: Kaffir lime leaf, lemongrass, galangal root, and Thai basil are ingredients that are integral components in Thai cuisine. Find them at the natural foods store or an ethnic market to add the greatest authenticity to your Thai dishes.

Tofu: Tofu is processed soybean curd and has its origins in ancient China. It comes in several forms, including super-firm, extra-firm, firm, soft, and silken. You can even find sprouted tofu. The sprouting makes the tofu easier to digest while the flavor is much the same. The recipes indicate which type is called for. You can even find sprouted tofu. The sprouting makes the tofu easier to digest while the flavor is much the same.

Transition condiments: Vegan mayonnaise, butter, and cheese, sour cream, and cream cheese. These I don't recommend consuming on a regular basis. Use in moderation to satisfy a craving for their less healthy dairy alternatives.

Truffle oil: Truffles are a highly sought-after edible fungi in the mushroom family that grow underground around tree roots. Truffle oil is available in different varieties, including oil that is infused with black or white truffles, each with its own unique flavor.

Vanilla beans: Fresh vanilla beans add a gourmet touch to smoothies and desserts. Try the Tahitian and Mexican varieties.

Vegan cheese: Chao cheese by Field Roast is my current favorite. I also like Daiya or Follow Your Heart, and Kite Hill. Miyokos creamery is another favorite for artisan vegan cheese. Visit miyokos kitchen.com to order. I like to say that "no cheese will remain unconquered," meaning that soon any animal-based cheese will be available plant-based. Keep your eyes open for a vegan cheese shop to open in a town near you!

Vegan mayonnaise: Try Vegenaise, Just Mayo, or make your own (page 113).

Vegan sausages: Tofurky and Field Roast have good products.

Vinegars. Coconut vinegar and raw apple cider vinegar are my go-to vinegars. There are many other varieties to choose from.

Wheat-free tamari: A by-product of the miso-making process, this is my recommended soy sauce for all the recipes in the book.

Other special foods to consider keeping on hand include granola, pasta sauce, tomato paste, curry paste (check out Thai Kitchen's product), and cans or asceptic packages of your favorite beans. Other condiments to stock up include catsup, different varieties of mustard, and horseradish. You can also pick up a healthy salad dressing or two, though making our own is always best!

Natural Sweeteners

The consumption of refined white sugar and high-fructose corn syrup is increasingly linked to many health problems, including emotional disorders, obesity, diabetes, and tooth decay. It is believed that because refined sugars are missing the nutrients that are contained in naturally sweet whole foods, the body is drained of

~~~~~~~~~~~~~~~~~~~~~~~~~~~~~~~~

Chef's Tips and Tricks

Date Syrup ♥

Enjoy this fruit-based sweetener to replace maple syrup, agave nectar, or other concentrated sweeteners.

Makes about 1 cup syrup
1/4 cup pitted dates
1 cup water

1. Combine the dates and water in a strong blender and blend until smooth. Store in a glass jar in the refrigerator for up to 4 days.

~~~~~~~~~~~~~~~~~~~~~~~~~~~~~~~~

its own store of minerals and nutrients in its efforts to metabolize the sugar.

Vegan Fusion natural food preparation makes use of various naturally occurring and minimally processed sweeteners. You can replace traditional white sugar with raw cane sugar or organic sugar at a one-to-one ratio without making any changes to your recipes. You can also replace the white sugar with any of the sweeteners that follow. These sweeteners are superior to white sugar, but it is still believed that most of them need to be used in moderation.

The following chart indicates how much of a sweetener is needed to replace 1 cup of white, refined sugar. The chart indicates how much liquid to delete from the recipe to maintain its consistency if the sweetener is a liquid.

Sweetener	Replace 1 cup of refined sugar with	Reduce liquids by
Agave nectar: A natural extract from this famous Mexican cactus, with a low glycemic index. There currently is some controversy surrounding agave and its similarity to high-fructose corn syrup.	¾ cup	⅓
Barley malt syrup: Roughly half as sweet as honey or sugar. Made from sprouted barley and has a nutty, caramel flavor. Contains gluten.	¾ cup	¼
Brown rice syrup: A relatively neutral-flavored sweetener that is roughly half as sweet as sugar or honey. It's made from fermented brown rice.	1 cup	¼
Blackstrap molasses: This syrup is a liquid by-product of the sugar-refining process. It contains many of the nutrients of the sugar cane plant. Has a strong, distinct flavor.	½ cup	¼
Coconut crystals: This air-dried coconut nectar creates a nutrient-rich granulated sugar that is our recommended sugar for the recipes in this book. It has a dark, rich flavor with a lower glycemic index than cane sugar. Manufactured by Coconut Secret.	1 cup	0
Coconut nectar: A mildly flavored sweetener manufactured by Coconut Secret that is a wonderful replacement for agave nectar. It has a low glycemic index and is loaded with vitamins, minerals, amino acids, and other nutrients.	¾ cup	⅓
Date sugar: A granulated sugar produced from drying fresh dates.	⅔ cup	0
Fruit syrup: The preferred method of sweetening involves soaking then blending raisins and dates with filtered water to create a sweet syrup. Try ½ cup of raisins with 1 cup of water and experiment to find desired sweetness.	1 cup	¼
Lucuma powder: A raw, low-glycemic sweetener with a slight maple flavor. Comes from the lucuma fruit, grown in the Peruvian Andes and referred to as the "gold of the Incas."	1 cup	0
Maple syrup: Forty gallons of sap from the maple tree are needed to create 1 gallon of pure maple syrup. It is mineral rich and graded according to color and flavor. Grade A is the mildest and lightest; Grade C is the darkest and richest. Good for baking.	¾ cup	¼
Stevia (powdered): Stevia is a plant that originates in the Brazilian rainforest. The powdered form is between 200 and 400 percent sweeter than white sugar. It is noncaloric, does not promote tooth decay, and is said to be an acceptable form of sugar for diabetics and those with blood sugar imbalances. For baking conversions, please visit http://www.ehow.com/how_2268348_substitute-stevia-sugar-baking.html.	1 teaspoon	0
Sucanat: Abbreviation for "sugar cane natural." It is a granular sweetener that consists of evaporated sugar cane juice. It has about the same sweetness as sugar. It retains most of the vitamins and minerals of the sugar cane.	1 cup	0

continues

continued

Sweetener	Replace 1 cup of refined sugar with	Reduce liquids by
Xylitol: A naturally occurring sugar substitute found in the fibers of fruits and vegetables, such as berries, corn husks, oats, plums, and mushrooms. Originally extracted from birch trees in Finland in the nineteenth century. Said to promote dental health and to be a safe sweetener for diabetics because of its low glycemic index.	1 cup	0
Yacón: This tuber is a distant relative of the sunflower. From the Andean region of South America, mineral-rich yacón syrup has a dark brown color and is used as a low-calorie sweetener.	¾ cup	⅓

CHAPTER 7

How One Recipe Can Equal Thousands + Easy Cooking Techniques

A journey of a thousand miles begins with one step.
—LAO-TZU

This chapter gives you the tips and techniques that will enable you to rock the house (the kitchen at least) with your new found culinary prowess. Refer to this chapter to refresh yourself on the basics of vegan natural food preparation.

Top Ten Tips for Efficient Food Preparation

Before getting started, here are some tips to make your experience in the kitchen more efficient and enjoyable. Remember, with practice, everything becomes easier!

1. Commit to trying new ingredients. Experiment with one new ingredient a week. This will allow you to expand your repertoire and further refine your palate with the new flavors and textures you will be experiencing. Ask at the grocery store or research online to see how to incorporate the ingredient in your meals.

2. Invite a friend to help in the kitchen. Preparing food together can be a bonding experience and can make the process more fun. You can also learn from each other and grow in your culinary ability.

3. Read each recipe carefully and understand the process involved. Understand when multitasking is necessary, rather than waiting for each step to be complete before moving on to the next step.

4. Before beginning any preparation, create a clean work area and gather all of your necessary ingredients and kitchen gear.

5. Having the proper tools is essential to being able to whip food up quickly. Work up to a fully stocked kitchen.

6. Although the recipes are designed to taste their best by

following the exact measurements, eventually you will learn to discover acceptable approximations. With baking, however, measurements need to be precise because leavening is involved.

7. Some herbs, such as parsley, cilantro, or dill, don't need to be plucked from the thin part of their stems before mincing or chopping. Just keep them bundled together and chop into the whole bunch at once. The thin parts of the stems generally have the same flavor, and once minced, basically taste the same.

8. Cut stacks of veggies rather than each individual piece. Don't separate celery stalks when you can cut into the whole bunch at once. The same goes for heads of lettuce and cabbage. Stack tomato, potato, or onion slices and cut them simultaneously.

9. You don't need to peel carrots, cucumbers, potatoes, or beets unless specified; just wash them well. This is not only quicker, but also helps preserve the nutritional content of the food.

10. To help cut down on preparation time, set aside an hour or so on one of your least busy days for advance prepping. Having prepped ingredients on hand makes it easier to create meals on the go. You can cut vegetables and store them in a glass container in the fridge. You can also cook a squash, grain, or pot of beans. You can then use these foods in recipes over the next few days. Consider preparing a pot of rice in a rice cooker in the morning and using it for the evening meal.

Composting

The Cycle of Life

Curious what to do with all of the scraps that don't make it into your soup stock? Consider composting. Composting is the method of breaking down food waste, grass trimmings, and leaves to create nutrient-rich and fertile soil. It's the next step we can take toward creating a more sustainable method of growing our food.

Compost contains nitrogen and micronutrients to keep the soil healthy and can be used as a mulch and soil amendment. When the soil is healthy, plant yields are higher and fertilizers and pesticides aren't as necessary.

Composting completes the cycle of life from seed to table and back to the earth. Many communities sponsor composting programs and can give you all the tools and instructions you need to succeed. Check out www.compostguide.com for a complete guide to composting.

With these tips in mind, also remember to have fun! Preparing and eating food is one of life's greatest pleasures. No matter where you are on your culinary journey, with the appropriate tools, ingredients, and attitude, and with lots of practice, you will soon be experiencing this joie de vivre in the comfort of your own kitchen.

About the Recipes and Vegan Fusion Cuisine

Vegan Fusion is a style of cuisine that celebrates the culinary contributions from around the world. This means that I often combine ingredients from different ethnic foods in the same dish or menu. Vegan Fusion cuisine also represents a return to the natural methods of growing food and utilizes organic ingredients whenever possible.

Each recipe offers information on key nutrients contained in the dish, as well as nutritional information. It is important to remember when looking at the nutritional information that optional ingredients and variations are not included in the nutritional analysis of the recipe.

Throughout the book, you will see the following icons:

♥ indicates a recipe that is 95 percent or more raw, or can be easily adapted to raw. See page 66 for information on raw foods.

Ⓖ indicates a gluten-free recipe or variation.

♦ indicates a recipe or variation of a recipe that is made without the addition of processed oil.

📖 Template Recipes: recipes that particularly lend themselves to numerous variations.

About the Template Recipes

The template recipe style of recipe development will greatly expand your creativity in the kitchen. To view recipes as a template, you look at a recipe in the most general form possible and break it down into its component parts. Once we have broken down the recipe into its parts, we can alter any one—or all of them—to create a new recipe. The cool thing about this is that even when we leave every other part of the recipe the same, altering one component creates a new flavor profile for the entire dish.

Throughout the book, I have highlighted those recipes that lend themselves to this approach more than others. In other recipes, I simply list suggestions for how to create variations. The Creamy Asparagus Soup with Corn (page 250) is a shining example of a template recipe.

First, instead of viewing it as "asparagus soup," look at it as a "creamy vegetable soup." This way we know that even if we are out of asparagus, this soup can still be an option.

The component parts are the following:

Base: In this case, vegetable stock or water, onion, celery, and garlic
Main vegetable component: Asparagus
Creaminess component: Cashews
Herb/spices component: Dill, crushed red pepper flakes
Vegetable added after blending component: Corn

After breaking this down into its parts, our asparagus soup recipe now becomes a template for hundreds of recipes:

- Change the base by experimenting with different types of vegetable stock.
- Change the main veggie component by replacing the asparagus with broccoli, cauliflower, zucchini, or any combination of vegetables you desire.
- To create creaminess, you can replace the cashews with macadamia nuts, sunflower seeds, pumpkin seeds, Brazil

nuts, hazelnuts, blanched almonds—any of which can be raw or toasted. You can also replace them with coconut milk, soy milk, rice milk, almond milk, or other plant-based milks.

- The herb component can be altered by replacing the dill with any herb or herb combination of your choosing, such as cilantro, basil, or parsley.
- To create ethnic flair, you can add Mexican spices, such as chili powder and cumin; Indian spices, such as curry powder; or Italian spices, such as oregano, thyme, or rosemary.
- Once your soup is blended, you can then add any vegetables of your choosing. Replace the corn with chopped broccoli, mushrooms, asparagus, red bell pepper, or any combination.

I think you get the idea!

As you follow the recipes in the book, keep this idea of a template recipe in mind and look over the variations to give you ideas on how you can create your own unique spin on the recipe.

The Monk Bowl

The Monk Bowl, introduced to me by my business partner Bo Rinaldi, consists of combining a grain, a green, and a protein in one meal. It is another perfect example of a template recipe, and is an intuitive way to look at meal creation that allows for so much variety and flavor combinations. Revolutionary in its simplicity, the Monk Bowl is an easy, delicious way to introduce healthful eating.

Monk Bowl template recipe:

- Grain component: Rotate through different types of rice, millet, quinoa, brown rice pasta, and so on.
- Green component: Change it up to serve your favorite vegetable or vegetables—raw, steamed, roasted, grilled, sautéed.
- Protein component: Legumes, tofu or tempeh. The tofu or tempeh can be roasted, sautéed, or grilled and made with various marinades. Legumes can be boiled, refried or made into patties. Dried spices (see page 85) can be added to your legumes to create even more variety.

Most Monk Bowls can be prepared from beginning to end within 20 to 30 minutes. One of my main go-to meals is a Monk Bowl with quinoa, steamed vegetables, and roasted tempeh or tofu, served with a side salad. I love adding a simple topping of hemp or flax oil, wheat-free tamari, and nutritional yeast. You can get more creative by serving yours with any number of different sauces or dressings, such as peanut, barbecue, sweet-and-sour, or the others in this book. See the Simple One-Pot Meal (page 266) for another example of a Monk Bowl.

Storage of Prepared Foods

As for the shelf life of the dishes in *Healing the Vegan Way*, I generally recommend enjoying the food the day it is prepared and for the next day or two after that. Some recipes, such as dressings or baked goods, may last a bit longer. Please check daily to ensure freshness. Store most leftovers in a glass container in the refrigerator.

Techniques

As you get ready to prepare these dishes, some of the ingredients may be unfamiliar, or there may be certain cooking methods or techniques that you haven't mastered. Read on to learn how to work with certain ingredients, and you'll be cooking like a pro in no time.

Basic Knife Cuts

Refer to this section as you prepare the recipes if you have any questions about how to cut the ingredients.

Mince: The finest that can be cut by hand, to mince is to chop a food into very small pieces. Used with garlic, ginger, fresh herbs.

Dice: Slightly larger than mince, ¼-inch uniform pieces. Good for carrots, onions, zucchini, potatoes, peppers.

Chop: Larger than diced; usually ½ inch in diameter. Try with carrots, zucchini, potatoes, beets, peppers, onions, eggplant, tomatoes.

Slice: Many types are possible: thin or thick, half-moon shape, rings, or diagonal. Works with onion, cabbage, cucumber, zucchini, carrots, eggplant, peppers, beets, tomatoes.

Chiffonade: Thin ribbon strips of herbs, such as basil, mint, or sage. To chiffonade, form a stack of a few leaves of the herb, roll like a burrito, and cut thin slices to form the ribbons.

Cube: Chopped into uniform squares. Can vary in size. Try carrots, eggplant, zucchini, beets, jicama, potatoes.

Julienne: Long, thin strips (à la matchsticks) about ⅛-inch wide. Used with carrots, zucchini, peppers. Try using different-colored bell peppers like red, orange, and green.

Shred: Cut into thin strips, either by hand or using a grater or food processor. Try carrots, beets, zucchini, jicama, cabbage.

Cooking Grains

Follow these steps and you will always have perfectly cooked grains.

1. Rinse the grain thoroughly and drain the excess water.
2. Bring the measured amount of grain and liquid (either vegetable stock—page 108—or water) to a boil. You may wish to add a small amount of sea salt. (The advantages of adding the salt at this stage, rather than after the grain is cooked, are that the salt flavor will be more uniformly distributed if you add it before cooking, and it prevents the necessity of stirring the salt into the cooked grain, which can create a mushy texture.)
3. Cover with a tight-fitting lid, lower the heat to low, and simmer for the recommended time. As the grain is being steamed, do not lift the lid until the grain is finished cooking.

Cooking times may vary, depending upon altitude and stove cooking temperatures. The grain is generally finished cooking when it is chewy and all the liquid is absorbed.

Enhance the flavor of your grain dishes by adding such ingredients as minced garlic or ginger, diced onion, a couple of bay

Grain Cooking Chart

Grain	Liquid per cup of grain	Approx. cooking time	Approx. yield (cups)
Amaranth: Ancient grain of Aztecs, higher in protein and nutrients than most grains	2 ½ cups	25 minutes	2 ½ cups
Barley, pearled: Good in soups and stews. Contains gluten.	3 cups	45 minutes	3 ½ cups
Buckwheat: Hearty, nutty flavor. When toasted, it's called kasha and takes less time to cook. Also used as a breakfast cereal.	2 cups	15 minutes	2 ½ cups
Cornmeal: Made from ground corn—a staple of Native Americans; use in corn bread or grits.	3 cups	20 minutes	3 ½ cups
Couscous: A North African staple made from ground semolina. Contains gluten.	1 ½ cups	15 minutes	1 ½ cups
Farro: An ancient variety of wheat with a nutty flavor that is high in fiber, iron, protein, zinc, niacin, and folate. Wonderful as the base for risottos. Contains gluten.	2 ¾ cups; drain excess if necessary	30 minutes for whole grain, less for pearled and semipearled	2 cups
Kamut: An ancient variety of wheat that many with wheat allergies are able to tolerate. Contains gluten.	3 cups	1 hour	3 cups
Millet: A highly nutritious grain that is used in casseroles, stews, and cereals. Especially tasty with flax oil.	2 ½ cups	20 minutes	3 cups
Oats: A versatile grain that is popular as a cereal, for baking, and for milks. Look for certified gluten-free varieties, if needed.			
Steel-cut	3 cups	30 to 40 minutes	3 cups
Groats	3 cups	1 hour	3 cups
Rolled	3 cups	10 minutes	3 cups
Quick	2 cups	5 minutes	2 cups
Polenta: A type of cornmeal; used in Italian cooking. To cook, bring liquid to a boil. Lower the heat to a simmer and whisk in the polenta, stirring until done.	3 cups	10 minutes	3 cups
Quinoa: Ancient grain of the Incas. High in protein and nutrients. Has a delicate, nutty flavor.	2 cups	20 minutes	2 ½ cups
Rice: Rice has a high nutrient content and is a staple in many of the world's cultures. Basmati rice has a nutty flavor and is used in Indian cooking.			
Brown basmati	2 cups	35 to 40 minutes	2 ¼ cups
White basmati	1 ½ cups	20 minutes	2 cups
Brown long-grain	2 cups	45 minutes	3 cups
Brown short-grain	2 cups	45 minutes	3 cups
Wild	3 cups	1 hour	4 cups
Jasmine	1 ¾ cups	20 minutes	3 ½ cups
Sushi	1 ¼ cups	20 minutes	3 cups

Grain Cooking Chart (*continued*)

Grain		Liquid per cup of grain	Approx. cooking time	Approx. yield (cups)
Rye: A staple grain throughout Europe. Used as a cereal or ground to make breads, including pumpernickel. Contains gluten.				
	Berries	4 cups	1 hour	3 cups
	Flakes	3 cups	20 minutes	3 cups
Spelt: An ancient form of wheat. It contains more protein and nutrition than wheat. Contains gluten.		3 ½ cups	1 ½ hours	3 cups
Teff: From Ethiopia, the smallest grain in the world, and the main ingredient for injera flatbread		3 cups	20 minutes	1 ½ cups
Wheat: A primary bread grain. Bulgur is used in Middle Eastern dishes, such as tabbouleh. Cracked may be used as a cereal. Contains gluten.				
	Whole	3 cups	2 hours	2 ¾ cups
	Bulgur	2 cups	15 minutes	2 ½ cups
	Cracked	2 cups	25 minutes	2 ½ cups

leaves or kaffir lime leaves, or crushed lemongrass while cooking. If you wish to use a rice cooker, Miracle puts out a stainless-steel version. Steer clear of aluminum or nonstick rice cookers.

Cooking Legumes

Before you cook dried legumes, pick over them thoroughly, removing any stones or debris. This improves digestibility and reduces gas. Dried legumes, except split peas, should be soaked before cooking, and they can take some time to soften, which is why many people soak their legumes overnight. If you forget to soak them overnight, a quick method is to bring the legumes and four times the amount of water to a boil, remove from the heat, cover, and allow to sit for a few hours. Soaking improves digestibility and reduces gas. Other methods for improving digestibility include adding some fennel seeds, a handful of brown rice,

or a few strips of the sea vegetable kombu (rinse well before using) to the legumes while cooking.

After soaking or boiling legumes, discard the soak water, add the measured amount of vegetable stock (page 108) or filtered water to a heavy-bottomed pot, bring to a boil, cover, lower the heat to a simmer, and cook until tender. Do not add salt to the cooking liquid; it can make the legumes tough. Legumes are done cooking when they are tender but not mushy. They should retain their original shape.

Please see the following legume cooking chart. Note that the times in the chart are for cooking dried legumes. Please reduce the cooking time by 25 percent when legumes are soaked.

Working with Tofu

Tofu is sold in a number of different forms, including superfirm, extra-firm, firm, soft,

Legume Cooking Chart

Legume	Liquid per cup legume	Approx. cook time	Approx. yield
Adzuki/aduki beans: Tender red bean used in Japanese and macrobiotic cooking	3 ¼ cups	45 minutes	3 cups
Anasazi beans: Means "the ancient ones" in Navajo language; sweeter and meatier than most beans	3 cups	2 hours	2 cups
Black beans (turtle beans): Good in Spanish, South American, and Caribbean dishes	4 cups	1 ¼ hours	2 ½ cups
Black-eyed peas: A staple of the American South	4 cups	1 ¼ hours	2 cups
Chickpeas (garbanzo beans): Used in Middle Eastern and Indian dishes. Pureed cooked chickpeas form the base of hummus.	4 cups	3 to 4 hours	2 cups
Great northern beans: Large white beans	4 cups	1 ½ hours	2 cups
Kidney beans: Medium-size red beans. The most popular bean in the United States, also used in Mexican cooking.	4 cups	1 ½ hours	2 cups
Lentils: Come in green, red, and French varieties. A member of the pea family used in Indian dal dishes and soups.	3 cups	45 minutes	2 ¼ cups
Lima beans: White beans with a distinctive flavor and high in nutrients			
Regular limas	3 cups	1 ½ hours	1 ¼ cups
Baby limas	3 cups	1 ½ hours	1 ¾ cups
Mung beans: Grown in India and Asia. Used in Indian dal dishes. May be soaked and sprouted and used in soups and salads.	3 cups	45 minutes	2 ¼ cups
Navy beans (white beans): Hearty beans used in soups, stews, and cold salads.	4 cups	2 ½ hours	2 cups
Pinto beans: Used in Mexican and Southwestern cooking. Used in soups and as refried beans in burritos.	4 cups	2 ½ hours	2 cups
Split peas: Come in yellow and green varieties. Do not need to be soaked. Used in soups and Indian dals.	3 cups	45 minutes	2 ¼ cups
Soybeans: Versatile, high-protein beans widely used in Asia. May be processed into tofu, tempeh, miso, soy milk, soy sauce, and soy cheese.	4 cups	3+ hours	2 cups

and silken. There is even a sprouted tofu, which is said to be easier to digest. Each different form lends itself to a particular type of food preparation. The recipes will specify which form of tofu is required for the dish.

Silken style: Blend and use to replace dairy products in puddings, frostings, dressings, creamy soups, and sauces.

Soft: Use cubed in soups or pureed in sauces, spreads, or dips.

Medium and firm styles: Use scrambled, grated in casseroles, or cubed in stir-fries.

Superfirm and extra-firm styles: Use grilled or baked as cutlets, or cubed and roasted. It may also be steamed and used in steamed vegetable dishes.

Leftover tofu should be rinsed and covered with water in a glass container in the refrigerator. Change water daily. Use within 3 or 4 days. Firm and extra-firm tofu may be frozen for up to 2 months. Frozen tofu, once defrosted, has a spongy texture that absorbs marinades more than does tofu that has not been frozen.

How to press tofu: Some recommend pressing tofu to remove excess water, create a firmer tofu, and to help the tofu absorb marinades more effectively. Pressing is generally not needed for the superfirm and many extra-firm varieties. If you would like to press your tofu, place the block of tofu on a clean surface, such as a plate, baking sheet, or casserole dish. Place a clean plate on top of the tofu and weigh down with a jar or other weight. Allow it to press for 15 to 45 minutes, draining the liquid periodically. You can also purchase

a tofu press on one of the websites listed in the Additional Resources section.

To make tofu cutlets: Slice a block of extra-firm tofu into thirds or fourths. If you wish, you can then cut these cutlets in half to yield six or eight cutlets per pound. You can also cut the tofu diagonally to create triangular cutlets. Cutlets can be marinated and then roasted or grilled.

To make tofu cubes: To make medium-size cubes, slice the tofu as you would for three or four cutlets. Then make four cuts along the length and three cuts along the width of the tofu. You can make the cubes larger or smaller by altering the number of cuts.

Working with Tempeh

Tempeh is a cultured soy product that originates in Indonesia, and tastes best when thoroughly cooked before consuming. Many different varieties of tempeh are created by mixing the soy bean with grains, such as millet, wheat, or rice, together with sea vegetables and seasonings. Tempeh is high in protein, and has a heavier, courser texture than tofu. It usually has a mild, slightly fermented flavor.

Its color is usually tan with a few dark gray spots. For storage, tempeh may be frozen or refrigerated.

There are many brands of tempeh on the market. One of my favorites is Turtle Island. It is typically available in an 8-ounce package. Several varieties come in a thick, square block; others, as a thinner rectangle. Some recommend steaming the tempeh before using in dishes, to remove the bitterness and help it absorb marinades more effectively. To do so, place a steamer basket in a large pot with about 1 inch of water over high heat. Cover, bring to a boil, and add the tempeh. Lower the heat to medium and cook covered for 10 minutes. Store leftover tempeh in a sealed glass container in the refrigerator for up to 3 days.

To make tempeh cutlets: You can slice the square block in half to create a thinner block and then cut it in half or into triangles. The longer block may also be sliced into thinner cutlets. These cutlets may then be cut into cubes.

Roasting Tofu and Tempeh

Tofu and tempeh cubes can be marinated, roasted, and then stored for a couple of days in a glass container in the refrigerator, to be used in salads, stir-fries, or on their own as a snack. With tofu, it is best to use extra-firm or superfirm varieties, for optimal texture.

To roast tofu and tempeh cutlets, and cubes, follow these three simple steps:

1. Preheat an oven or toaster oven to 375°F. Cut the tofu or tempeh into cutlets or cubes as mentioned earlier.

2. Place the cubes in a marinade of your choosing. A simple marinade can consist of a spritz of tamari, a small amount of melted coconut oil, and a small amount of water. Allow the cubes to sit for a few minutes and up to overnight. If marinating overnight, store in an airtight container in the refrigerator. If you follow an oil-free diet, you can omit the oil and add vegetable stock (page 108) or additional water.

3. Place on a well-oiled baking sheet or casserole dish. Roast until golden brown, 15 to 20 minutes, stirring the cubes occasionally to ensure even cooking. Because brands and oven temperatures differ, check periodically to attain your desired level of doneness. If making cutlets, you can flip after 10 minutes. Try a convection oven or use a broil setting, for a crispier crust. If using the broil setting, the cubes will cook faster than roasting.

Working with Seitan

Originating in ancient China, seitan is also referred to as "meat of wheat." The nemesis of the gluten intolerant, it is pure wheat gluten dough that has been cooked in a broth with different types of seasonings (so, those with gluten intolerance should choose another protein). Seitan can be used as an animal product replacement in virtually any dish. Several brands are available on the market. Experiment with them all to find your favorite. If you are ambitious and wish to make your own, go to www.about.com and enter "making seitan," which gives step-by-step instructions.

Chef's Tips and Tricks

Toaster Oven

I prefer to use the toaster oven for small quantities of up to 14 ounces of tofu or 8 ounces of tempeh. This amount conveniently fits in the baking tray. Take note that food tends to cook faster in a toaster oven than in a regular oven. Depending on the toaster, you can typically roast the tofu or tempeh in 15 minutes instead of 20. Not only is it more time-efficient, it is more energy-efficient—no need to heat up your whole oven for a small batch!

Seitan comes in different shapes and sizes (cubes, strips, or pieces) and has a chewy texture. For the best flavor, you can sauté the seitan, with a small amount of diced onion and minced garlic, in a little coconut oil over medium-high heat for 3 minutes, stirring frequently. Add a splash of wheat-free tamari or other soy sauce, and mix well before adding to the recipes.

Grilling

Don't tell the raw food police, but grilling creates a smoky, deep, and rich flavor. Try grilling tempeh and tofu cutlets, as well as many vegetables, such as portobello mushrooms, corn, onions, baby bok choy, carrots, bell peppers, asparagus, zucchini, coconut meat, or eggplant. You can even grill fruit, such as pineapple slices, peaches, apples, or pears. If you wish for added flavor, place the food in a marinade (see page 107) from a few minutes to overnight before grilling. Baste or brush lightly with oil, brushing occasionally and grilling until char marks appear and the food is heated thoroughly, flipping periodically. If using a gas grill, avoid placing food over a direct flame.

Another grilling option is to use a stovetop grill. Kitchen supply stores sell cast-iron and nonstick pans that are flat, straddle two burners, and have a griddle on one side and a grooved side for grilling. The flavor is similar and you get the signature char marks.

Steam or Water Sautéing

Steam or water sautéing may be used if you wish to eliminate the use of heated oils in your diet. Water or vegetable stock (page 108) is used instead of oil in the initial cooking stages for dishes that are sautéed. Place a small amount of water or stock in a heated pan, add the vegetables, and follow the recipes as you would if using oil. Add small amounts of water at a time, if necessary, to prevent sticking. Lemon juice and or a splash of wheat-free tamari may also be mixed in with the water, for added flavor.

Toasting Spices, Nuts, and Seeds

Toasting is one of my favorite methods for bringing out a deeper flavor of ingredients. There are two techniques I commonly use.

1. Dry sauté pan. For this method, place a dry sauté pan over high heat and allow the pan to heat up. Add the food to the pan, and cook until the food turns golden brown, stirring constantly. This method is good for spices, grains, and small quantities of nuts or seeds. If you wish, you can use an oil sauté for seeds or nuts by placing a small amount of high-heat oil, such

as coconut, in the pan before adding the seeds or nuts.

2. Oven. Preheat your oven to 350°F. Place the food on a dry baking sheet and leave in the oven until golden brown, stirring occasionally and being mindful to avoid burning. This method is best for nuts, seeds, and shredded coconut. Nuts become crunchier after cooling down. If you have more time, you can enhance the flavor even more by roasting at lower temperatures for longer periods of time. For instance, nuts roasted at 200°F for 45 minutes, have a richer, toastier flavor than those roasted at a high temperature for shorter periods of time.

CHAPTER 8

Easy Pantry Basics

The most indispensable ingredient of all good home cooking:
love for those you are cooking for.
—SOPHIA LOREN

First things first. This chapter will provide you with simple recipes and condiments that can be used to enhance the flavor of the remaining recipes in the book. Some, such as Plant-Based Milk (Template Recipe, page 104), Gluten-Free Flour Mix (page 105), or Soup Stock (page 108), can form the base of other dishes. Others, such as the ethnic spice blends (pages 105–107), will allow you to create a world of ethnic cuisine with the flick of a finger.

Having Balsamic Reduction (page 109) or Raw Brazil Nut Parmesan (page 111) on hand allows you to add new texture and flavor profiles to your creations. You will gain instant street cred with your guests when they learn you created your own Homemade Catsup (page 110), Vegan Mayonnaise (page 113), or Turmeric Hot Sauce (page 109).

In the recipes, you will notice a prep time, cooking time, and total time. In many instances, prepping will take place while some cooking is occurring, so the total time will not necessarily equal the total prep time and cooking time.

I suggest taking time on your least busy day to prepare some of these recipes for use during the week and you will bring your meals to the next level of awesomeness!

Brazil Nut Milk ♥ⓖ◆▱

YIELD: 4 CUPS MILK

Prep time: 10 minutes, Soak time: 20 minutes,
Total time: 30 minutes, Serving size: 1 cup,
Number of servings: 4

Looking for a break from the typical plant-based milks? Give your beverage a taste of the tropics by using Brazil nuts as the base. Selenium is a key nutrient found in abundance in Brazil nuts. It is essential for thyroid function as well as helping the body produce glutathione, an antioxidant enzyme that fights free radicals. A complete protein, Brazil nuts also contain brain-healthy polyunsaturated fats. Store this rich and creamy milk in a glass jar in the refrigerator and enjoy on its own as a refreshing beverage or as a base for any smoothies, soups, and sauces that call for plant-based milk.

1 cup Brazil nuts
3½ cups water
3 pitted Medjool dates, or desired sweetener
  to taste (optional)
Pinch of sea salt
Pinch of ground cinnamon

1. Place the Brazil nuts in a bowl with ample water to cover. Allow to sit for 20 minutes, or up to 6 hours. Rinse and drain well.

2. Transfer to a blender along with the 3½ cups of fresh water and the dates, salt, and cinnamon and blend well.

3. Pour through a fine-mesh strainer or nut-milk bag (see page 82).

4. Store the milk in a glass jar in the refrigerator for up to 3 days.

Notes: This recipe also works for rice milk. Just follow the ratios, using uncooked brown rice and water. It's a convenient way to save on packaging; it's fresh and tastes better!

Nut, seed, and rice milks will last for 3 to 4 days when stored in a glass jar in the refrigerator.

Nutrition Facts per serving (259 g) for an unstrained milk: Calories 270, Fat Calories 195, Total Fat 22 g, Saturated Fat 5 g, Cholesterol 0 mg, Sodium 8 mg, Total Carb 18 g, Dietary Fiber 4 g, Sugars 13 g, Protein 5 g

TEMPLATE RECIPE
Plant-Based Milk

Nut or seed component: Replace the Brazil nuts with any seed or nut of your choosing, such as almonds, hazelnuts, macadamia nuts, pumpkin seeds, cashews, sesame seeds, dried coconut, or sunflower seeds. See chart on opposite page for soaking times, if you choose to soak.

Spice component: Add pinch of ground nutmeg, cardamom, and/or allspice.

You can add 1 vanilla bean along with dates, or ¾ teaspoon of pure vanilla extract after straining.

Superfood component: Add maca powder, hemp seeds, or cacao nibs or powder to taste, after the milk has been blended and strained. Return to the blender and blend to mix well. (See page 44 for more about superfoods.)

Sweetener component: Replace the dates with sweetener of choice, such as coconut nectar or pure maple syrup (see page 89).

Soaking Chart

Soaking nuts and seeds improves their digestibility and makes more nutrients available. Even soaking for 15 minutes will produce some benefit, so don't hesitate to soak, even if you do not have the time to follow the times below.

Rinse the nuts or seeds well and place them in a bowl or jar with water in a ratio of 1 part nuts or seeds to 3 or 4 parts water. Allow them to sit for the recommended time before draining, rinsing, and using in recipes.

Nut/Seed	Soak Time
Almonds	4 to 6 hours
Brazil nuts	4 to 6 hours
Cashews	1 to 2 hours
Hazelnuts	4 to 6 hours
Macadamia nuts	1 to 2 hours
Pecans	4 to 6 hours
Pine nuts	1 to 2 hours
Walnuts	4 to 6 hours
Pumpkin seeds	1 to 4 hours
Sesame seeds	1 to 4 hours
Sunflower seeds	1 to 4 hours

~~~~~~~~~~~~~~~~~~~~~~~~~~~~~

Gluten-Free Flour Mix Ⓖ ◉

Use this blend to replace wheat flour in the recipes.

1 part sorghum flour
1 part fine brown rice flour
1 part tapioca flour, or ½ part potato starch (not potato flour) and ½ part tapioca flour (the same as tapioca starch) or arrowroot powder

1. Combine these gluten-free flours and starches in the above ratio, to obtain the necessary quantity of flour substitute.

2. When using this mix to replace wheat flour, add ¼ teaspoon of xanthan or guar gum for each cup of flour for cookies, and ½ teaspoon per cup of flour for cakes and brownies.

ETHNIC SPICE BLENDS

Spice blends allow you to simply create ethnic variations to your dishes. Start by adding a small amount of the blend and increase the quantity to taste. Remember that it will take some time for the flavors to absorb, so use sparingly at first.

Italian Spice Mix Ⓖ ◉

MAKES ½ CUP SPICE MIX

3 tablespoons dried basil
2 tablespoons dried marjoram
1 tablespoon dried oregano
1 tablespoon dried sage
2 teaspoons dried thyme
1 teaspoon garlic powder

1. Place all the ingredients in a medium-size bowl and mix well. Store in a glass jar and use within 1 month.

Indian Spice Mix^{G●}

MAKES ABOUT ½ CUP SPICE MIX

3 tablespoons curry powder
2 tablespoons ground cumin (optionally toasted; see page 101)
1 tablespoon ground coriander
1 tablespoon brown mustard or fennel seeds
1 teaspoon ground ginger
½ teaspoon ground cardamom
¼ teaspoon ground cloves

1. Place all the ingredients in a medium-size bowl and mix well. Store in a glass jar and use within 1 month.

Mexican Spice Mix^{G●}

MAKES ABOUT ½ CUP SPICE MIX

¼ cup chili powder
2 tablespoons ground cumin (optionally toasted; see page 101)
1 tablespoon dried oregano
½ teaspoon ground cinnamon
½ teaspoon chipotle chile powder

1. Place all the ingredients in a medium-size bowl and mix well. Store in a glass jar and use within 1 month.

Moroccan Spice Mix^{G●}

MAKES ABOUT ½ CUP SPICE MIX

2 tablespoons ground cumin
2 tablespoons ground coriander
1 ½ tablespoons paprika
1 tablespoon ground turmeric
1 teaspoon ground ginger
1 teaspoon ground cinnamon
1 teaspoon ground allspice
½ teaspoon cayenne pepper

1. Place all the ingredients in a medium-size bowl and mix well. Store in a glass jar and use within 1 month.

Ethiopian Spice Mix, also called Berbere^{G●}

MAKES ABOUT ½ CUP SPICE MIX

2 tablespoons paprika
2 tablespoons ground ginger
1 tablespoon ground coriander
1 ½ teaspoons allspice
1 ½ teaspoons ground cinnamon
1 ½ teaspoons fenugreek
¾ teaspoon ground nutmeg
¾ teaspoon ground cloves
¾ teaspoon cayenne pepper

1. Place all the ingredients in a medium-size bowl and mix well. Store in a glass jar and use within 1 month.

Herbes de Provence Spice Mix^{G●}

Create your own blend of this classic French herb combination. Feel free to leave out an ingredient or two (or three), if necessary. You can even experiment with different quantities of the same ingredients, based upon your personal preference.

MAKES ABOUT ¾ CUP SPICE MIX

2 tablespoons dried thyme

2 tablespoons dried summer savory

2 tablespoons dried marjoram

1 tablespoon dried rosemary

1 tablespoon dried tarragon

1 tablespoon dried oregano

1 tablespoon dried basil

1 tablespoon dried sage

2 teaspoons crushed culinary-grade
   lavender flowers

2 teaspoons dried fennel seeds

1. Place all the ingredients in a medium-size bowl and mix well. Store in a glass jar and use within 1 month.

MARINADES

Creating marinades is a key technique in vegan food preparation, especially when working with tofu, which will take on the flavor of the marinade. Place vegetables and tofu in the marinade for a minimum of ten minutes. The longer they sit in the marinade, the more of its flavors they will acquire. These are simple marinades that make enough for 14 ounces of tofu or tempeh or two servings of vegetables.

Use the following marinades as a starting point to create a vast array of flavorful marinades. Some of my favorite marinade ingredients to add include toasted sesame oil, mirin, stone-ground or Dijon mustard, brown rice vinegar, horseradish, minced garlic or ginger, pure maple syrup, balsamic vinegar, red or white wine, sherry, liquid smoke, truffle oil, and a variety of spices and herbs.

Maple Balsamic Marinade **G**

MAKES ABOUT ½ CUP MARINADE

¼ cup filtered water

3 tablespoons wheat-free tamari or other
   soy sauce

2 tablespoons olive oil or melted coconut oil
   (optional)

1 tablespoon pure maple syrup or agave
   nectar

2 teaspoons balsamic or red wine vinegar

1 teaspoon minced garlic, or peeled and
   minced fresh ginger

1 tablespoon minced fresh herbs (optional)

Pinch of cayenne pepper

1. Place all the ingredients in a medium-size bowl and whisk well.

Lemon Dijon Marinade **♥ G**

MAKES ABOUT ½ CUP MARINADE

¼ cup freshly squeezed lemon juice

¼ cup filtered water

2 tablespoons minced fresh herbs (try dill,
   thyme, oregano, and parsley)

1 ½ teaspoons Dijon or stone-ground
   mustard

½ teaspoon sea salt

¼ teaspoon freshly ground black pepper

1 tablespoon olive oil (optional)

⅛ teaspoon cayenne pepper or crushed red
   pepper flakes

1. Place all the ingredients in a medium-size bowl and whisk well.

VARIATION

🌢 For an oil-free version, omit the oil.

SOUP STOCK

Soup stock is at the foundation of any good soup or stew. In fact, you can use the stock when cooking grains or in other recipes where water is called for to create another layer of flavor. Why purchase a store-bought brand when it is so easy to create your own?

For a simple soup stock, save the clippings and scraps of vegetables used in preparing other recipes. Place them in a large, thick-bottomed stockpot over low heat with water to cover and simmer until all the veggies are completely cooked. Cook until the liquid is reduced to 75 to 50 percent of the original volume. The vegetables' flavor will be imparted to the broth. Experiment with different vegetables and herbs until you discover your favorite combinations. In general, you are looking to create a relatively neutral stock that can be used for all of your soup needs. Strain well, and add salt and freshly ground pepper to taste to the liquid.

Try using trimmings from potatoes, celery, carrots, tomatoes, onions, parsley, mushrooms, parsnip, zucchini, leeks, corn cobs, and garlic. Many avoid using vegetables that become bitter, such as bell peppers, radishes, turnips, broccoli, cauliflower, and Brussels sprouts. As far as herbs go, the only one I use freely is parsley. You can use a few sprigs of other herbs, such as thyme, fennel, oregano, dill, basil, or marjoram. Keep in mind that too much of these herbs can overpower the stock. Also be sure to add toward the end of the cooking process to avoid bitterness. The stock may be frozen and defrosted for future use. You can even pour the broth into ice cube trays, freeze, and use as needed.

If you find that you do not have so many trimmings to use, you can keep a bag or small bucket in the freezer to save the trimmings.

Once you have enough accumulated to fill a stockpot, get your soup stock going.

Nutritional Information

When looking at the nutritional information for the following recipes, please remember that this information pertains to the recipe as written, without optional ingredients or variations. Any recipe that contains beans is using the nutritional profile of freshly cooked beans. If you are opting for canned beans, please use a sodium-free variety or rinse the beans well to reduce the sodium.

When plant-based milks are used in a recipe, the nutritional analysis was done with the first milk listed.

CONDIMENTS AND ACCOMPANIMENTS

Salt-Free Seasoning ♥ⓖ◗

YIELD: ¼ CUP SEASONING

Prep time: 5 minutes, Total time: 5 minutes, Serving size: 1/2 teaspoon, Number of servings: 24

Are you on a sodium-restricted diet? Perhaps your health professional has advised against any added salt for health reasons, but you still want to turn to it for taste reasons. You may know by now that flavor doesn't have to come from salt itself, but that nature provides it through other means, such as the naturally salty celery and sea vegetables. Here is a homemade seasoning to turn to under these circumstances or anytime you are looking for a unique seasoning for your culinary creations.

¼ cup kelp granules
1 teaspoon celery seeds
1 teaspoon onion powder
1 teaspoon garlic powder
½ teaspoon freshly ground black pepper

1. Place all the ingredients in a bowl and whisk well.

Nutrition Facts per serving (12 g): Calories 10, Fat Calories 0, Total Fat 0 g, Saturated Fat 0 g, Cholesterol 0 mg, Sodium 25 mg, Total Carb 2 g, Dietary Fiber less than 1 g, Sugars 0 g, Protein 1 g

Balsamic Reduction

YIELD: ½ CUP BALSAMIC REDUCTION

Prep time: 5 minutes, Cook time: 30 minutes, Total time: 35 minutes, Serving size: 1 teaspoon, Number of servings: 24

Balsamic vinegar is a reduction itself—of white sweet grapes boiled down to a syrup. Balsamic hails from Italy, where it is produced in the regions of Modena and Reggio. It has a rich, complex flavor with a hint of sweetness from the grapes. Reduce it even further via the addition of another grape product—heart-heathy red wine. Drizzle this over salads and for garnishing your culinary creations!

1 cup balsamic vinegar
¼ cup red wine (try Chianti)
2 tablespoons white balsamic vinegar
(optional)

1 tablespoon coconut sugar, Sucanat, or organic sugar (optional)

1. Place all the ingredients in a saucepan over medium-high heat.

2. Cook for 30 minutes, or until the liquid is reduced in half, stirring occasionally and being careful not to boil.

3. Allow the mixture to cool before transferring to a squeeze bottle. Store in the fridge for up to 2 weeks.

Nutrition Facts per serving (78 g): Calories 70, Fat Calories 0, Total Fat 0 g, Saturated Fat 0 g, Cholesterol 0 mg, Sodium 15 mg, Total Carb 11 g, Dietary Fiber 0 g, Sugars 10 g, Protein 0 g

Turmeric Hot Sauce

YIELD: 1 CUP HOT SAUCE

Prep time: 10 minutes, Cook time: 15 minutes, Total time: 25 minutes, Serving size: 1 teaspoon, Number of servings: 48

Add some heat to your favorite recipes with an antioxidant-rich hot sauce. Fresh turmeric is finding more and more uses in the healthy living community due to the numerous benefits of its bright yellow component, curcumin, which greatly aids the digestive system and calms inflammation. Jalapeños rank as medium on the Scoville scale of pepper heat (see page 179), which is indicative of their capsaicin content, another potent anti-inflammatory, rendering this sauce not only flavorful but also potentially beneficial to those with pain and other inflammatory issues.

¾ cup seeded and chopped red or green jalapeño pepper

½ cup plus 2 tablespoons water

⅓ cup peeled and thinly sliced carrot

2 tablespoons peeled and thinly sliced fresh turmeric (see Chef's Tips and Tricks)

1 garlic clove

1 ½ teaspoons peeled and minced fresh ginger (see Chef's Tips and Tricks)

1 teaspoon raw apple cider vinegar

1 large pitted date

1 tablespoon freshly squeezed lemon or lime juice

¼ teaspoon freshly ground black pepper

1. Place the jalapeño, ginger, and turmeric in a small pot over medium-high heat. Cook for 2 minutes, stirring constantly.

2. Add the water and carrot and cook until the carrot is just soft, about 10 minutes, stirring frequently.

3. Transfer to a blender with the remaining ingredients and blend well.

Nutrition Facts per serving (3 g): Calories 0, Fat Calories 0, Total Fat 0 g, Saturated Fat 0 g, Cholesterol 0 mg, Sodium 0 mg, Total Carb less than 1 g, Dietary Fiber less than 1 g, Sugars 0 g, Protein 0 g

VARIATIONS

Add 2 teaspoons of coconut oil along with the jalapeños.

♥ For a raw hot sauce, place all the ingredients in a blender and blend well.

Homemade Catsup ⓖ ◆

YIELD: 1 CUP CATSUP

Prep time: 10 minutes, Total time: 10 minutes, Serving size: 1 tablespoon, Number of servings: 16

Maybe you've heard people say, "Sugar is in everything, even catsup!" Indeed, catsup or ketchup is notorious for its sneaky high sugar content. Not so this version, which is made with unrefined sweeteners or fruit, but still has all the flavor and tomato-originating lycopene intact—and you get the warm-fuzzy feel of calling it homemade. Very simple to make—doesn't even require a blender—this catsup is perfect on Millet Black Bean Veggie Burgers (page 269), Magnificent Mushroom Burgers (page 270), and Parsnip Fries (page 199).

¼ cup plus 3 tablespoons water

6 ounces tomato paste

1 tablespoon raw apple cider vinegar

1 teaspoon agave nectar or Date Syrup (page 88)

¾ teaspoon onion powder

¾ teaspoon garlic powder

¼ teaspoon sea salt, or to taste

¼ teaspoon celery seeds

¼ teaspoon allspice powder

¼ teaspoon freshly ground black pepper

1. Place all the ingredients in a bowl and whisk well.

Nutrition Facts per serving (19 g): Calories 10, Fat Calories 0, Total Fat 0 g, Saturated Fat 0 g, Cholesterol 0 mg, Sodium 50 mg, Total Carb 3 g, Dietary Fiber less than 1 g, Sugars 2 g, Protein 1 g

Raw Brazil Nut Parmesan♥ⓖ♦

YIELD: 2 CUPS PARMESAN

Prep time: 5 minutes, Total time: 5 minutes, Serving size: 1 tablespoon, Number of servings: 32

Commercial Parmesan cheese is not only not vegan, it is also not vegetarian. Parmigiano-Reggiano, its official Italian name, is made from milk, salt, and rennet—a natural enzyme from a calf's intestine. Bypass all that in favor of this definitely veg and vegan nut-based Parm that is simple to make but complexly bold in flavor and surprisingly versatile: it can be sprinkled on anything! With a Brazil nut base, you'll also get selenium, necessary for all of us and especially pertinent for those with depression. Sprinkle on steamed veggies, salads (especially the Caesar, page 181), or over pasta in the Broccoli Rabe Penne Pasta (page 292).

1 cup raw Brazil nuts
2 tablespoons nutritional yeast
¾ teaspoon garlic flakes
¾ teaspoon onion flakes
¼ teaspoon sea salt, or to taste
⅛ teaspoon freshly ground black pepper

1. Place all the ingredients in a food processor and process until finely ground.

2. Store in a glass jar in the refrigerator for up to 7 days.

Nutrition Facts per serving (8 g) : Calories 30, Fat Calories 25, Total Fat 3 g, Saturated Fat 1 g, Cholesterol 0 mg, Sodium 20 mg, Total Carb 1 g, Dietary Fiber less than 1 g, Sugars 0 g, Protein 1 g

Herb Croutonsⓖ

YIELD: 3 CUPS CROUTONS

Prep time: 10 minutes, Cook time: 20 minutes, Total time: 30 minutes, Serving size: 1/4 cup, Number of servings: 12

The word crouton comes from the French word for "crust." Croutons have resourceful and practical origins as a use for day-old bread, crisped by baking with oil and added to soups. Nowadays, croutons are available in many flavor varieties and often accompany salads. The addition of nutritional yeast here, besides adding some B vitamins, adds a cheesy flavor not always found in the usual crouton. Enjoy sprinkled on your soups and salads when looking for that extra crunch!

2 tablespoons olive or melted coconut oil
¾ teaspoon dried oregano
¼ teaspoon dried thyme
1 teaspoon garlic powder
½ teaspoon onion powder
1 ½ teaspoon nutritional yeast
¼ teaspoon sea salt, or to taste
⅛ teaspoon freshly ground black pepper
⅛ teaspoon crushed red pepper flakes
6 cups cubed vegan bread (½-inch cubes; try gluten-free)

1. Preheat the oven to 375°F. Place all the ingredients, except the bread, in a bowl and stir well.

2. Add the bread and toss well.

3. Transfer to a baking sheet and bake for 20 minutes, or until golden brown.

VARIATIONS

For Herbed Bread Crumbs, allow the cooked croutons to cool. Once cooled slightly, transfer to a food processor and gently pulse until crumbs are formed.

◆For an oil-free version, replace the oil with ¼ cup of water or vegetable stock (see page 108). Bake until the moisture is removed.

Nutrition Facts per serving (39 g): Calories 90, Fat Calories 25, Total Fat 3 g, Saturated Fat 1 g, Cholesterol 0 mg, Sodium 180 mg, Total Carb 13 g, Dietary Fiber 3 g, Sugars 1 g, Protein 3 g

Coco Bacon🄶◆

YIELD: 3 CUPS COCONUT BACON

Prep time: 5 minutes, Cook time: 10 minutes, Total time: 15 minutes, Serving size: 1/8 cup, Number of servings: 24

Give Babe a break and impress your friends and dinner guests with this bacon substitute, which has all the elements of its animal based counterpart: crispiness, saltiness, smokiness, sweetness, and fat, though in this version a much healthier and digestible fat. Use sprinkled on salads or on Wasabi Garlic Twice-Baked Potatoes (page 209), Smoky Split Pea Soup (page 254), or on top of your Garden Veggie Scramble (page 128).

3 cups large dried coconut flakes
1 tablespoon wheat-free tamari or other soy sauce
1 tablespoon water

1 teaspoon pure maple syrup
¼ teaspoon liquid smoke (see page 85)
1 teaspoon olive or coconut oil (optional)

1. Preheat the oven to 375°F. Place all the ingredients in a bowl and mix well. Transfer to a lightly oiled baking sheet and bake for 5 minutes. Stir well, being careful not to break up too many flakes.

2. Bake for an additional 5 minutes, or until golden brown.

3. Allow to cool slightly before serving.

VARIATION

◆For an oil-free version, omit the oil.

Nutrition Facts per serving (12 g): Calories 50, Fat Calories 25, Total Fat 3 g, Saturated Fat 3 g, Cholesterol 0 mg, Sodium 70 mg, Total Carb 6 g, Dietary Fiber 1 g, Sugars 4 g, Protein 0 g

Vegan Sour Cream🄶

YIELD: ¾ CUP SOUR CREAM

Prep time: 5 minutes, Total time: 5 minutes, Serving size: 1 tablespoon, Number of servings: 12

Did you know it takes only one or two steps to take mayonnaise to sour cream, plant-based style? Just add tangy lemon and a pinch of salt, and taste the difference! You can use homemade Vegan Mayonnaise (page 113), or store-bought, such as Vegenaise. Serve a dollop on your Mexican favorites, such as Tempeh Fajitas (page 279) or Mushroom Cauliflower Tacos (page 277).

¾ cup Vegan Mayonnaise (page 113)
1 tablespoon freshly squeezed lemon juice

½ teaspoon fresh dill (optional)
Pinch of sea salt

1. Place all the ingredients in a bowl and whisk well.

Nutrition Facts per serving (23 g): Calories 80, Fat Calories 80, Total Fat 9 g, Saturated Fat 1 g, Cholesterol 0 mg, Sodium 45 mg, Total Carb 0 g, Dietary Fiber 0 g, Sugars 0 g, Protein 0 g

Raw Cashew Sour Cream ♥ Ⓖ

YIELD: 1 ¾ CUPS SOUR CREAM

Prep time: 35 minutes, Total time: 35 minutes, Serving size: 1 tablespoon, Number of servings: 28

It may take you just about as long to make this homemade raw version of sour cream as it does to run to the store to purchase it. Multitalented cashews provide the creaminess, and lemon steps up to the plate to provide the sour. This sour cream delivers on essential minerals and vitamin C. Enjoy on top of Raw Carrot Brazil Nut Soup (page 245) or Walnut Taco Salad (page 187).

1 cup raw cashew pieces
2 tablespoons plus 2 teaspoons freshly squeezed lemon juice
½ to ¾ cup water
2 teaspoons olive oil (optional)
1 teaspoon minced fresh dill (optional)
¼ teaspoon sea salt, or to taste

1. Place the cashews in a bowl with ample water to cover. Allow to sit for 25 minutes, or up to 3 hours.

2. Rinse and drain well.

3. Place in a blender with all the remaining ingredients, including the ½ cup of fresh water, and blend until creamy. Add additional water, if necessary, to reach your desired consistency. This will be determined by the strength of your blender.

VARIATION

♦ For an oil-free version, omit the oil.

Nutrition Facts per serving (13 g): Calories 45, Fat Calories 30, Total Fat 10 g, Saturated Fat 0 g, Cholesterol 0 mg, Sodium 20 mg, Total Carb 3 g, Dietary Fiber 0 g, Sugars 1 g, Protein 1 g

Vegan Mayonnaise Ⓖ

YIELD: 2 ¼ CUPS MAYONNAISE

Prep time: 15 minutes, Total time: 15 minutes, Serving size: 1 tablespoon, Number of servings: 36

Making homemade mayo is not only simple but also helps you avoid the preservatives of store-bought mayonnaise. Try this clean version with just these few household staples. The main ingredient—multifaceted, mildly flavored safflower oil—is made from safflower seeds, which are very similar to sunflower seeds and contain a wealth of vitamin E and monounsaturated fat. While this is certainly not an oil-free or fat-free condiment, many of us still enjoy the flavor and texture of mayonnaise on occasion. Why not save on the packaging and make your own? Use wherever vegan mayonnaise is called for.

1 ½ cups safflower oil
¾ cup soy milk (see note)

2 teaspoons raw coconut nectar or agave
 nectar (optional)
¾ teaspoon Dijon mustard
¼ teaspoon sea salt, or to taste
2 teaspoons freshly squeezed lemon juice

1. Combine all the ingredients, except
   the lemon juice, in a blender and blend
   until smooth.

2. Slowly add the lemon juice through the
   top while blending, until the mixture
   thickens.

*Note: Some brands of soy milk will emulsify better
than others. For best results, shake the soy milk well
and use at room temperature.*

VARIATION

◆ For an oil-free version, replace the oil
with 1 cup soaked and drained raw cashew
pieces or macadamia nuts. Add additional milk if necessary to reach desired
consistency.

Nutrition Facts per serving (17 g): Calories 80, Fat
Calories 80, Total Fat 9 g, Saturated Fat 1 g, Cho-
lesterol 0 mg, Sodium 20 mg, Total Carb 0 g, Dietary
Fiber 0 g, Sugars 0 g, Protein 0 g

Roasted Garlic Spread Ⓖ

YIELD: ½ CUP GARLIC SPREAD

Prep time: 10 minutes, Cook time: 15 minutes,
Total time: 25 minutes, Serving size: 1 tablespoon,
Number of servings: 8

Garlic, a superfood and a member of the
onion family, has been called on throughout
history, including by Hippocrates, as a cura-
tive for respiratory and digestive symptoms,
parasites, and fatigue. Today it is also used
for blood system and heart conditions, such
as artery hardening, high cholesterol, high
blood pressure, and heart disease. Garlic lov-
ers will enjoy this exceptional spread on toast
along with the Okra Bruschetta (page 162).
Wonderful in Nori Rolls (page 263) and Raw
Collard Veggie Rolls (page 260).

1 cup peeled garlic cloves (about 40 cloves)
1 tablespoon plus 1 teaspoon olive oil
⅛ teaspoon sea salt, or to taste
Pinch of freshly ground black pepper
1 tablespoon chiffonaded fresh basil
½ teaspoon fresh minced marjoram
2 teaspoons nutritional yeast
Pinch of crushed red pepper flakes
¼ teaspoon balsamic vinegar
¼ teaspoon truffle oil (optional)

1. Preheat the oven to 400°F. Place the
   garlic, 1 tablespoon of the olive oil, and
   the salt and black pepper in a small
   baking dish and toss well.

2. Bake until the garlic is just soft and
   slightly browned, about 15 minutes.

3. Transfer to a small food processor and
   process until just pureed.

4. Add the remaining ingredients, including the remaining teaspoon of olive oil,
   and process for 30 seconds.

VARIATIONS

◆ For an oil-free version, replace the oil
with ¼ cup of water or vegetable stock
(see page 108).

Add 1 tablespoon of finely chopped fresh flat-leaf parsley, and ½ teaspoon each of fresh thyme and oregano.

Replace the basil with fresh cilantro or minced dill.

Add 2 teaspoons of an ethnic spice blend, such as Mexican (page 106), Indian (page 106), or Moroccan (page 106).

Nutrition Facts per serving (24 g): Calories 40, Fat Calories 15, Total Fat 2 g, Saturated Fat 0 g, Cholesterol 0 mg, Sodium 40 mg, Total Carb 5 g, Dietary Fiber 0 g, Sugars 0 g, Protein 1 g

CHAPTER 9

Breakfast

The best way to ensure an energizing day is to begin with a healthy, nutrient-rich, plant-strong breakfast. In this chapter, you will find an assortment of recipes to choose from. Power up your day with the Açai Power Bowl (page 120). For a lighter start, enjoy the Simple Breakfast Chia Pudding (page 117), Trifecta Stewed Dried Fruit (page 121), or Sunflower Seed Fig Puree (page 118) topped with fresh fruit. You can go even lighter by enjoying a superfood smoothie from Chapter 10.

For a hardier breakfast, go with the Garden Veggie Scramble (page 128) and Herb-Roasted Potatoes (page 214), or Purple Potato Tempeh Hash (page 130). Have a granola craving? I provide two different granola recipes—one cooked (Pepita Pecan Granola, page 124) and one raw (Raw Apricot Fennel Granola, page 121), so you can compare both versions. Going gourmet? Enjoy the Sun-Dried Tomato Fennel Breakfast Tart (page 129). If you find yourself too busy in the morning for breakfast, check out the Quicker and Easier Overnight Oatmeal recipe (page 127).

Be a champion and start your day the right way!

Simple Breakfast Chia Pudding ♥ ⓖ ♦ ▱

YIELD: 2 ½ CUPS PUDDING

Prep time: 5 minutes, Soaking time: 15 minutes,
Total time: 15 minutes, Serving size: 1/2 cup,
Number of servings: 5

This filling pudding, topped with berries or other fresh fruit, optimizes the seeds versatility by adding one of my favorite spice combos of cinnamon and cardamom. Chia seeds are a superfood of the moment finding their way into any meal of the day, given their omega-3 fatty acids, protein content, and energy supply. You can save time in the morning by preparing the pudding in the evening and placing in the fridge overnight.

PUDDING

¼ cup chia seeds

1 ¼ cups water

Pinch of ground cinnamon

Pinch of ground cardamom

1 ¼ cups soy, rice, or almond milk
   (for homemade, see Plant-Based Milk,
   page 104)

Sweetener (optional)

TOPPINGS

Fresh fruit, such as chopped plums, sliced
   bananas, berries, chopped apple, or pear

Nuts and seeds

Dried fruit

1. Prepare the pudding: Place the chia seeds in a bowl with the water, cinnamon, and cardamom. Stir well. Allow to sit until the water is absorbed, about 15 minutes.

2. Meanwhile prepare your fruit (peel, slice, or rinse as necessary).

3. Transfer the mixture to individual bowls. Top with soy milk and sweetener to taste, if using, and stir well. Add the toppings before serving.

Nutrition Facts per serving (131 g) not including fruit: Calories 75, Fat Calories 40, Total Fat 4.5 g, Saturated Fat 1 g , Cholesterol 0 mg, Sodium 25 mg, Total Carb 6 g, Dietary Fiber 5 g, Sugars 0 g, Protein 4 g

TEMPLATE RECIPE
Chia Pudding

- -

Pudding component: Replace the water with different plant-based milks (for homemade, see Plant-Based Milk, page 104). Blend the milk with 3 tablespoons of raw cacao powder or cacao nibs (see Choco-Chia Pudding, page 295). Add a pinch of other spices, such as allspice or nutmeg.

Topping component: Experiment with different dried fruits, nuts, and seeds.

Sweetener component: See the sweetener chart on page 89 for different sweeteners. Try coconut nectar, Date Syrup (page 88), or pure maple syrup.

QUICKER AND EASIER

One of my favorite quick and easy breakfasts: gluten-free toast, topped with a drizzle of flax or hemp oil, a spread of tahini or almond butter, and a sprinkle of nutritional yeast.

Rainbow Fruit and Crème ⊙◆

YIELD: 4 ½ CUPS FRUIT AND CRÈME

Prep time: 10 minutes, Total time: 10 minutes, Serving size: 1 cup, Number of servings: 4

Perhaps you've heard the advice to "eat the colors of the rainbow" to glean optimal nutrient content and variety. When it comes to finding a rainbow of colors and nutritional benefits in just one bowl, this recipe has you covered, from the antioxidants in berries, to the fiber in mango and papaya, potassium in bananas, and iron content of the dates, just to name a few. Enjoy with a glass of Choco Maca Elixir (page 145) or Citrus Magic (page 137).

1 cup peeled, seeded, and chopped papaya
  (½-inch pieces)
1 cup peeled, pitted, and chopped mango
  (½-inch pieces)
1 cup sliced banana
½ cup blueberries
½ cup raspberries
¼ cup peeled and diced kiwi
½ cup Cashew Cream (page 297)
¼ cup chopped hazelnuts (optional), toasted
  (see page 101)

1. Combine the fruit in an artistic fashion in four bowls.

2. Top with a dollop of cashew cream and chopped hazelnuts, if using.

VARIATIONS

Experiment with different fruits, such as peach, pear, plum, apple, apricot, pomegranate seeds, or dried figs.

Superfood it up by adding cacao nibs, goji berries, chia seeds, or ground flaxseeds.

Nutrition Facts per serving (214 g): Calories 275, Fat Calories 85, Total Fat 10 g, Saturated Fat 2 g, Cholesterol 0 mg, Sodium 5 mg, Total Carb 47 g, Dietary Fiber 6 g, Sugars 30 g, Protein 6 g

Sunflower Seed Fig Puree ♥⊙◆▱

YIELD: 3 ½ CUPS PUREE

Prep time: 10 minutes, Soak time: 20 minutes or more, Total time: 30 minutes or more, Serving size: 1/2 cup, Number of servings: 7

A surprisingly rich yet light breakfast puree awaits! Sunflower seeds pack a potent nutrient punch for their small size. Best eaten raw, the seeds are a great source of polyunsaturated oil and contain fiber and hormone-balancing lignans. Combining the vitamin C and antioxidants of fresh fruit and the glucose-stabilizing properties of cinnamon, this puree is an excellent way to fuel your morning. Serve this raw breakfast puree with fresh fruit, dried fruit, nuts, and seeds. For best results, allow the figs and sunflower seeds to soak for 4 to 6 hours, or up to overnight. Start your soaking the night before. Remember to save the fig soak water and to discard the sunflower seed soak water.

12 figs (try Black Mission, Calimyrna, or
  Turkish)
2 ½ cups water
½ cup raw sunflower seeds
⅛ teaspoon ground cinnamon
Sweetener (optional) (see page 89)
Fruit, nuts, or seeds, to serve

1. Place the figs and water in a bowl or jar and allow to sit for at least 20 minutes, or up to overnight.

2. Place the sunflower seeds in another bowl or jar with ample water to cover. Allow to sit for 20 minutes, or up to overnight.

3. Rinse and drain the sunflower seeds well. Discard the sunflower seed soak water. Place the sunflower seeds in a blender.

4. Add the figs, fig soak water, and cinnamon and blend well, adding sweetener to taste, if desired. Pour into bowls and top with fruit, nuts, or seeds.

Nutrition Facts per serving (30 g): Calories 130, Fat Calories 70, Total Fat 8 g, Saturated Fat 1 g, Cholesterol 0 mg, Sodium 0 mg, Total Carb 12 g, Dietary Fiber 3 g, Sugars 7 g, Protein 4 g

TEMPLATE RECIPE
Raw Breakfast Seed and Fruit Puree

Dried fruit component: Replace the figs with other dried fruit, such as apricots, prunes, or raisins.

Seed component: Replace the sunflower seeds with any nut or seed of your choosing, such as sesame, pumpkin, or almond.

Sweetener component: Add three pitted dates along with the figs for a sweeter puree. You can also add coconut nectar, pure maple syrup, or sweetener of choice (see page 89) to taste after pureeing.

Raw Pumpkin Seed and Sunseed Yogurt ♥ Ⓖ ◗

YIELD: 4 CUPS YOGURT

Prep time: 15 minutes, Soak time: 3 hours, Culturing time: 10 hours, Total time: 13.25 hours , Serving size: 1/2 cup, Number of servings: 8

Get your tang on with this seed-based yogurt that combines the health benefits of two of the most healthful ingredients on the block: pumpkin and sunflower seeds. The culturing process takes place on its own. No need to track down probiotic powders, though, as an option, adding half of an acidophilus capsule will accelerate the process. Sunflower seeds deliver selenium, magnesium, copper, vitamin E, and antioxidants in a tiny package. In a slightly bigger package, pumpkin seeds provide fiber, protein, iron, potassium, phosphorus, zinc, and also magnesium. Sweeten this yogurt to taste and top with fresh fruit.

½ cup raw pumpkin seeds
½ cup raw sunflower seeds
1 ½ cups water

1. Place the pumpkin seeds and sunflower seeds in a large bowl with ample water to cover 2 inches above the seeds.

2. Allow to sit for 3 to 4 hours. Drain and rinse the seeds well. Discard the soak water. Transfer to a strong blender with the 1 ½ cups of fresh water and blend well. Place in a mason jar and cover with a cheesecloth or sprout bag secured with a rubber band (see page 82).

3. Allow to sit overnight in a warm place (68° to 72°F). The mixture should have a bubbly texture with liquid (the

whey) on the bottom. Poke a chopstick through the mixture to the bottom of the jar and carefully pour out the whey. The remaining mixture is the yogurt.

VARIATIONS

Replace the seeds with sesame seeds, hemp seeds, cashews, macadamia nuts, or pine nuts.

Add ½ teaspoon of ground cinnamon and ¼ teaspoon of ground cardamom after the mixture cultures, and mix well.

Nutrition Facts per serving (55 g): Calories 60, Fat Calories 50, Total Fat 5.5 g, Saturated Fat 1 g, Cholesterol 0 mg, Sodium 0 mg, Total Carb 1 g, Dietary Fiber 1 g, Sugars 0 g, Protein 3 g

Açai Power Bowl🅖💧

YIELD: 2 CUPS GRANOLA AND FRUIT

Prep time: 20 minutes, Total time: 20 minutes, Serving size: 1 cup, Number of servings: 2

Açai, with its varied and debated pronunciations, is a dark purple berry with Brazilian origins. In the Amazon it is blended with manioc root and eaten as a porridge. Here it is mostly found frozen. When blended with water, frozen açai turns into a slushie or a sorbet consistency and makes a super summer treat with granola and fruit. Açai is low in sugar and high in iron, fiber, calcium, and vitamin A, with high levels of antioxidants. Top these bowls with a dollop of almond butter or tahini, and coconut yogurt or plant-based milk.

1 cup granola, store-bought or homemade (pages 121 and 124)
⅓ cup frozen açai

¼ cup water, juice, or plant-based milk (for homemade, see page 104)
1 medium-size banana, sliced
2 strawberries, sliced
2 tablespoons raw cacao nibs
2 teaspoons hemp seeds
2 tablespoons unsweetened shredded coconut or large coconut flakes (optional) (optionally toasted, see page 101)

1. Divide the granola between two bowls.

2. Place the açai and water in a blender and blend until smooth. Pour over the granola.

3. Top with the fruit, cacao nibs, hemp seeds, and coconut flakes, if using, before serving.

VARIATIONS

Change up the granolas, juices, or plant-based milk, fruit, and toppings for a multitude of açai experiences.

♥ For a raw version, use Raw Apricot Fennel Granola (page 121).

Nutrition Facts per serving (215 g) made with water and a low-fat granola: Calories 315, Fat Calories 105, Total Fat 12 g, Saturated Fat 5 g, Cholesterol 0 mg, Sodium 105 mg, Total Carb 51 g, Dietary Fiber 10 g, Sugars 19 g, Protein 8 g

Trifecta Stewed Dried Fruit⊙◊

YIELD: 2 CUPS FRUIT

Prep time: 10 minutes, Cook time: 15 minutes, Total time: 25 minutes, Serving size: 1/2 cup, Number of servings: 4

This trifecta takes advantage of a powerful trio of sweet and comforting dried fruits: prunes, apricots, and figs, supplying maximal fiber, potassium, and antioxidant carotenoids, such as vitamin A. When dried, the nutrients in these fruits are more concentrated. Rehydrating them in orange juice brings the vitamin C content up even higher, and Chinese-origin star anise adds surprising benefits besides being flavorful: it is antiviral, antifungal, and antibacterial. Serve with a dollop of Cashew Cream (page 297) or vegan yogurt.

1 cup freshly squeezed orange juice
½ cup water
¾ cup pitted prunes
¼ cup dried apricots
4 dried figs
1 star anise
1 cinnamon stick
⅓ cup slivered almonds

1. Place all the ingredients, except the almonds, in a small pot over medium heat.

2. Cook, stirring occasionally, for 20 minutes, or until all of the fruit is rehydrated and plump.

3. Remove the star anise and cinnamon stick. Top with the slivered almonds before serving.

VARIATIONS

Replace the orange juice with the fruit juice of your choosing.

Replace the almonds with pumpkin seeds, sesame seeds, or chopped pecans or hazelnuts.

Nutrition Facts per serving (123 g): Calories 185, Fat Calories 40, Total Fat 5 g, Saturated Fat 0 g, Cholesterol 0 mg, Sodium 0 mg, Total Carb 37 g, Dietary Fiber 5 g, Sugars 23 g, Protein 4 g

Raw Apricot Fennel Granola♥⊙◊

YIELD: 6 CUPS GRANOLA

Prep time: 30 minutes, Dehydrating time: 26 hours, Total time: 26.5 hours, Serving size: 1/2 cup, Number of servings: 12

This sweet and crunchy homemade granola beats any bagged version. Gluten-free, pseudocereal buckwheat is a grainlike seed that is very filling and an ally of the cardiovascular system, since its flavonoid rutin maintains blood flow and prevents platelet clotting. Sunflower seeds are excellent sources of vitamins B_1 and E and copper, while dried apricot never disappoints in its delivery of fiber and potassium. Enjoy with a variety of plant-based milks and top with fresh fruit of your choosing for a colorful way to start the day.

DRY

1 cup raw buckwheat groats
1 cup raw sunflower seeds
1 cup raw cashew pieces

WET

½ cup dried apricots

⅓ cup pitted Medjool dates (see page 125)

1 cup water or fruit juice (try orange, apple, or pineapple)

1 teaspoon orange zest (optional)

½ teaspoon ground cinnamon

¼ teaspoon ground cardamom

½ teaspoon pure vanilla extract

1 ½ teaspoons fennel seeds

Pinch of sea salt

TO SERVE

Toppings of choice such as sliced fresh fruit, chopped dried fruit, chopped nuts or seeds

Plant-based milk of choice (for homemade, see page 104)

1. Prepare the dry ingredients: Place the buckwheat groats, sunflower seeds, and cashews in a bowl with ample water to cover. Allow to sit for 30 minutes, or up to 4 hours. Rinse and drain well. Return to the bowl.

2. Meanwhile, prepare the wet ingredients: Place the apricots, dates, and water in another bowl and allow to sit for 30 minutes. Transfer to a blender along with the orange zest, if using, cinnamon, cardamom, vanilla, and salt and blend until pureed. Transfer to the dry mixture and mix well. Add the fennel seeds and mix well.

3. Pour the mixture onto two Teflex or ParaFlexx dehydrator sheets. Dehydrate at 145°F for 2 hours. Lower the temperature to 115°F and dehydrate for 12 hours.

4. Flip the dehydrator sheet onto the dehydrator tray, and dehydrate for an additional 12 hours, before removing.

5. Add toppings and plant-based milk of choice and enjoy!

VARIATIONS

For a cooked version, place the granola on a well-oiled baking sheet, and bake at 300°F for 70 minutes, or until dry, stirring occasionally to prevent sticking.

To view this recipe as a template, check out the template recipe box for the Pepita Pecan Granola (page 124).

Nutrition Facts per serving (66 g): Calories 290, Fat Calories 160, Saturated Fat 2.5 g, Cholesterol 0 mg, Sodium 20 mg, Total Carb 28 g, Dietary Fiber 5 g, Sugars 8 g, Protein 10 g

Banana Date Breakfast Muffins⬥

YIELD: 10 MUFFINS

Prep time: 15 minutes, Cook time: 30 minutes, Total time: 45 minutes, Serving size: 1 muffin, Number of servings: 10

Banana and dates are a sweet combo bursting with health benefits. Besides potassium, bananas contain tryptophan, which is converted into serotonin for happy moods. Easily digested dates are stellar energy boosters—fibrous and full of iron, magnesium, and potassium, too! Enjoy these oil- and processed sugar-free treats warm out of the oven along with your Açai Power Bowl (page 120).

Oil, for pan (optional)

WET

1 ½ cups mashed banana

¼ cup diced Medjool dates (see page 125)

1 teaspoon pure vanilla extract

1 tablespoon chia seeds or ground flaxseeds
   mixed with 3 tablespoons water

½ teaspoon lemon zest (optional)

DRY

½ cup spelt or gluten-free flour

½ cup rolled oats (try gluten-free)

½ cup dried unsweetened shredded coconut

1 teaspoon baking powder

¾ teaspoon ground cinnamon

⅛ teaspoon sea salt

⅛ teaspoon ground cardamom

⅛ teaspoon ground nutmeg (optional)

1. Preheat the oven to 350°F. Lightly oil
   ten wells of a muffin tin or line with
   muffin papers.

2. Place the wet ingredients in a food processor and process until smooth. Place
   the dry ingredients in another bowl and
   whisk well. Add the wet to the dry and
   mix well.

3. Using a ¼-cup measuring cup or scoop,
   pour the batter into the prepared muffin tin.

4. Place in the oven and bake for
   30 minutes.

VARIATIONS

Add ½ cup of vegan chocolate chips.
Decadent: top with vegan butter before
serving.

Add ½ cup of pitted and chopped dates,
raisins, or currants, for extra sweetness.

Add ½ cup chopped nuts, such as raw
walnuts or pecans.

Ⓖ For a gluten-free version, replace the
spelt flour with the Gluten-Free Flour Mix
(page 105) and use certified gluten-free
rolled oats.

Nutrition Facts per serving (68 g): Calories 180, Fat
Calories 75, Total Fat 9 g, Saturated Fat 7 g, Chole-
sterol 0 mg, Sodium 70 mg, Total Carb 25 g, Dietary
Fiber 5 g, Sugars 9 g, Protein 3 g

Lemon Blueberry Pancakes

YIELD: 8 PANCAKES

Prep time: 15 minutes, Cook time: 15 minutes,
Total time: 30 minutes, Serving size: 1/4 cup
pancake batter, Number of servings: 8

These vegan pancakes are a long way from
Aunt Jemima's yet with the same comfort
food feeling. The flaxseeds substitute seam-
lessly for eggs, and flour made from spelt—
one of the oldest crops in history—helps
regulate the body's metabolism, improve
digestion, and lower blood sugar and cholesterol. Blueberries add bursts of color and
flavor, and are high in antioxidants, combating
free radicals right and left. Serve with a side
of Coco Bacon (page 112) and Herb-Roasted
Potatoes (page 214).

WET

1 tablespoon ground flaxseeds

3 tablespoons water

1 ¾ cups almond, soy, or rice milk
   (for homemade, see Plant-Based Milk,
   page 104)

3 tablespoons freshly squeezed lemon juice

½ teaspoon pure vanilla extract

½ teaspoon lemon zest

½ cup blueberries

DRY

1 ¼ cups flour (try white spelt)

1 teaspoon baking powder

½ teaspoon baking soda

½ teaspoon sea salt

½ teaspoon ground cinnamon

¼ teaspoon ground cardamom, nutmeg, or allspice

Coconut oil, for cooking

1. Preheat a griddle over high heat.

2. Place the flaxseeds and water in a small bowl and mix well. Allow to sit for 10 minutes.

3. Meanwhile, place all the remaining wet ingredients in a bowl and mix well. Place the dry ingredients in a separate bowl and mix well.

4. Add all the wet ingredients, including the ground flaxseeds and water, to the dry ingredients and mix well.

5. Grease the griddle with a small amount of coconut oil. Pour ¼ cup of batter onto the griddle to create eight 4-inch-diameter pancakes. Cook until bubbles form and the sides begin to dry, about 3 minutes. Waiting for this to happen helps prevent the pancakes from sticking. Carefully flip. Cook for an additional 3 minutes before serving.

VARIATIONS

Replace the blueberries with raspberries, blackberries, strawberries, goji berries, or sliced bananas.

Add ¼ cup of vegan chocolate chips along with the wet ingredients.

Ⓖ For a gluten-free version, use the Gluten-Free Flour Mix (page 105).

Nutrition Facts per serving (97 g): Calories 120, Fat Calories 20, Total Fat 2 g, Saturated Fat 1 g, Cholesterol 0 mg, Sodium 170 mg, Total Carb 22 g, Dietary Fiber 4 g, Sugars 3 g, Protein 5 g

Pepita Pecan Granola ♦ ⧉

YIELD: 6 CUPS

Prep time: 15 minutes, Cook time: 40 minutes, Total time: 55 minutes, Serving size: 3/4 cup, Number of servings: 8

Starting with a crunch and ending with a wave of sweetness, this versatile granola is a treasure chest of minerals, thanks to the pecans—these flavorful nuts are loaded with manganese, copper, magnesium, and zinc. They are also high in healthy fats. Oats, a granola staple, have more dietary fiber than any other grain, specifically a fiber called beta glucan, which is efficient in lowering dangerous types of cholesterol. Both pecans and oats contain iron as well, and the vitamin C in the orange juice in this granola helps absorption of nonheme iron, the iron found in plant foods. Serve over coconut yogurt or with the addition of a plant-based milk and fresh fruit.

DRY

2 cups rolled oats (try gluten-free)

¾ cup spelt flour

½ cup raw pumpkin seeds

½ cup chopped raw pecans

½ teaspoon ground cinnamon

¼ teaspoon ground cardamom

¼ teaspoon ground nutmeg

⅛ teaspoon sea salt

WET

1 teaspoon orange zest (optional)

¾ cup freshly squeezed orange juice

¾ cup pitted Medjool dates

¼ cup applesauce

1 ½ teaspoons pure vanilla extract

Oil, for pan (optional)

1. Preheat the oven to 350°F. Combine all the dry ingredients in a large bowl and mix well.

2. Combine all the wet ingredients in a blender and blend until smooth. Add the wet to the dry and mix well.

3. Transfer to a well-oiled or parchment paper–lined baking sheet. Bake for 20 minutes. Remove from the oven, carefully stir well, and return to the oven. Bake for 10 minutes. Remove from the oven, carefully stir well, and return to the oven. Bake until golden brown, about 10 minutes.

4. Allow to cool completely before placing in a glass storage container. Granola will continue to dry out as it cools.

VARIATIONS

G For a gluten-free version, use the Gluten-Free Flour Mix (page 105) and certified gluten-free rolled oats.

Chef's Tips and Tricks

Medjool dates are the moistest variety. If using other varieties, such as Deglet, soak the pitted dates in the orange juice for 20 minutes, or until soft.

A large variety of dates are grown, mostly in the Middle East, and more than 20 different varieties can be ordered online, but in shops and bulk sections one of four varieties of dates will most commonly be found. Dried dates are sun-ripened on the tree, and fresh or soft dates are also available at times. Dates freeze very well if needed.

Medjool dates are usually the largest, softest, and sweetest, and are great for everything from smoothies to baking to making date paste. A certain moistness in them often makes soaking unneeded.

Deglet Noor dates are lighter in color than Medjool and also tend to be less moist and need more soaking for any kind of blending use. However, as such, they are easy to cut up into bits. Great for energy bars or baking. They are the go-to variety for almost any store or supermarket and therefore easily found. Similar in flavor and texture to Deglets are Zahidis. The sweetest and gooiest are Khadrawy.

Less commonly available and a lighter brown, Thoory dates are quite firm and dry.

Smaller in size, Halawi dates can be used in a recipe that calls for caramel, due to their caramel-like flavor.

Nutrition Facts per serving (89 g): Calories 270, Fat Calories 95, Total Fat 11 g, Saturated Fat 1.5 g, Cholesterol 0 mg, Sodium 25 mg, Total Carb 38 g, Dietary Fiber 6 g, Sugars 12 g, Protein 9 g

TEMPLATE RECIPE
Homemade Granola

- -

Dry component: Replace the pecans and pepitas with nuts and seeds of your choosing, such as hazelnuts, almonds, walnuts, sunflower seeds, or sesame seeds. Experiment with different flours.

Wet component: Replace the applesauce with ¼ cup of coconut oil or grapeseed oil. Replace the dates with pure maple syrup or sweetener of choice (see page 89). Replace the orange juice with other fruit juices, such as pineapple, tangerine, peach, or nectarine. Add 1 teaspoon of orange zest.

Add-in component: Add ½ cup of unsweetened shredded coconut and/or ½ cup of dried fruit, such as raisins, currants, crystalized ginger, chopped apricots, papaya, or banana. Add ½ cup of hemp seeds and/or cacao nibs.

Multigrain Grits 🅖 ◐

YIELD: 4 CUPS GRITS

Prep time: 5 minutes, Cook time: 20 minutes, Total time: 25 minutes, Serving size: 1 cup, Number of servings: 4

Some like it sweet and some like it savory. Creamy down-home goodness, courtesy of mineral-rich grits, is enhanced with complete-protein quinoa, and high-fiber oats to yield a powerhouse mix of grains. Once this base is made, follow the variations to take it in a sweet or savory direction that strikes your

fancy. The sweet version can replace your morning bowl of oatmeal. The savory version is perfect for brunch, and even the base of a Monk Bowl (see pages 100, 267). Enjoy with Galactic Green Juice (page 135) or Gold Milk (page 144).

BASE RECIPE

4 ½ cups water

¼ teaspoon sea salt

½ cup corn grits

½ cup uncooked quinoa (try rainbow blend), rinsed and drained (see pages 95, 144)

½ cup rolled oats (try gluten-free)

FOR SAVORY

Soy, rice, almond, or hemp milk (for homemade, see Plant-Based Milk, page 104)

1 garlic clove, pressed or minced

¼ teaspoon sea salt

⅛ teaspoon freshly ground black pepper

¼ teaspoon crushed red pepper flakes

¼ cup thinly sliced green onion

FOR SWEET

Soy, rice, almond, or hemp milk (for homemade, see Plant-Based Milk, page 104)

Tahini, almond butter, peanut butter, or other nut or seed butter

¼ teaspoon ground cinnamon

⅛ teaspoon ground nutmeg

Dried fruit, nuts, and seeds

Fresh fruit (banana, berries, sliced pears, apples, peaches)

1. Prepare the base recipe: Place the water in a 1-quart pot over medium-high heat. Add the salt, grits, and quinoa and cook for 15 minutes, stirring occasionally.

2. Add the oats, mix well, and cook for 5 minutes, stirring occasionally.

3. Add the sweet or savory fixings and enjoy.

VARIATION

G For a gluten-free version, use certified gluten-free rolled oats.

Nutrition Facts per serving (352 g) for base recipe: Calories 230, Fat Calories 25, Total Fat 3 g, Saturated Fat 0 g, Cholesterol 0 mg, Sodium 160 mg, Total Carb 342 g, Dietary Fiber 4 g, Sugars less than 1 g, Protein 8 g

Iron-Rich Morning Glory Steel-Cut Oats **G** ●

YIELD: 3 CUPS OATS

Prep time: 5 minutes, Cook time: 30 minutes, Total time: 35 minutes, Serving size: 3/4 cup, Number of servings: 4

This hearty oatmeal delivers iron in four delicious doses: oats, dates, raisins, and black-strap molasses. Steel-cut oats in their least processed form, just chopped whole oat groats, have a nuttier and chewier feel than rolled or quick oats. They'll provide a steady energy boost with complex carbohydrates. Top with additional fresh fruit, a sprinkle of hemp seeds or ground flaxseeds, and cacao nibs, and serve with plant-based milk and sweetener of your choosing. Can also be served with a dollop of coconut or soy yogurt.

2 ½ cups water
¾ cup steel-cut oats
Pinch of sea salt
¼ cup pitted and diced dates
¼ cup raisins
⅛ teaspoon ground cinnamon
1 tablespoon blackstrap molasses
1 banana, sliced

1. Place the water, oats, and salt in a 1-quart pot over medium-high heat. Cook for 15 minutes, stirring occasionally, lowering the heat to medium to prevent boiling over.

2. Add the dates, raisins, and cinnamon and cook for 10 minutes, stirring occasionally. Add the molasses and banana and cook for 5 minutes, or until the oats are soft, stirring occasionally.

VARIATIONS

Replace the dates and raisins with dried fruit of your choosing.

Replace the banana with other fresh fruit, such as mango, peach, blackberries, or strawberries.

QUICKER AND EASIER

Overnight Oatmeal **G** ●

Strapped for time in the mornings? The night before, try combining 1/2 cup of quick-cooking rolled oats, 2 tablespoons of chia seeds, a pinch each of cinnamon and ground cardamom, 1 teaspoon of pure vanilla extract (optional), and 1 1/3 cups of plant-based milk, such as almond, soy, or hemp (for homemade, see Plant-Based Milk, page 104) in a bowl or jar and mix well. Cover and place in the refrigerator overnight. In the morning, you can enjoy cold or heat in a pan for a few minutes, add desired sweetener to taste (see page 89), and top with additional plant-based milk, fresh and dried fruit, and nuts and seeds of your choosing, such as hemp seeds or pumpkin seeds.

Nutrition Facts per serving (195 g): Calories 225, Fat Calories 20, Total Fat 2 g, Saturated Fat 0 g, Cholesterol 0 mg, Sodium 40 mg, Total Carb 49 g, Dietary Fiber 5 g, Sugars 22 g, Protein 6 g

TEMPLATE RECIPE
Garden Scramble

- -

Base: Replace the tofu with tempeh, seitan, or Beyond Meat (see page 84).

Veggie component: Add 1 cup of seeded and diced bell pepper and/or diced zucchini along with the mushrooms.

Herb component: Replace the basil with fresh cilantro, parsley, or 2 teaspoons of fresh dill.

Ethnic component: For a Mexican Scramble, add 1 cup of cooked black beans (see page 98), 2 tablespoons of chopped fresh cilantro, and 2 teaspoons of chili powder, and replace the tomato with salsa (such as Smoky Salsa, page 151).

For an Indian Scramble, add 2 tablespoons of chopped fresh cilantro, 1 tablespoon of curry powder, and 1 teaspoon of ground cumin.

For an Italian Scramble, add ½ cup of diced olives, ½ cup of thinly sliced sun-dried tomatoes, 2 tablespoons of chiffonaded fresh basil, and ½ teaspoon of minced fresh rosemary.

Garden Veggie Scramble^G

YIELD: 4 CUPS SCRAMBLE

Prep time: 10 minutes, Cook time: 15 minutes, Total time: 25 minutes, Serving size: 1 cup, Number of servings: 4

This ultimate savory veggie breakfast features tofu, which has ultrastrong protein power, and scrambles up fluffy with veggies, such as mushrooms. Your choice of spinach, arugula, or kale delivers vitamins A, C, K, folate, potassium, magnesium, manganese, and iron. Enjoy as well the immunity-boosting powers of onion and garlic. If you are feeling decadent, add 3/4 cup of grated vegan mozzarella-style cheese along with the arugula. For a hardy breakfast, enjoy with Herb-Roasted Potatoes (page 214) and a cup of Choco Maca Elixir (page 145).

2 teaspoons coconut oil
½ cup diced yellow onion
3 garlic cloves, pressed or minced
1 cup diced cremini mushrooms
14 ounces extra-firm tofu, crumbled
½ teaspoon ground turmeric
1 cup chopped tomato (½-inch pieces)
¼ teaspoon sea salt, or to taste
⅛ teaspoon freshly ground black pepper, or
    to taste
1 cup spinach, arugula, or stemmed and
    shredded kale
1 tablespoon chiffonaded fresh basil
1 tablespoon nutritional yeast
1 teaspoon wheat-free tamari or other soy
    sauce (optional)

1. Place a large sauté pan over medium-high heat and melt the coconut oil. Add

the onion and cook for 1 minute, stirring frequently. Add the garlic and cook for 1 minute, stirring frequently. Add the mushrooms and cook until they begin to soften, about 3 minutes, stirring frequently and adding small amount of water, if necessary, to prevent sticking.

2. Add the tofu and turmeric and cook until the tofu begins to brown, about 5 minutes, stirring frequently. Lower the heat to medium, add the tomato, and cook until it begins to soften, about 3 minutes, stirring frequently.

3. Add the remaining ingredients and cook until the arugula is wilted, about 2 minutes, stirring frequently. Serve warm.

VARIATION

🌢For an oil-free version, omit the oil and use the water sauté method (see page 101).

Nutrition Facts per serving (243 g): Calories 145, Fat Calories 70, Total Fat 7.5 g, Saturated Fat 2.5 g, Cholesterol 0 mg, Sodium 160 mg, Total Carb 8 g, Dietary Fiber 3 g, Sugars 3 g, Protein 12 g

Sun-Dried Tomato Fennel Breakfast Tart🅖

YIELD: 1 PIE

Prep time: 20 minutes, Cook time: 30 minutes, Total time: 50 minutes, Serving size: 1 slice, Number of servings: 8

With a crunchy crust and a creamy, savory filling, this breakfast tart is for when you are ready to indulge. This plant-based version of a traditional cheese tart takes advantage of various protein leaders—almonds, garbanzo flour, and cashews—and combines them with fennel's subtle sweetness and sun-dried tomato's intense, concentrated saltiness, for an exquisite flavor. You can't beat fennel for its light, bright flavor and affinity for gently soothing the belly. You can also get your morning vitamin C from this mineral- and fiber-rich bulbous plant. Enjoy this tart on those special occasions and gourmet brunches. Feeling hungry? Serve with Purple Potato Tempeh Hash (page 130) and a cup of Warming Herbal Chai (page 133).

CRUST

1 cup slivered almonds

1 ¼ cups garbanzo flour

¼ teaspoon sea salt

2 tablespoons melted coconut oil

¼ cup water

Oil, for pan

FILLING

1 cup raw cashew pieces

¾ cup water

¼ cup diced shallot

3 garlic cloves, pressed or minced

¼ cup diced sun-dried tomato

¼ cup finely chopped fennel

3 tablespoons chiffonaded fresh sorrel or basil

2 tablespoons nutritional yeast

1 tablespoon freshly squeezed lemon juice

¼ teaspoon smoked paprika or cayenne pepper

½ teaspoon sea salt, or to taste

⅛ teaspoon freshly ground black pepper

¼ cup thinly sliced red onion

1. Prepare the crust: Preheat the oven to 350°F. Place the almonds in a food processor and process until finely ground. Transfer to a bowl with the remaining crust ingredients and mix well. Form into a ball. The dough should be slightly moist. Add up to 2 tablespoons of additional water, if necessary. Roll out to slightly more than ¼ inch thick with a rolling pin and place in a well-oiled 8-inch tart pan. You can also press dough with your hands directly into the pan. Finish the edges by pinching with your thumb and index finger. Bake for 10 minutes. Remove from the oven.

2. Meanwhile, prepare the filling: Place the cashews in a bowl with ample water to cover. Allow to sit for 20 minutes. Rinse and drain well. Transfer to a blender with the ¾ cup of fresh water and blend until creamy. Transfer to a bowl. Add the shallot, garlic, sun-dried tomato, fennel, sorrel, nutritional yeast, lemon juice, smoked paprika, salt, and black pepper and mix well. Taste and add additional salt, if necessary.

3. Pour into the tart shell. Top with the red onion, place in the oven, and bake for 30 minutes, or until golden brown. Allow to cool slightly before slicing.

VARIATIONS

Replace the almonds with pecans or hazelnuts.

Replace the cashews with macadamia nuts.

Add ½ cup of corn, seeded and diced bell peppers, or diced mushrooms.

Try sautéing the red onion until just soft before adding to this dish.

◆ Replace the oil with additional water or mashed banana.

Nutrition Facts per serving (98 g): Calories 340, Fat Calories 210, Total Fat 23.5 g, Saturated Fat 6 g, Cholesterol 0 mg, Sodium 160 mg, Total Carb 23 g, Dietary Fiber 5 g, Sugars 5 g, Protein 12 g

Purple Potato Tempeh Hash ⓖ

YIELD: 4 CUPS HASH

Prep time: 20 minutes, Cook time: 15 minutes, Total time: 35 minutes, Serving size: heaping 3/4 cup, Number of servings: 5

If you are looking for a filling breakfast that provides sustained energy, this is your dish. This fiber-packed hash is savory, smoky and slightly sweet thanks to the purple potatoes. Purple potatoes have their origins in Peru and Bolivia and have more antioxidants than other potato varieties, making their potassium content even more valuable for heart health. Superfilling tempeh, a perfect source of quality protein, and high B-vitamin greens round out this meal nicely. Serve as a side for Multigrain Grits (page 126) or Iron-Rich Morning Glory Steel-Cut Oats (page 127).

1 ½ cups chopped purple sweet potato (½-inch pieces)
2 teaspoons coconut oil
1 thinly cup sliced yellow onion
2 tablespoons minced garlic
8 ounces tempeh, cut into ½-inch pieces
1 cup seeded and diced red bell pepper

¼ teaspoon liquid smoke (see page 85), or
    1 teaspoon smoked paprika (optional)
1 tablespoon wheat-free tamari or other
    soy sauce
½ teaspoon paprika
Pinch of sea salt, or to taste
⅛ teaspoon freshly ground black pepper
⅛ teaspoon cayenne pepper
1 tablespoon nutritional yeast (optional)
1 cup arugula, shredded kale, or chard

1. Place a steamer basket in a pot with ½ inch of water over medium-high heat. Bring to a boil. Add the potato and cook until just tender, about 10 minutes. Remove from the heat.

2. Meanwhile, place the oil in a sauté pan over medium-high heat. Add the onion and garlic and cook for 3 minutes, stirring frequently. Add the tempeh and bell pepper and cook for 5 minutes, stirring frequently, adding small amounts of water, if necessary, to prevent sticking.

3. Add the liquid smoke, if using, soy sauce, paprika, salt, black pepper, cayenne, and nutritional yeast, if using, and cook for 3 minutes, stirring frequently.

4. Add the arugula and cook for 1 minute, stirring frequently. Add the cooked potato and gently stir well before serving.

VARIATIONS

Replace the purple potatoes with sweet potatoes or other potatoes.

Replace the tempeh with tofu, seitan, or Beyond Meat (see page 84).

Add 1 teaspoon of seeded and diced jalapeño pepper along with the onion.

Add 1 cup of thinly sliced mushrooms along with the onion.

Add 1 cup of grated vegan cheese along with the arugula.

◆ For an oil-free version, use the water sauté method (see page 101).

Nutrition Facts per serving (163 g): Calories 170, Fat Calories 60, Total Fat 7 g, Saturated Fat 2.5 g, Cholesterol 0 mg, Sodium 240 mg, Total Carb 18 g, Dietary Fiber 2 g, Sugars 3 g, Protein 11 g

CHAPTER 10

Teas, Elixirs, Juices, and Smoothies

Welcome to the world of liquid nutrition! Here you'll find a full spectrum of beverages to enjoy as complements to your meal or for between-meal energy bursts. Using my patented template recipe format, this chapter actually contains thousands of variations (at least 2,495 on last count). While many drinks are introduced, please remember to consume plenty of the king of beverages—water! Many consider dehydration as a leading cause of malaise. So, drink it up! Starting your day with a glass of water with a small amount of freshly squeezed lemon juice is an amazing way to get your digestive juices flowing. You can also enhance your water-drinking experience by adding fresh herbs and fruit (see Herb and Fruit Water, page 140).

Drinking teas and juices have been part of healing protocols for hundreds of years. Try the Digestive Tea (page 133) on its own or after a nice meal. Energize the herbal way with a glass of Warming Herbal Chai (page 133). Looking for a potent immunity boost?

Imbibe a Ginger Turmeric Shooter (page 140) or Flu Buster (page 140).

Experience the healing qualities of fruits and vegetables in juices, such as the Ultimate Hangover Cure (page 135), Rehydrating Watermelon Chiller (page 136), and Kale Kolada (page 143).

Using plant-based milks as a base for other drinks will open up a universe of possibilities. Start your journey with the Choco-Maca Elixir (page 145) and the Sesame Hemp Revitalizer (page 146). Discover the healing qualities of turmeric in this vegan version of an ancient Ayurvedic (see page 26) beverage, Gold Milk (page 144).

Smoothies are the perfect way to introduce superfoods, such as spirulina, hemp seeds, maca, turmeric, açai, cacao nibs, and more. Check out classic smoothies, such as the Tropical Smoothie (page 146) and Berry Green Smoothie (page 147), or enjoy a satisfying snack with the High-Protein Vanilla Almond Shake (page 148).

I lift up my glass to you as you enjoy your healthy libations. To life!

Note: The nutritional analysis for juices includes the foods in their whole form, including the juice and pulp (the latter of which is not consumed in the juice). For nut and seed milks, including the quinoa milk, the nutritional analysis is for the unstrained ingredients.

Digestive Tea⊕♦

YIELD: 3 CUPS TEA

Prep time: 5 minutes, Cook time: 25 minutes, Total time: 30 minutes, Serving size: 1 cup, Number of servings: 3

With lemongrass, ginger, and fennel, this tea helps soothe the stomach and promote digestion. Lemongrass contributes a lemon-scented aromatic compound called citral, which is a well-known digestive antimicrobial now being studied for its anticancer potential. Ginger is a key support for nausea and other stomach upsets, and mint soothes and promotes normal digestion, as well as being a trusted palate cleanser. Fennel is a master at eliminating indigestion. You can reuse the herbs for a second, though less strong, batch of tea.

3 ½ cups water
2 lemongrass stalks
½ inch fresh ginger, sliced
2 teaspoons fennel seeds
1 mint sprig (about 15 leaves)

1. Place the water in a pot over high heat. Bring to a boil. Lower the heat to medium.

2. Meanwhile, carefully cut the very bottom portion off the lemongrass. Cut off the top portion, leaving a 6-inch stalk.

Place on a cutting board and carefully smash with the side of a strong knife or a clean glass measuring cup to open the stalk so that its flavor will infuse.

3. Add the lemongrass to the pot along with the ginger and fennel seeds, and cook for 20 minutes. Do not boil.

4. Add the mint leaves, turn off the heat, and steep for 5 minutes. Strain well before serving. Serve warm or iced.

VARIATIONS

Replace the lemongrass with the juice of 1 lemon.

Add 2 tablespoons of licorice root along with the lemongrass.

Nutrition Facts per serving (14 g): Calories 10, Fat Calories 0, Total Fat 0 g, Saturated Fat 0 g, Cholesterol 0 mg, Sodium 0 mg, Total Carb 1 g, Dietary Fiber 1 g, Sugars 0 g, Protein 0 g

Warming Herbal Chai⊕♦

YIELD: 3 ¾ CUPS CHAI

Prep time: 5 minutes, Cook time: 25 minutes, Total time: 30 minutes, Serving size: 1 1/4 cups, Number of servings: 3

Cinnamon, cardamom, and ginger often are used as supporting spices in a main dish, but in this warming chai they take starring roles and work harmoniously to enhance one another's benefits. All three have compelling digestive and immunity-boosting qualities. Ginger additionally offers antioxidant support; cardamom is a reliable detoxifier and mood enhancer; and cinnamon adds anti-inflammatory and antibacterial effects, as well as helping regulate insulin and even improve memory. The flavors produce a beverage both stimulating and comforting at the same time. Add plant-based milk (see page 104) and sweetener (see page 89) of choice to taste.

5 ¼ cups water

1 inch fresh ginger, thinly sliced

10 cardamom pods (1 teaspoon seeds, ½ teaspoon ground)

2 cinnamon sticks

1 star anise

½ teaspoon whole black peppercorns

½ teaspoon whole cloves (optional)

½ teaspoon allspice berries (optional)

Pinch of ground nutmeg (optional)

1. Place the water in a pot over high heat and bring to a boil.

2. Add all the remaining ingredients, lower the heat to medium-low, and cook for 25 minutes.

3. Strain well before serving.

VARIATION

For a caffeinated option, add two bags of yerba mate tea or 2 tablespoons of black tea, and steep for 5 minutes before straining.

Nutrition Facts per serving (400 g): Calories 10, Fat Calories 5, Total Fat 0 g, Saturated Fat 0 g, Cholesterol 0 mg, Sodium 15 mg, Total Carb 6 g, Dietary Fiber 1 g, Sugars 0 g, Protein 0 g

Chef's Tips and Tricks

Juicing Tips

To peel or not to peel? Be sure to peel any nonorganic produce used in juicing. The skin can be left on organic produce, including ginger and turmeric. It is highly recommended to use organic produce in all juices (and smoothies), to minimize exposure to harmful chemicals. Please see page 60 for more information on organics.

Always remember to remove the seeds from apples before juicing. A substance called amygdalin, in the apple seeds, can turn into a poisonous hydrogen cyanide in your intestines. You would need to consume a large amount of seeds to have an effect; still, better to err on the side of caution.

For maximum nutritional benefit, it is recommended to enjoy fresh juices within 20 minutes of preparing. The exception to this is if you are cold-pressing your juices, in which case you can enjoy them within a few days.

Smoothies are also best enjoyed within 20 to 30 minutes for maximum nutritional benefits, though preparing a smoothie in the evening for the next day's breakfast is a convenient way to save time in your busy morning, while still receiving some of the benefits of the drink.

Ultimate Hangover Cure ♥ⓖ◆

YIELD: 2 CUPS HANGOVER CURE

Prep time: 10 minutes, Total time: 10 minutes,
Serving size: 1 cup, Number of servings: 2

After a night of overindulging, these plant friends can come to the rescue to help your body to put itself back together again. The electrolytes in coconut water are ideal for countering the dehydrating effects of alcohol that can cause headache and belly distress. Cilantro is known as a powerful, cleansing, liver detoxifier. Apple helps to restore lost B vitamins, soothe an irritated digestive tract, and also acts as a great detoxifier. Lime juice adds a little vitamin C and sweetness, and actually helps with water absorption. Even if your hangover is not from alcohol, but from the stress of overexertion or illness, you'll find this a restorative refresher to get back on track.

½ cup chopped fresh cilantro
2 cups cored and chopped green apple
2 tablespoons freshly squeezed lime juice
1 cup coconut water
½ teaspoon spirulina (optional)
Pinch of sea salt (optional)

1. Place the cilantro, then apple, through a juicer.

2. Add the lime juice, coconut water, spirulina, if using, and salt.

3. Stir well before serving.

Nutrition Facts per serving (276 g): Calories 90, Fat Calories 10, Total Fat 1 g, Saturated Fat 0.5 g, Cholesterol 0 mg, Sodium 130 mg, Total Carb 23 g, Dietary Fiber 5 g, Sugars 16g, Protein 2 g

Galactic Green Juice ♥ⓖ◆▱

YIELD: 2 ½ CUPS JUICE

Prep time: 10 minutes, Total time: 10 minutes,
Serving size: 1 1/4 cups, Number of servings: 2

Cucumber, the ultimate hydrator, pairs with mineral and water packed celery and the dark leafy green power of kale. The synergistic trio of lemon, apple, and cayenne adds cleansing health benefits as well as a perfect balance of tart, sweet, and spicy. Enjoy a burst of vitamins C and K, and plenty of antioxidant action with this supersatisfying beverage. Enjoy along with your main meal and with Nori Rolls (page 263) or Jamaican Patties (page 280).

1 large cucumber, cut into ½-inch pieces
    (3 cups chopped)
1 cup chopped celery (½-inch pieces)
2 cups loosely packed stemmed kale
1 peeled and quartered lemon
1 green apple, cored
Pinch of cayenne pepper

1. Place all the ingredients, except the cayenne, through a juicer.

2. Add the cayenne to the juice and stir well before serving.

Nutrition Facts per serving (394 g): Calories 120, Fat Calories 10, Total Fat 1 g, Saturated Fat 0 g, Cholesterol 0 mg, Sodium 75 mg, Total Carb 29 g, Dietary Fiber 7 g, Sugars 15 g, Protein 4 g

Green component: Replace the kale with other green vegetables, such as chard, dandelion greens, spinach, or romaine lettuce.

Herb component: Add a small handful of fresh parsley, cilantro, or basil.

Fruit component: Replace the green apple with other fruit, such as other types of apple, or pear, grapes, or peach.

1. Place all the ingredients in a blender and blend well. Serve chilled.

VARIATIONS

Add ½ teaspoon of food-grade rose water for a Watermelon Rose Chiller.

Replace the lime juice with freshly squeezed lemon juice.

Replace the watermelon with other melon, such as cantaloupe, honeydew, or Crenshaw.

Nutrition Facts per serving (227 g): Calories 55, Fat Calories 0, Total Fat 0 g, Saturated Fat 0 g, Cholesterol 0 mg, Sodium 100 mg, Total Carb 13 g, Dietary Fiber 1 g, Sugars 10 g, Protein 1 g

Rehydrating Watermelon Chiller ♥ⓖ♦

YIELD: 4 CUPS CHILLER

Prep time: 10 minutes, Total time: 10 minutes, Serving size: 1 cup, Number of servings: 4

Watermelon and cucumber top every list of most hydrating fruits and veggies, with 92 and 96 percent water, respectively. Combined with nature's electrolyte, coconut water, refreshing lime, and cooling mint, this drink may be as good as it gets for rehydrating after a good workout, or when enjoying the outdoors on a warm day.

3 ½ cups cubed watermelon
1 cup coconut water or water
½ cup peeled, seeded, and chopped
    cucumber (½-inch pieces)
2 tablespoons fresh mint
2 tablespoons freshly squeezed lime juice
Pinch of sea salt

Digest Aid Juice ♥ⓖ♦

YIELD: 2 CUPS JUICE

Prep time: 15 minutes, Total time: 15 minutes, Serving size: 1 cup, Number of servings: 2

Soothing cucumber juice has an impressive water content, and also raises stomach pH and thereby is a helpful aid for such issues as acid reflux. The absorption of iron from spinach is enhanced by the vitamin C content of anti-inflammatory pineapple and lemon juice, while fennel provides further digestive support by reducing fullness. Enjoy between meals or first thing in the morning when you want a digestive system boost.

1 inch fresh ginger
2 ½ cups chopped cucumber (1-inch pieces)
1 ½ cups loosely packed spinach
1 ½ cups cored and chopped green apple
    (1-inch pieces)

½ cup chopped pineapple (1-inch pieces)

¼ cup chopped fennel bulb

2 tablespoons freshly squeezed lemon juice

1 tablespoon aloe vera juice (optional)

1. Place the ginger, cucumber, spinach, apple, pineapple, and fennel through a juicer.

2. Transfer to a jar with the lemon juice, and aloe vera juice, if using, and stir well before serving.

VARIATIONS

Replace the apple with pear, peach, or nectarine.

Replace the lemon juice with freshly squeezed lime or orange juice.

Replace the spinach with kale, chard, or romaine lettuce.

Nutrition Facts per serving (316 g): Calories 105, Fat Calories 10, Total Fat 1 g, Saturated Fat 0 g, Cholesterol 0 mg, Sodium 30 mg, Total Carb 26 g, Dietary Fiber 4 g, Sugars 17 g, Protein 2 g

Sunrise Carrot Juice ♥ⓖ◆

YIELD: 2 ½ CUPS JUICE

Prep time: 10 minutes, Total time: 10 minutes, Serving size: 1 1/4 cups, Number of servings: 2

Carrots' benefits for the eyes are due to their plentiful beta-carotene, which provides the orange color and is converted to vitamin A during digestion. Parsley is a highly nutritious culinary herb, and when juiced delivers quality carotenoids, flavonoids, and phytonutrients, being especially rich in chlorophyll.

Enjoy along with your Broccoli Dill Quiche (page 274) or Jamaican Patties (page 280).

1 inch fresh ginger

¼ cup chopped and loosely packed fresh flat-leaf parsley

4 ½ cups chopped carrots (½-inch pieces)

½ cup chopped beet (½-inch pieces)

1 cup chopped celery (½-inch pieces)

½ cup water or coconut water

1. Place all the ingredients, except the coconut water, through a juicer.

2. Add the coconut water to the juice and stir well before serving.

VARIATIONS

Replace the beet and celery with other vegetables, such as cucumber, kale, or spinach.

Replace the ginger with garlic or fresh turmeric.

Replace the parsley with fresh cilantro or basil, or 2 tablespoons of fresh dill.

Nutrition Facts per serving (385 g): Calories 145, Fat Calories 10, Total Fat 1 g, Saturated Fat 0 g, Cholesterol 0 mg, Sodium 275 mg, Total Carb 34 g, Dietary Fiber 10 g, Sugars 18 g, Protein 4 g

Citrus Magic ♥ⓖ◆

YIELD: 3 CUPS JUICE

Prep time: 10 minutes, Total time: 10 minutes, Serving size: 1 cup, Number of servings: 3

Pineapples contain a generous fiber, water, and vitamin C content, and are a well-known food source of an enzyme called bromelain, which reduces both sinus congestion and joint pain. With additional vitamin C plus folate in the orange, and all of the astounding benefits of turmeric and ginger, you will certainly feel the magic. Have a glass before your morning meal.

4 cups chopped pineapple (½-inch pieces)

1 ½ cups freshly squeezed orange juice

1 tablespoon peeled and minced fresh turmeric

1 tablespoon peeled and minced fresh ginger

1. Place all the ingredients in a blender and blend well.

VARIATIONS

Replace all or some of the pineapple with papaya, mango, or peach.

Replace the orange juice with fruit juice of choice, such as apple or pear.

Add a banana to thicken it up.

Try adding a superfood, such as 1 tablespoon of maca powder, spirulina, or chlorella.

Add 1 ½ tablespoons of a high-quality oil, such as hemp or flaxseed.

Nutrition Facts per serving (348 g): Calories 175, Total Fat 0 g, Saturated Fat 0 g, Cholesterol 0 mg, Sodium 5 mg, Total Carb 44 g, Dietary Fiber 4 g, Sugars 32 g, Protein 2 g

Green Master Cleanse ⓖ ◈

YIELD: 2 CUPS CLEANSE

Prep time: 5 minutes, Total time: 5 minutes, Serving size: 1 cup, Number of servings: 2

A twist on the popular Master Cleanse, which contains water, lemon juice, maple, and cayenne pepper, the green in this beverage comes from spirulina, a sea alga that is one of the oldest life forms on Earth and as such may have been the world's first superfood—it is composed of 55 to 75 percent protein alongside a wide array of other nutrients. The beautiful dark green superpowder can be taken directly in water. Here it is sweetened with mineral-rich maple syrup and enhanced with a lemony tang and cayenne's circulation friendly heat! The result is both cleansing and nourishing at the same time. Enjoy as a light beverage to sustain you between meals.

1 ½ cups water

¼ cup freshly squeezed lemon juice

1 tablespoon pure maple syrup

½ teaspoon spirulina powder

⅛ to ¼ teaspoon cayenne pepper

1. Place all the ingredients in a jar and mix well. Serve chilled or at room temperature.

VARIATIONS

Replace the maple syrup with sweetener of choice, such as coconut nectar or agave nectar (see page 89).

Add 1 teaspoon of maca powder along with the spirulina.

Replace the lemon juice with freshly squeezed lime or orange juice.

Nutrition Facts per serving (41 g): Calories 35, Fat Calories 0, Total Fat 0 g, Saturated Fat 0 g, Cholesterol 0 mg, Sodium 10 mg, Total Carb 9 g, Dietary Fiber 0 g, Sugars 7 g, Protein 1 g

Juices vs. Smoothies

Juices are made with a juicer that extracts fiber from the fruits and vegetables. Smoothies are blended in a blender, keeping all the fiber. The differences don't end there: here are the pros and cons to help you decide whether to break out your juicer or blender or what to order on your next visit to a juice bar.

Juicing has multiple advantages. The nutrients from the vegetables and the fruits are very easily absorbed into the system without the need for the body to work on their digestion. For many, this results in a swift sensation of an energy lift. Juicing is also a great way to get your veggies in, because even some less favorite veggies are palatable when juiced with a little fruit or other vegetables, and 1 to 2 pounds of produce can fit into a single juice serving. Juicing is not only well known for its instant supply of nutrients, but has been effective in healing. Juice cleanses that last from one to ten or more days are said to supply abundant energy, a refreshed feeling, and reputed disease curing. Fasting and juicing clinics report remarkable effects in changing a person's health and lifestyle for the positive.

Some drawbacks to juicing include the need to drink quickly, often within 20 minutes of the juicing process, unless the juice is pressed, which results in a longer shelf life. This is to maximize nutrient intake because, after exposure to light and air, nutrients degrade as time passes. Juicing can be time consuming in terms of cleaning the juicer after each use and shopping for produce, and the expense of getting a quality juicer that does not heat and oxygenate the finished product too much. Losing the fiber can be seen as a con because not only is fiber needed in the diet, but it is possible that fiber helps counter the negative effects of oxalates from the greens. There is always the waste factor of what to do with the fiber, although some turn it into veggie burgers or compost it. Compared to smoothies, juices sometimes have fewer nutrients because they are not profiting from the bonus nutrients in the seeds or peel of some fruits and vegetables.

Smoothies are a great way to deliver superfoods into the system and are often filling enough to substitute a meal. Unlike juices, smoothies can include some kind of good fat, such as avocado or a nut butter, which satiates. (Of course, you can always blend the avocado or nut butters with your juice . . . enjoying both juice and smoothie at once.) Because ingredients are blended, all fiber and its benefits are retained. One benefit of retaining the fiber is that it helps regulate blood sugar and can prevent against a blood sugar spike. Smoothies are less prone to oxidation, and while it is recommended to drink within 20 to 30 minutes for maximum nutrition, many of them can be kept airtight for up to two days in the fridge. Self-made smoothies are more universally available because more people already have a blender in the home.

Some say that blending the ingredients loses some of the nutrients to heat and oxidation, which is a smoothie con. In some cases the smoothies can be overkill—too much food in one sitting and at times overly abundant in sugars and healthy fats. There is some concern about bad food combinations in smoothies where digestion and absorption is compromised.

Chewing: The absence of chewing is a point raised by those who believe it is healthier to chew food instead of drinking it. The digestive enzymes in saliva are very important to a healthy digestive process, and subsequently, nutrient absorption. Ayurveda proposes that each bite should be chewed thirty-two times, one time for each tooth. Thereby the recommendation to "chew your juice/smoothie" is a good one: keeping it in the mouth as long as possible to expose each sip to these enzymes in the saliva.

Herb and Fruit Water

Add a new dimension to your water drinking by placing a few sprigs of fresh herbs or a few slices of fruit in your glass or pitcher. This adds a subtle flavor to the water, which makes it easier to drink larger quantities. You will also receive the benefits of the micronutrients of whatever ingredient you place in the water. Some favorites include such herbs as rosemary, basil, dill, mint (be sure to crush the leaves first, to release the flavor and natural oils), fennel, and lemongrass. Fruit to add includes orange, lemon, lime, strawberries, even blueberries. Cucumber slices are also a favorite. Experiment with single ingredients and combos.

Ginger Turmeric Shooter ♥ⓖ◉

YIELD: ¼ CUP SHOOTER

Prep time: 10 minutes, Total time: 10 minutes, Serving size: 1/8 cup, Number of servings: 2

Ginger and turmeric are in the same family. Both have powerful healing quantities and both are big on nutrition. Orange/yellow turmeric is a widely known and researched antibacterial and anti-inflammatory plant. Turmeric is now showing promise in preventing Alzheimer's, which has a low incidence in India, where the root is used abundantly. Ginger and cayenne are both great at enhancing overall circulation and relieving sinus congestion, sore throat, nausea, and muscle pain. Enjoy a fiery shot whenever you are experiencing low energy. Follow with a glass of Citrus Magic (page 137) for a double whammy.

4 inches fresh ginger (or enough to yield 1 ounce juice)
4 inches fresh turmeric (or enough to yield 1 ounce juice)
Pinch of cayenne pepper

1. Place the ginger and turmeric through a juicer.

2. Add the cayenne and stir well. Drink within 15 minutes.

Add 1 cup of freshly squeezed orange or grapefruit juice, along with the optional addition of 1 tablespoon of cold-pressed olive, flaxseed, or hemp oil.

Nutrition Facts per serving (26 g): Calories 60, Fat Calories 15, Total Fat 1.5 g, Saturated Fat 0 g, Cholesterol 0 mg, Sodium 7 mg, Total Carb 11 g, Dietary Fiber 3 g, Sugars 1 g, Protein 1 g

Try squeezing the juice of 1/2 lemon into a large glass of water as your first beverage of the day, to hydrate the lymphatic system and get your digestive juices flowing.

Flu Buster ♥ⓖ◉

YIELD: ¼ CUP FLU BUSTER

Prep time: 15 minutes, Total time: 15 minutes, Serving size: 1/8 cup , Number of servings: 2

Starting to feel low energy as flu season approaches? To speed along recovery, concoct this combo of antiviral powerhouses. Ginger, turmeric, and wheatgrass all have strong antiviral properties, and ginger is antinausea, to boot. Wheatgrass is truly one of nature's superfoods, providing an abundance of minerals; vitamins, including vitamins A, C, and K; protein; and up to 70 percent chlorophyll, which is a crucial blood builder.

2 inches fresh ginger
1 lemon, skin removed
2 inches fresh turmeric
Leaves from 2 mint sprigs (optional)
1 ounce wheatgrass, store-bought or home
    juiced (see page 82)
Pinch of cayenne pepper

1. Place the ginger, lemon, turmeric, and mint leaves, if using, through a juicer.

2. Add the wheatgrass and cayenne and stir well before drinking.

VARIATIONS

Replace the lemon with lime, orange, or grapefruit.

Toss in a few cloves of garlic along with the ginger.

Nutrition Facts per serving (53 g): Calories 100, Fat Calories 5, Total Fat 0.5 g, Saturated Fat 0 g, Cholesterol 0 mg, Sodium 0 mg, Total Carb 16 g, Dietary Fiber 7 g, Sugars 1 g, Protein 6 g

QUICKER AND EASIER

Noni Shot

Looking for another quick immunity boost? Try a noni shot. The noni berry grows on a tree called canary wood and comes in powdered, pulp, or juice form. It has been used historically to treat menstrual cramps, urinary tract infections, arthritis, and diabetes. Recent studies have shown that the antioxidants and anti-inflammatory content of the noni fruit may prevent stroke, and that drinking the juice may reduce pain sensations. Cholesterol lowering and antibacterial (specifically *E. coli* fighting) properties have also resulted from noni consumption. The juice is high in vitamin C, while the noni pulp also contains niacin, iron, and potassium.

Basil Rose Lemonade ♥☻◆

YIELD: 2 CUPS LEMONADE

Prep time: 15 minutes, Total time: 15 minutes, Serving size: 1 cup, Number of servings: 2

Here is a creative twist on traditional lemonade with added enhancers in the form of basil, rosemary, and rose water. Basil is considered one of the healthiest herbs—with outstanding quantities of vitamins A and K. Basil also acts as an anti-inflammatory. Lemon juice is known to help with kidney stones, reduce strokes, and lower body temperature. Rose water, made throughout ancient history by distilling rose petals, is rich in flavonoids and antioxidants.

Enjoy as an afternoon refresher or with such meals as Millet Black Bean Veggie Burgers (page 269) or Sloppy Joes (page 281).

1 ½ cups water
¼ cup plus 1 tablespoon freshly squeezed
    lemon juice
2 ½ tablespoons finely chopped fresh basil
⅛ teaspoon minced fresh rosemary
¼ teaspoon rose water (see Chef's Tips and
    Tricks)
2 ½ tablespoons agave nectar, coconut
    nectar, pure maple syrup, or desired
    sweetener to taste

1. Place all the ingredients in a blender and blend well. Serve chilled.

VARIATIONS

Replace the lemon juice with freshly squeezed lime juice.

Replace the water with coconut water.

For lavender rose lemonade, omit the basil and rosemary, and infuse 1 tablespoon of culinary-grade lavender flowers in ¼ cup of hot water for 15 minutes. Strain well and add the water to the above recipe.

Nutrition Facts per serving (67 g): Calories 90, Fat Calories 0, Total Fat 0 g, Saturated Fat 0 g, Cholesterol 0 mg, Sodium 0 mg, Total Carb 23 g, Dietary Fiber 0 g, Sugars 19 g, Protein 0 g

Açai Spritzer ♥ⓖ◗

YIELD: 2 CUPS SPRITZER

Prep time: 5 minutes, Total time: 5 minutes, Serving size: 1 cup, Number of servings: 2

A delightful refresher especially in the heat of a summer afternoon, enjoy this hydrator while reaping the benefits of the açai berry—superfood extraordinaire du jour. The berries contain antioxidants, fiber, and heart-healthy fats. Sit and sip on a porch with a breeze and imagine the berries escorting out any damaging oxidizing agents.

16 ounces chilled sparkling water
½ cup açai (1 [3.5-ounce] frozen packet, defrosted)
2 tablespoons raw agave nectar, coconut nectar, pure maple syrup, or desired sweetener to taste (page 89)

> ### Chef's Tips and Tricks
>
> #### Culinary-Grade Lavender and Rose Water
>
> Lavender flowers and rose water, make wonderful fragrant additions to your culinary creations. Be sure you are purchasing a food-grade variety, as some brands of lavender contain higher amounts of camphor oil or are sprayed with chemicals and are best used for potpourri. Likewise, some brands of rose water are higher in rose oil and are more suited for use as perfume. The package should indicate whether it is for culinary uses. Lavender flowers purchased in the bulk spice or tea section of a natural foods store are generally culinary grade, though it does not hurt to ask!

¼ teaspoon ground cinnamon
⅛ teaspoon ground nutmeg
Pineapple or star fruit slices

1. Place all the ingredients, except the pineapple or star fruit, in a jar or pitcher and stir well.

2. Pour into glasses and garnish with the pineapple or star fruit slices before serving.

VARIATIONS

Replace the açai with frozen and blended blueberries, raspberries, or strawberries.

Replace the sparkling water with coconut water.

Nutrition Facts per serving (307 g): Calories 90, Fat Calories 25, Total Fat 2.5 g, Saturated Fat 1 g, Cholesterol 0 mg, Sodium 10 mg, Total Carb 16 g, Dietary Fiber 1 g, Sugars 13 g, Protein less than 1 g

Kale Kolada ♥ⓖ◊

YIELD: 3 CUPS KOLADA

Prep time: 15 minutes, Total time: 15 minutes,
Serving size: 1 cup, Number of servings: 3

Originating in the tropical Americas, pineapple is now cultivated throughout the world and is a part of many cuisines. (Did you know you can replant the pineapple top to generate a new pineapple in one and half to two years?) Of course, pineapple is also one of the bases of the ever-popular piña colada. Try this healthy three-ingredient version of the classic treat for a dose of electrolytes in sweet coconut water, high fiber, vitamin K, and iron-rich earthy kale, and a wide array of vitamins and minerals in juicy pineapple. Break out the umbrella toothpicks and serve this at your next pool party along with Watermelon Gazpacho (page 243) and Grilled Plantain Kebabs (page 166).

2 ½ cups tightly packed stemmed and chopped kale
2 ½ cups chopped pineapple
1 ¼ cups coconut water

1. Juice the kale.

2. Transfer to a blender with the pineapple and coconut water, and blend well.

VARIATIONS

Depending upon your juicer, you can juice the pineapple as well as the kale. Add the coconut water and stir well. Note that some juicers do not extract the pineapple juice so easily, so blending may be your best option.

Replace the kale with spinach.

Replace the pineapple with other fruit, such as mango, strawberries, or peaches.

Replace the coconut water with water and add desired sweetener to taste (page 89).

Replace the coconut water with other fruit juice, such as orange or grapefruit.

Nutrition Facts per serving (293 g): Calories 120, Fat Calories 10, Total Fat 1 g, Saturated Fat 0 g, Cholesterol 0 mg, Sodium 130 mg, Total Carb 27 g, Dietary Fiber 5 g, Sugars 17 g, Protein 3 g

Quinoa Milk ♥ⓖ◊

YIELD: 3 CUPS MILK

Prep time: 15 minutes, Total time: 15 minutes,
Serving size: 1 cup, Number of servings: 3

Want to drink a complete protein? Quinoa is one of the few foods to contain all the essential amino acids. Actually a seed instead of a grain, quinoa not only delivers huge on protein, but also magnesium, manganese, folate, and phosphorus. All this in a homemade milk with a delightful light and nutty flavor. Use this as a base for your smoothies, poured over granola, or in creamy vegan soups, such as Ital Roasted Squash and Sweet Potato (page 251). The milk will last up to 3 days stored in a glass jar in the refrigerator.

¾ cup uncooked quinoa
3 cups water
Pinch of sea salt (optional)

1. Place the quinoa in a fine-mesh strainer or seed/nut-milk bag (see note). Rinse and drain well.

2. Transfer to a blender along with the water and salt, and blend until creamy.

3. Pour through the strainer or a sprout bag (see page 82). Store the liquid in a glass jar.

Note: To sprout quinoa and improve its digestibility, once rinsed, place in a bowl with water to cover. Allow to sit for 2 hours or longer. Rinse and drain well. Return to the bowl. Cover with a towel and allow to sit for up to 6 hours or overnight. Rinse and drain well before using in the recipe.

VARIATIONS

Add desired sweeteners to taste (see page 89).

Replace ½ cup of the quinoa with nuts or seeds, such as sunflower seeds, hemp seeds, almonds, Brazil nuts, macadamia nuts, cashews, or pecans.

Nutrition Facts per serving (51 g) for an unstrained milk: Calories 155, Fat Calories 25, Total Fat 2.5 g, Saturated Fat 0 g, Cholesterol 0 mg, Sodium 0 mg, Total Carb 27 g, Dietary Fiber 3 g, Protein 6 g

Gold Milk🄖

YIELD: 2 CUPS MILK

Prep time: 10 minutes, Cook time: 5 minutes, Total time: 15 minutes, Serving size: 1 cup, Number of servings: 2

A traditional beverage from Ayurvedic cuisine (see page 26), sweet and velvety gold milk is a potent and delicious way to incorporate the many incredible benefits of superfood turmeric into your diet. The oil and spices used traditionally here are known to help increase absorption of its medicinal

properties, as well as add extra nutrients. Enjoy warm or cold. Store the turmeric paste in a glass jar in the refrigerator for up to ten days. Create different variations by altering the milk and sweetener. Enjoy as part of an Indian feast with Creamy Lentil Saag (page 290) and Golden Rice (page 204).

TURMERIC PASTE
¼ cup ground turmeric
½ teaspoon freshly ground black pepper
¼ teaspoon ground cinnamon
⅛ teaspoon ground cardamom
Pinch of cayenne pepper
½ cup water

MILK
2 cups soy, rice, coconut, or almond milk (for homemade, see Plant-Based Milk, page 104)
1 tablespoon turmeric paste
1 teaspoon coconut oil (optional)
Pure maple syrup, coconut nectar, or agave nectar to taste

1. Create the turmeric paste: Place the turmeric, black pepper, cinnamon, cardamom, and cayenne in a small saucepan over medium heat. Add the water and stir well until a thick paste is formed. Allow to cool and place in a small glass bowl.

2. Prepare the milk: For a warm beverage, place the soy milk in a small saucepan over low heat. Stir occasionally and be sure not to burn. For a cold beverage, place the soy milk in a blender.

3. Add 1 tablespoon of the turmeric paste to the soy milk and stir or blend well. Add the coconut oil, if using (omit for

the cold version), and sweeten to taste before serving.

VARIATIONS

♦ For an oil-free version, omit the oil.

Add 2 teaspoons of the turmeric paste to your smoothies for an added nutrient boost.

Nutrition Facts per serving (261 g): Calories: 100, Fat Calories: 50 g, Total Fat 5 g, Saturated Fat 1 g, Cholesterol 0 mg, Sodium 90 mg, Total Carb 16 g, Dietary Fiber 4 g, Sugars 4 g, Protein 8 g

Choco-Maca Elixir ♥Ⓖ♦

YIELD: 3 CUPS ELIXIR

Prep time: 10 minutes, Total time: 10 minutes, Serving size: 1 cup, Number of servings: 3

Maca is a root vegetable eaten in Peru and used in powder form for its superfood benefits: to augment energy and stamina and to increase libido. In this soothing chocolaty elixir, it is paired with cacao, which has phenylethylamine that increases alertness and concentration, so the drinker can expect top physical and mental achievements! Cacao is also distinguished as having the highest concentration of antioxidants, by weight, of any superfood. Serve over ice or warmed over low heat.

3 cups almond, soy, or rice milk
  (for homemade, see Plant-Based Milk,
  page 104), or coconut beverage
¼ cup unsweetened cocoa powder or cacao
  powder
1 tablespoon maca powder
¼ teaspoon ground cinnamon

¼ teaspoon ground cardamom or nutmeg
Sweetener of choice (see page 89)

1. Place all the ingredients, except the sweetener, in a blender and blend well.

2. Add sweetener to taste and blend well before serving. Serve as is or over ice.

VARIATIONS

For a thicker beverage, add 1 fresh or frozen banana, three pitted dates, and 2 teaspoons of chia seeds before blending.

Add ½ cup of ice to the blender for a chilled beverage.

♥ For a raw version, use raw cacao and raw seed or nut milk (for homemade, see Plant-Based Milk, page 104).

For a caffeinated experience, steep two bags of yerba mate tea in the almond milk over low heat for 8 minutes. Remove the tea bags and follow the recipe above.

Nutrition Facts per serving (256 g) not including sweetener to taste: Calories 85, Fat Calories 40, Total Fat 4.5 g, Saturated Fat 0.5 g, Cholesterol 0 mg, Sodium 185 mg, Total Carb 12 g, Dietary Fiber 4 g, Sugars 3 g, Protein 4 g

Sesame Hemp Revitalizer Ⓖ♦

YIELD: 3 CUPS REVITALIZER

Prep time: 15 minutes, Total time: 15 minutes, Serving size: 1/2 cup, Number of servings: 6

Sesame and hemp seeds are both small in size but deliver hefty nutritional benefits in this nutty and iron-rich beverage sure to revitalize your energy. Hemp seeds have premium quantities of protein, iron, magnesium, and zinc. Sesame seeds contain plentiful amounts of fiber, thiamine, vitamin B$_6$, calcium, and iron. For its part, blackstrap molasses has a low glycemic index and adds abundant iron, magnesium, and calcium.

3 ½ cups water

½ cup sesame seeds

¼ cup hemp seeds

3 tablespoons blackstrap molasses (see page 89)

3 pitted dates

¼ teaspoon ground nutmeg

1. Place all the ingredients in a blender and blend well. If you wish for a thinner beverage, pour through a strainer before serving.

VARIATIONS

Add ½ teaspoon of ground cinnamon, and a pinch each of ground cardamom and ground nutmeg.

For additional sweetness, you can add coconut nectar, pure maple syrup, or your sweetener of choice (page 89), to taste.

Replace the sesame seeds and hemp seeds with any combination of nuts and seeds, including pumpkin, almond, hazelnut, or cashews.

Nutrition Facts per serving (171 g): Calories 145, Fat Calories 80, Total Fat 9 g, Saturated Fat 1 g, Cholesterol 0 mg, Sodium 10 mg, Total Carb 14 g, Dietary Fiber 2 g, Sugars 8 g, Protein 4 g

Tropical Smoothie ♥ⓖ♦

YIELD: 4 CUPS SMOOTHIE

Prep time: 10 minutes, Total time: 10 minutes, Serving size: 1 cup, Number of servings: 4

The high fiber content of papaya, the energy-boosting potassium from the banana, plus the natural fruit sugar of vitamin A-rich mango and a splash of coconut goodness make this a supersatisfying sweet treat. Combine these fruits for a large dose of vitamin C and quick tropical escape. Follow the variation for adding greens and superfoods and you will take the nutrition to the next level.

3 cups chopped pineapple (½-inch pieces)

½ cup mango (½-inch pieces)

1 medium-size banana, (optionally frozen; see page 298)

1 cup chopped papaya (½-inch pieces)

½ cup coconut water or water

½ teaspoon freshly squeezed lime or lemon juice (optional)

1. Place all the ingredients in a blender and blend well.

VARIATIONS

Make it green: Add 1 cup of chopped kale, spinach, or arugula.

Superfood it up: Add maca powder, goji berries, cacao nibs, moringa powder, chlorella, spirulina, and/or hemp seeds (see Chapter 3 for more about superfoods).

Nutrition Facts per serving (248 g): Calories 130, Fat Calories 5, Total Fat 0.5 g, Saturated Fat 0 g, Cholesterol 0 mg, Sodium 35 mg, Total Carb 33 g, Dietary Fiber 4 g, Sugars 23 g, Protein 2 g

Berry Green Smoothie ♥ⓖ◐◇

YIELD: 4 CUPS SMOOTHIE

Prep time: 10 minutes, Total time: 10 minutes, Serving size: 1 cup, Number of servings: 4

The triad of berries, bananas, and greens combines well for a large dose of energy, nutrient density, and antioxidants in this powerhouse smoothie. With minerals in the bananas, concentrated phytonutrients in the greens, and flavonoids in the berries, this combination of ingredients is both filling and nutritionally satisfying. Adding the dates discussed in the variations creates a sweeter smoothie and gives an iron boost. Enjoy as part of your morning meal or as an afternoon energy boost.

10 ounces frozen berries (any variety) (about 2 ¼ cups)
2 large bananas
2 cups coconut water or water
2 large kale leaves, stemmed (1 cup chopped)
2 tablespoons raw cacao nibs (optional)

1. Place all the ingredients in a strong blender and blend until smooth. Enjoy within 20 minutes.

Nutrition Facts per serving (216 g): Calories 120, Fat Calories 5, Total Fat 1 g, Saturated Fat 0 g, Cholesterol 0 mg, Sodium 70 mg, Total Carb 30 g, Dietary Fiber 5 g, Sugars 17 g, Protein 2 g

---

TEMPLATE RECIPE
Green Smoothie

- -

Fruit component: Replace the berries with such fruit as pineapple, papayas, peaches, pears, nectarines, or mangoes.

Green component: Replace the kale with spinach, arugula, chard, romaine lettuce, or dandelion greens.

Liquid component: Replace the water with fruit juice, or plant-based milks such as almond, soy, rice, or hemp (for homemade, see Plant-Based Milk, page 104).

Superfood add-in component: Replace the cacao nibs or add hemp seeds, goji berries, chia seeds, moringa powder, chlorella, or spirulina (see pages 57–59 for more about superfoods).

Optional sweetener component: Add three pitted dates or 1 tablespoon of sweetener of choice, if necessary, for additional sweetening (see page 89).

Maca Horchata ♥ⓖ◐

YIELD: 4 CUPS HORCHATA

Prep time: 10 minutes, Soak time: 30 minutes, Total time: 40 minutes, Serving size: 1 cup, Number of servings: 4

Maca and rice horchata make a nice pair here, both having origins in Spanish-speaking countries. Although *horchata de arroz* (a beverage made from rice) is most widely known, the original was made from the sacred tiger nut, and called *horchata de chufa*—so feel free to get creative with the milk of your choice. Maca, a member of the radish family, has a mild flavor and an array of notable properties including quantities of vitamins B, C, and E, as well as reputed libido, energy, and stamina boosts. All of that infused into the sweet freshness of this beloved healthy carb beverage may lead you to a remarkable energy upgrade after imbibing. Enjoy this at your Mexican fiesta alongside Tempeh Fajitas (page 279) or Mushroom Cauliflower Tacos (page 277).

½ cup uncooked short-grain brown rice

4 ½ cups water

½ teaspoon ground cinnamon

1 teaspoon pure vanilla extract

Pinch of sea salt

3 tablespoons agave nectar, coconut nectar, pure maple syrup, or desired sweetener to taste (see page 89)

1 ½ teaspoons maca powder

1. Place the brown rice in a bowl with 2 cups of the water. Allow to sit for 30 minutes, or up to overnight.

2. Transfer to a blender and blend well. Pour through a fine strainer, such as a sprout bag (see page 82) or cheesecloth. Discard the rice. Return the liquid to the blender.

3. Add the remaining ingredients, including the remaining 2 ½ cups of fresh water, and blend well. Serve over ice or chill before serving.

VARIATIONS

You can replace the rice with nuts, such as almonds, cashews, or Brazil nuts.

Nutrition Facts per serving (71 g): Calories 210, Fat Calories 15, Total Fat 1.5 g, Saturated Fat 0 g, Cholesterol 0 mg, Sodium 44 mg, Total Carb 46 g, Dietary Fiber 3 g, Sugars 17 g, Protein 5 g

High-Protein Vanilla Almond Shake♥ⓖ◗

YIELD: 4 CUPS SHAKE

Prep time: 10 minutes, Total time: 10 minutes, Serving size: 1 cup, Number of servings: 4

A double dose of almonds plus hemp in this superpotent shake provide a valuable source of protein, minerals, and fiber. Cacao phytonutrients add a natural chocolaty energy spike that blends well with the vanilla and creamy banana in this delicious combo of flavors. The shake is rounded out by the high concentration of brain-boosting omega-3s in the hemp seeds, and the memory-enhancing properties of energizing maca root powder.

2 cups vanilla almond milk (for homemade, see Plant-Based Milk, page 104)

3 tablespoons almond butter

2 medium-size peeled and frozen bananas

2 tablespoons hemp seeds

2 teaspoons maca powder

Seeds of 1 vanilla bean, or 1 teaspoon pure vanilla extract

2 tablespoons raw cacao nibs

Sweetener to taste, such as pitted dates, maple, coconut nectar, or agave nectar (optional, see page 89)

1. Place the almond milk, almond butter, bananas, hemp seeds, maca powder, and vanilla bean seeds in a strong blender and blend until smooth.

TEAS, ELIXIRS, JUICES, AND SMOOTHIES

2. Add the cacao nibs and blend for
   30 seconds.

VARIATIONS

Replace the almond milk with macadamia,
cashew, or hemp milk (for homemade, see
Plant-Based Milk, page 104).

Replace the almond butter with tahini or
cashew butter.

Add superfoods, such as 1 tablespoon of
spirulina and/or chia seeds.

Nutrition Facts per serving (207 g): Calories 215,
Fat Calories 115, Total Fat 13 g, Saturated Fat 2.5 g,
Cholesterol 0 mg, Sodium 97 mg, Total Carb 22 g,
Dietary Fiber 6 g, Sugars 9 g, Protein 7 g

CHAPTER 11

Savory Snacks and Appetizers

Keeping yourself satiated throughout the day with healthy food is the key to reaching any of your health goals. That is where the art of the snack comes in. Homemade spreads, such as Glorious Guacamole (page 151), Smoky Salsa (page 151), or White Bean Artichoke Dip with Arugula (page 155) can be a between-meal lifesaver when enjoyed with gluten-free crackers or fresh veggies, such as carrots, celery, and cucumber. Munching on the Curried Crispy Chickpeas (page 154) as a between-meal snack is also highly satisfying.

Those interested in raw food appetizers will appreciate the inclusion of the flavorful Avocado Mousse–Stuffed Tomatoes (page 152), Truffled Cashew Cheese (page 159), and Pecan Veggie Pâté (page 169).

The recipes in this section can be used as a starter for your main meal.

Try the Lemon Garlic Steamed Artichokes (page 153), Veggie Lettuce Boats (page 160), or Okra Bruschetta (page 162) to get the party started. You can also combine a number of appetizer selections to create a tapas-style meal, where guests share small plates to create a full meal. Enjoy sharing Black Bean Tostones (page 167), Grilled Plantain Kebabs (page 166), Quinoa Amaranth Cakes (page 168), or Curried Garbanzo Cakes with Poppy Seeds (page 164).

If you're seeking oil-free dishes, this is just a friendly reminder to look for the oil-free icon, which points out the oil-free alternative if the main recipe does contain oil.

Oh, and don't forget to sample a variety of sauces from Chapter 13 to enhance these dishes.

Smoky Salsa ♥ⓖ◆

YIELD: 2 CUPS SALSA

Prep time: 20 minutes, Total time: 20 minutes,
Serving size: 1/4 cup, Number of servings: 8

The smoky flavor in this salsa is provided by chipotle chile powder—made from dried and smoked red jalapeño peppers. These add bonus vitamins A and B_6, riboflavin, iron, and potassium to the antioxidant blend of tomato, onion, garlic, and cilantro in a smoky, spicy, sweet combo that energizes metabolism as well. Enjoy this salsa on its own as dip for chips, or in a Mexican fiesta meal with rice and Spicy Pinto Beans (page 206), Glorious Guacamole (page 151), Garlicky Greens (page 191), and Vegan Sour Cream (page 112).

2 cups chopped tomato (½-inch pieces)
¼ cup diced red onion
1 large clove garlic, pressed or minced
1 ½ tablespoons freshly squeezed lime juice
1 tablespoon finely chopped fresh cilantro
¼ teaspoon seeded and diced jalapeño
**   pepper**
½ teaspoon sea salt, or to taste
⅛ teaspoon freshly ground black pepper
¼ teaspoon chipotle chile powder (optional)

1. Combine all the ingredients in a bowl and mix well. If you wish, let sit for up to 20 minutes, to allow the flavors to meld, before serving.

VARIATIONS

Replace some or all of the tomatoes with chopped mango.

Replace the tomato with grilled pineapple (see page 101).

Add 1 cup of cooked and drained black beans.

Add 1 cup of raw or roasted corn (see page 192).

Nutrition Facts per serving (78 g): Calories 10, Fat Calories 0, Total Fat 0g, Saturated Fat 0 g, Cholesterol 0 mg, Sodium 150 mg, Total Carb 3 g, Dietary Fiber less than 1 g, Sugars 2 g, Protein 1 g

Glorious Guacamole ♥ⓖ◆

YIELD: 1 ¼ CUPS GUACAMOLE

Prep time: 15 minutes, Total time: 15 minutes,
Serving size: 1/4 cup, Number of servings: 5

What a glorious way to celebrate avocado's perks: monounsaturated fats, protein, potassium, dietary fiber, and vitamins B_6, C, and K. Its creamy goodness is enhanced by nutrient-packed garlic, onions, pepper and spices, and a little lime for sweetness. If you are not serving the guacamole immediately, you can leave the avocado pit in the dip to keep it staying greener longer. Serve on its own as a dip for crudités or chips, You can also add a dollop to such dishes as Mexican Seitan-Stuffed Peppers (page 291), Mushroom Cauliflower Tacos (page 277), or Tempeh Fajitas (page 279).

1 ½ cups mashed avocado (about 2 medium-
**   size avocados)**
3 tablespoons minced red onion
1 large garlic clove, pressed or minced
½ teaspoon seeded and diced jalapeño pepper
2 tablespoons freshly squeezed lime juice
1 tablespoon plus 1 teaspoon finely chopped
**   fresh cilantro**
¼ teaspoon chili powder

⅛ teaspoon chipotle chile powder or
   additional chili powder
¼ teaspoon sea salt, or to taste
⅛ teaspoon freshly ground black pepper

1. Combine all the ingredients in a bowl
   and mix well.

VARIATION

Add ½ cup of diced tomato or salsa of
choice.

Nutrition Facts per serving (80 g): Calories 80, Fat
Calories 60, Total Fat 7 g, Saturated Fat 1 g, Chole-
sterol 0 mg, Sodium 130 mg, Total Carb 6 g, Dietary
Fiber 3 g, Sugars less than 1 g, Protein 1 g

Avocado Mousse–Stuffed Tomatoes ♥ⓖ◊

YIELD: 4 TOMATOES

Prep time: 25 minutes, Total time: 25 minutes,
Serving size: 1 stuffed tomato, Number of
servings: 4

Avocado and tomatoes are a classic combo,
appearing in salad combos worldwide. Take
this dynamic duo to the next level by stuffing the lovely red tomatoes, rich in lycopene
and vitamin C, with an elegant avocado
mousse—all the while gleaning the benefits of
the health promoting fats of avocado, which
help ensure proper carotenoid absorption
and overall nutrient metabolism. Enjoy with
whatever tomatoes are fresh and in season as
a between-meal snack or before your meal of
Millet Black Bean Veggie Burgers (page 269)
or Black Bean Grits (page 272).

4 small tomatoes
Cilantro sprigs

AVOCADO MOUSSE

1 cup mashed avocado
2 tablespoons freshly squeezed lime juice
2 teaspoons minced fresh cilantro
1 small garlic clove, pressed
¼ teaspoon seeded and minced jalapeño
   pepper
Pinch of chili powder
Pinch of chipotle chile powder
¼ teaspoon sea salt, or to taste
Pinch of freshly ground black pepper

1. With a paring knife, cut a circular hole
   around the stem of each tomato. Scoop
   out the inside with a spoon and discard.

2. Prepare the avocado mousse: Place all
   the mousse ingredients in a food processor and process until creamy. Scoop
   into the tomatoes and top with cilantro
   sprigs before serving.

For an Avocado Cream Sauce, soak ½ cup of raw cashew pieces in a bowl with ample room to cover. Drain and rinse well. Place in a blender with ½ cup of water and blend until creamy. Add to the food processor with the mousse ingredients and process well.

Nutrition Facts per serving (163 g): Calories 80, Fat Calories 50, Total Fat 6 g, Saturated Fat 1 g, Cholesterol 0 mg, Sodium 155 mg, Total Carb 8 g, Dietary Fiber 4 g, Sugars 3 g, Protein 2 g

Lemon Garlic Steamed Artichokes with Simple Dipping Sauce ⓖ

YIELD: 2 LARGE ARTICHOKES

Prep time: 10 minutes, Cook time: 40 minutes, Total time: 50 minutes, Serving size: 1/3 artichoke, Number of servings: 6

It is well worth working your way through the tough exterior of an artichoke to get to the health benefits inside. Besides fiber, artichokes provide plenty of vitamins A and K, folate, and antioxidants. While reveling in the sensual flavor experience, you profit from the reputed cancer-fighting component allicin in garlic, and the antibacterial and antiviral components of tangy lemon. Serve with the simple dipping sauce included in this recipe, or switch it up with Cilantro Mint Chutney (page 229), Creamy Mexican Dipping Sauce (page 234), or Zesty Chimichurri Sauce (page 231).

1 lemon, sliced
6 garlic cloves
3 bay leaves (optional)

2 large artichokes

SIMPLE ARTICHOKE DIPPING SAUCE (MAKES ½ CUP)

3 tablespoons olive oil
2 tablespoons freshly squeezed lemon juice
2 tablespoons water
1 tablespoon nutritional yeast (optional)
1 garlic clove, pressed or minced
1 teaspoon minced fresh flat-leaf parsley
½ teaspoon minced fresh thyme
⅛ teaspoon freshly ground black pepper
¼ teaspoon truffle oil (optional; see page 88)
Pinch of sea salt, or to taste
Pinch of crushed red pepper flakes

1. Place a steamer basket in a large pot with 2 inches of water over high heat. Add the lemon slices, garlic, and bay leaves, if using. Cover the pot, and bring to a boil.

2. Chop the very bottom off the stem of each artichoke, leaving about 1 inch of stem on the bud. Trim off the very bottom leaves of the artichokes. You can use culinary scissors to trim the pointy tips off the remaining leaves. Cut off and discard the top ½ inch of the artichokes, and place in the steamer basket.

3. Lower the heat to medium. Steam the artichokes until the bottom leaves are easily removed and the bottom is just soft, about 30 minutes.

4. Meanwhile, prepare the dipping sauce: Combine all the ingredients in a small bowl and whisk well.

5. Proceed to indulge. See the box on the opposite page for how to eat an artichoke.

For Grilled Artichokes, once the artichokes are steamed, preheat a grill to high. Slice the steamed artichoke in half, place on the grill. Baste with dipping sauce and grill until char marks appear, about 3 minutes on each side, depending upon the heat of the grill.

◆ For an oil-free version of the dipping sauce, replace the oil with vegetable stock (see page 108) or additional water, and omit the truffle oil.

Nutrition Facts per serving including sauce (83 g): Calories 95, Fat Calories 60, Total Fat 7 g, Saturated Fat 1 g, Cholesterol 0 mg, Sodium 75 mg, Total Carb 8 g, Dietary Fiber 3 g, Sugars 1 g, Protein 2 g

QUICKER AND EASIER

Use melted vegan butter or coconut oil as a dipping sauce. Add two pressed garlic cloves and a pinch of sea salt, freshly ground black pepper, and crushed red pepper flakes.

Curried Crispy Chickpeas⊙

YIELD: 3 CUPS CHICKPEAS

Prep time: 5 minutes, Cook time: 45 minutes, Total time: 50 minutes, Serving size: 1/4 cup, Number of servings: 12

Turn versatile chickpeas into a nutritional snack that anyone will enjoy munching on. The flavors of sesame, cumin, pepper, curry, and cayenne are not only tasty but boost the immune system with their healing properties. Chickpeas, also called garbanzo beans, are an excellent source of fiber, protein, iron, and the trace mineral manganese. Be sure to drain the chickpeas well before using in this recipe. Enjoy as a stand-alone snack or sprinkle on top of Creamy Lentil Saag (page 290) or Thai Curry Vegetables (page 289).

2 (15-ounce) cans chickpeas, drained and rinsed well, or 3 cups cooked (see page 98)

1 tablespoon sesame or coconut oil (optional; see variations)

2 ½ teaspoons curry powder

½ teaspoon ground cumin

¼ teaspoon sea salt, or to taste

⅛ teaspoon freshly ground black pepper

Pinch of cayenne pepper

1 teaspoon wheat-free tamari or other soy sauce

1 ½ tablespoons freshly squeezed lemon juice

1. Preheat the oven to 425°F. Place the chickpeas and sesame oil on a small baking sheet and toss well.

2. Bake for 45 minutes, or until crispy.

3. Place in a bowl along with the remaining ingredients and mix well to coat. Serve warm or cooled.

VARIATIONS

Replace the curry and cumin with 1 tablespoon of an ethnic spice blend, such as Italian (page 105), Moroccan (page 106), Mexican (page 106), or Ethiopian (page 106).

◆ For an oil-free version, replace the oil with water or vegetable stock (see page 108).

Nutrition Facts per serving (45g): Calories 80, Fat Calories 20 g, Total Fat 2 g, Saturated Fat 0 g, Cholesterol 0 mg, Sodium 80 mg, Total Carb 12 g, Dietary Fiber 3 g, Sugars 2 g, Protein 4 g

Broiled Artichoke Fritters◆

YIELD: 1 ½ CUPS FRITTERS

Prep time: 10 minutes, Cook time: 10 minutes,
Total time: 20 minutes, Serving size: 1/8 cup,
Number of servings: 10

Growing from flower buds in the sunflower family, artichokes have been used since early documented history to soothe digestion. These crunchy fritters are broiled rather than fried, making them a healthy version of familiar fried comfort foods. They are flavored with bright green herb parsley, another historical digestive aid, which also delivers plenty of vitamin A, C, and K and boosts the immune system. Serve with dipping sauces, such as Creamy Mexican Dipping Sauce (page 234), Raw Cashew Sour Cream (page 113), or Pesto (page 215).

1 (14-ounce) can artichoke hearts. quartered
    (1 ½ cups) (for lower sodium, use frozen
    and defrosted or fresh)
¼ cup plus 2 tablespoons bread crumbs
2 tablespoons yellow or blue cornmeal
1 tablespoon minced fresh flat-leaf parsley
½ teaspoon sea salt, or to taste
¼ teaspoon crushed red pepper flakes
⅛ teaspoon freshly ground black pepper

1. Drain the artichoke hearts well. Place
   the remaining ingredients in a bowl
   and mix well.

2. Preheat the oven broiler on LOW.

3. Coat each artichoke heart well with the
   bread crumb mixture and place on a
   baking sheet.

4. Cook until slightly browned, about
   7 minutes.

VARIATIONS

Replace the parsley with fresh dill or cilantro.

You can dip the artichokes in olive oil before coating with the bread crumb mixture. Use one hand for dipping in the oil, and the other hand for coating with the bread crumbs.

Go Indian by replacing the parsley with fresh cilantro, and adding 1 tablespoon of ground curry powder and 1 teaspoon of ground cumin.

Go Mexican by replacing the parsley with fresh cilantro, and adding 1 tablespoon of chili powder, 1 teaspoon of ground cumin, and ⅛ teaspoon of chipotle chile powder.

Ⓖ For gluten-free, use gluten-free bread crumbs (see page 112).

Nutrition Facts per serving (51g): Calories 35, Fat Calories 0, Total Fat 0 g, Saturated Fat 0 g, Cholesterol 0 mg, Sodium 155 mg, Total Carb 7 g, Dietary Fiber 1 g, Sugars 2 g, Protein 1 g

White Bean Artichoke Dip with ArugulaⒼ◆

YIELD: 1 ¾ CUPS DIP

Prep time: 15 minutes, Total time: 15 minutes,
Serving size: 1/8 cup, Number of servings: 14

This creamy and peppery dip is made from a base of white beans, which are a superfood because of their high vitamin, mineral, fiber, and protein content, and artichokes, which are packed with antioxidants and qualities known to help the liver to better process cholesterol. A little red pepper kick adds a nice circulatory effect, and goes well with the cheesy flavor supplied by the nutritional yeast, which has B vitamins, including some B_{12}. Serve as the beginning of a feast which may include Broccoli Rabe Penne Pasta with Oil-Free Cream Sauce (page 292), and Super Sprout Salad (page 173).

1 (15-ounce can) cannellini beans, drained and rinsed well, or 1 ½ cups cooked (see page 98)

1 cup chopped canned, jarred, or frozen and defrosted artichoke hearts, drained and rinsed well

1 tablespoon nutritional yeast

1 teaspoon rice vinegar (optional)

½ teaspoon sea salt, or to taste

¼ teaspoon minced garlic

¼ teaspoon freshly ground black pepper

¼ teaspoon crushed red pepper flakes

1 cup stemmed and chopped arugula or baby spinach

1 tablespoon chiffonaded fresh basil

1. Place the beans, artichoke hearts, nutritional yeast, rice vinegar, if using, salt, garlic, black pepper, and crushed red pepper flakes in a food processor and process until smooth.

2. Add the arugula and basil and process until smooth.

VARIATIONS

Add 1 to 2 tablespoons of olive oil.

Replace the cannellini beans with beans of your choosing, such as pinto, kidney, or black (see page 98).

Replace the arugula with spinach, chard, or kale.

Add additional herbs, such as 1 tablespoon of finely chopped fresh flat-leaf parsley and ½ teaspoon of minced fresh rosemary.

Replace the basil with fresh dill or cilantro.

Nutrition Facts per serving (52 g): Calories 30, Fat Calories 0, Total Fat 0 g, Saturated Fat 0 g, Cholesterol 0 mg, Sodium 90 mg, Total Carb 6 g, Dietary Fiber 2 g, Sugars 1 g, Protein 2 g

Sun-Dried Tomato Tapenade ♥ⓖ◆

YIELD: 1 CUP TAPENADE

Prep time: 15 minutes, Total time: 15 minutes, Serving size: 1 tablespoon, Number of servings: 16

This tangy and colorful tapenade features some nutritional heavy hitters. Sun-dried tomatoes' nutrients, such as potassium, iron, thiamine, riboflavin, and niacin, are well preserved by water removal. Olives provide cell protecting oleic acid along with a great variety of vitamins and minerals in each serving. Basil and thyme both top the nutrient-density list for herbs, with their range of antioxidants, potent anti-inflammatory oils, and vigorous antimicrobial properties, not to mention huge flavor. Serve as a spread on celery sticks, crackers, or sandwiches or in Raw Collard Veggie Rolls (page 260) or Nori Rolls (page 263).

½ cup sun-dried tomatoes

1 cup hot water

½ cup pitted and diced kalamata olives

1 large garlic clove

2 tablespoons chiffonaded fresh basil

1 tablespoon nutritional yeast (optional)

2 teaspoons freshly squeezed lemon juice

½ teaspoon fresh thyme

¼ teaspoon crushed red pepper flakes

1. Soak the sun-dried tomatoes in the hot water until soft, then drain well, reserving 2 tablespoons of the soak water.

2. Place in a food processor with all the remaining ingredients, including the 2 tablespoons of reserved soak water, and process until smooth.

VARIATIONS

Add additional herbs, such as 1 tablespoon of finely chopped fresh flat-leaf parsley, 1 teaspoon of fresh marjoram, 1 teaspoon of fresh oregano, and/or ½ teaspoon of minced fresh rosemary.

Experiment with different varieties of pitted olives.

Add 1 tablespoon of capers.

Nutrition Facts per serving (34 g): Calories 20, Fat Calories 10, Total Fat 1.5 g, Saturated Fat 0 g, Cholesterol 0 mg, Sodium 110 mg, Total Carb 1 g, Dietary Fiber 0 g, Sugars 2 g, Protein 0 g

Kalamata Rosemary Hummus 🅖 ⬜

YIELD: 3 ½ CUPS HUMMUS

Prep time: 15 minutes, Cook time: 20 minutes, Total time: 35 minutes, Serving size: 1/4 cup, Number of servings: 14

Mild, nutty chickpeas are practically synonymous with classic hummus. Big on protein and fiber, these legumes also contain a large percentage of daily requirements for folate, good for your nervous system, and manganese, good for bone health. Sesame tahini adds to the flavor as well as the nutrient profile as a good source of magnesium. Kalamata olives are a superb source of monounsaturated fats and vitamin E, while rosemary, an herb member of the mint family, offers iron, calcium, and vitamin B_6 even in small quantities. This recipe works best if you cook the chickpeas very well, until they are almost breaking apart, even if you are using canned beans. If you want to go the extra step, for the creamiest hummus, remove the skins from the beans before using. Serve with Homemade Pita Chips (page 158).

2 (15-ounce) cans chickpeas, drained and rinsed well, or 3 cups cooked (see page 98)

¼ cup tahini

3 tablespoons freshly squeezed lemon juice

3 tablespoons olive oil (optional) or water

2 large garlic cloves

2 teaspoons minced fresh rosemary

1 teaspoon ground cumin powder (optionally toasted; see page 101)

½ teaspoon sea salt, or to taste

¼ teaspoon freshly ground black pepper

Pinch of cayenne pepper

Pinch of chipotle chile pepper (optional)

3 tablespoons chopped and pitted kalamata olives

1. If using canned chickpeas, fill a medium-size pot with water and bring to a boil. Lower the heat to medium, add the beans, and cook for 20 minutes. Drain well.

2. Transfer to a food processor along with the remaining ingredients and process until smooth.

Chef's Tips and Tricks

The World of Olives

Olives take on a wide variety of culinary roles: they can be the base of a spread or tapanade, tossed into martinis, eaten stand-alone or in salads, or chopped and cooked into soups and other recipes. They are technically a fruit and naturally come with a pit.

If you've ever taken a moment to observe an olive bar, one thing that stands out is the variety of colors available. An olive's color is indicative of its ripeness when picked, ranging from a light green (taken off the tree unripe) through to a purple (medium ripe) and a rich black (very ripe). Hundreds of varieties are available, depending on their heredity, growing region, method of harvest (hand picked to ground collected), and the curing process (which turns them from the natural bitterness of their oleuropin content to a tasty, tart, chewy snack).

Here are some of the most popular and widely available olive types:

Kalamata: These olives are a dark purplish or light black, and originated in Greece. These are most appropriate in a recipe that asks for black olives.

Niçoise: Tossed into their eponymous salad, these olives are smallish and a purple variety, which hail from the south of France. They have a somewhat meatlike texture.

Picholine: Another French olive, these are small and green and a bit tart and crisp.

Manzanilla: This olive comes from Spain, is cured in brine, and is often stuffed with garlic or pimientos. It takes on a smoky flavor.

Gordal: Another Spanish variety, Gordal olives get their name from the Spanish word *gordo* (meaning "fat")—which accurately describes their size. They are ample, green, and firm.

Castelvetrano: An Italian variety, these olives are green, mild, slightly sweet, and chewy.

Cerignola: Another Italian specialty, Cerignola olives are a greenish yellow, large, and creamy.

Nyon: On the more bitter side, these French Provençal black olives have a wrinkled texture and a very classic olive flavor.

Gaeta: These olives are a light purple or brown and have a tart citrus flavor. Gaeta is a region on the west coast of Italy between Rome and Naples.

Alphonso: From Chile or Peru; try these large purple olives for a sour olive flavor that's big on meaty texture.

Mission: Mission olives come from California and are mostly used for olive oil production. However, they also make a good handy-sized snacking olive.

VARIATIONS

Create an indent in the hummus in the serving bowl. Add an additional ¼ cup of olive oil and 3 tablespoons of minced fresh flat-leaf parsley to the indentation. You can also add 2 teaspoons of chiffonaded fresh sage, 1 teaspoon of finely chopped oregano, and/or 1 teaspoon of fresh thyme.

Replace the kalamatas with another variety of olive.

While one of the secrets to the success of your hummus is to cook the chickpeas very well, if you are pressed for time, you can omit the cooking of the canned beans.

◆For an oil-free version, omit the oil and add water or mashed avocado.

Nutrition Facts per serving (69 g): Calories 100, Fat Calories 40, Total Fat 4.5 g, Saturated Fat 1 g, Cholesterol 0 mg, Sodium 140 mg, Total Carb 13 g, Dietary Fiber 3 g, Sugars 2 g, Protein 5 g

TEMPLATE RECIPE
Hummus, a.k.a. Bean Puree

Bean component: Replace the chickpeas with cannellini beans, black beans, or edamame.

Seasoning component: Replace the kalamata olives and rosemary with roasted red pepper, roasted garlic, or Caramelized Onions (page 162).

Ethnic component: Go Mexican by replacing the rosemary and kalamata olives with 2 tablespoons of minced cilantro and 1 tablespoon of chili powder. Create an Indian Hummus by replacing the rosemary and kalamata olives with 2 tablespoons of minced fresh cilantro and 1 tablespoon of curry powder.

QUICKER AND EASIER

Homemade Pita Chips

Follow these simple steps to create your own pita chips. Preheat the oven to 400°F. Place a small amount of olive oil or melted coconut oil in a bowl along with a sprinkle of salt, freshly ground black pepper, and optionally a pinch of Italian Spice Mix (page 105). Use a pastry brush to baste both sides of each piece of pita bread with the oil mixture. Slice each bread in half, then cut each half into four triangles. Place the triangles on a large baking sheet and bake until golden brown, about 10 minutes, depending upon the type of bread used.

◆For an oil-free version, simply slice the pita bread into triangles and toast until crispy.

Truffled Cashew Cheese ♥ⓖ▱

YIELD: 2 CUPS CHEESE

Prep time: 30 minutes, Total time: 30 minutes, Serving size: 2 tablespoons, Number of servings: 16

Here we have plant cheese at its finest, with the addition of the elegant and exotic truffle oil. Most truffle oils on the market are mixed with olive oil, thereby yielding the same health benefits as olive oil. (Steer clear of those brands of truffle oil that say "essence of truffle," as this is synthetic, designed to taste and smell like truffles, but without actual truffles.) Cashews are the star of the show in this plant-based cheese—offering up their sweetness, creaminess, and remarkable mineral content: copper, manganese, magnesium, and phosphorus. The cheese flavor comes from the addition of nutritional yeast and lemon juice. Herbs, spices, onions, and garlic top off the amazing taste and nutrient value of this incredible and impressive snack. Serve on the raw variation for Designer Seed and Nut Crust Pizzas (page 265), in Raw Collard Veggie Rolls (page 260), or stuffed in cherry tomatoes.

1 ½ cups raw cashew pieces

½ to ¾ cup water

2 tablespoons nutritional yeast

2 tablespoons diced green onion

1 ½ tablespoons freshly squeezed lemon juice

1 tablespoon finely chopped fresh flat-leaf parsley

1 tablespoon finely chopped fresh chervil (optional)

2 teaspoons minced fresh dill

1 teaspoon sea salt, or to taste

¼ teaspoon minced garlic

½ to ¾ teaspoon truffle oil

¼ teaspoon crushed red pepper flakes

⅛ teaspoon freshly ground black pepper

1. Place the cashews in a bowl with ample water to cover. Allow to sit for 25 minutes, or up to 3 hours.

2. Rinse, drain well, and transfer to a strong blender with the ½ cup to ¾ cup of fresh water. (The longer the cashews soak, the less water the recipe will need.) Blend until smooth, adding a small amount of additional water, if necessary, to reach a creamy consistency.

3. Transfer to a bowl along with the remaining ingredients and stir well. The flavors will mature with time.

VARIATION

◆For an oil-free version, omit the truffle oil.

Nutrition Facts per serving (50 g): Calories 120, Fat Calories 80, Total Fat 10 g, Saturated Fat 2 g, Cholesterol 0 mg, Sodium 150 mg, Total Carb 7 g, Dietary Fiber less than 1 g, Sugars 1 g, Protein 4 g

---

TEMPLATE RECIPE
Soft Plant-Based Cheeses

- -

Base component: Replace the cashews with macadamia nuts, Brazil nuts, hemp seeds, or blanched almonds.

◆**Seasoning component:** Replace the dill, parsley, and truffle oil with other fresh herbs, such as basil, sorrel, or cilantro.

Spice component: Add 1 tablespoon of an ethnic spice blend, such as Italian (page 105), Mexican (page 106), or Indian (page 106).

Add-on component: After blending, add 1 cup of vegetables, such as grated carrots or beets, julienned red cabbage, or diced colorful bell peppers. Reduce the salt and add ¼ cup of diced kalamata olives and/or sun-dried tomatoes.

Veggie Lettuce Boats♥Ⓖ

YIELD: 4 LEAVES

Prep time: 15 minutes, Total time: 15 minutes, not including making the cashew cheese, Serving size: 1 leaf, Number of servings: 4

For a light and crunchy snack with a flavorful, creamy, nut-based cheese, lay out the romaine and start assembling this salad-in-a-wrap. Romaine lettuce is not just a holder here; in fact, it is a prime source of dietary fiber, as well as vitamins B$_1$ and C, manganese, potassium, biotin, copper, and iron. Look for 4- to 6-inch-long leaves and be sure to assemble just before serving. Serve with a dipping sauce of choice, such as Sweet-and-Sour Sauce (page 236), Raw Tamarind Sauce (page 230), or Almond Dipping Sauce (page 233).

½ cup **Truffled Cashew Cheese (page 159)**
4 medium-size romaine lettuce leaves
½ seeded and julienned red bell pepper
½ seeded and julienned yellow bell pepper
1 small avocado, peeled, pitted, and thinly sliced
½ cup peeled and grated carrot
¼ cup sunflower sprouts
¼ cup chopped fresh cilantro

1. Place 2 tablespoons of the cheese in each romaine leaf.

2. Top each leaf with the remaining ingredients.

VARIATIONS

So many variations are possible. Stack your lettuce with other veggies, such as julienned red cabbage; grated beet, parsnip, or daikon; thinly sliced jicama or kohlrabi; or halved cherry tomatoes. Add fresh herbs, such as dill and/or parsley.

Replace the romaine with red leaf lettuce.

Get creative with add-ons, such as Simple Sauerkraut (page 176) or Quick Kimchi (page 178), Garlicky Greens (page 191) or grilled tofu or tempeh slices (see page 100).

● For an oil-free version, omit the truffle oil in the cashew cheese.

Nutrition Facts per serving (134 g): Calories 270, Fat Calories 180, Total Fat 20.5 g, Saturated Fat 3.5 g, Cholesterol 0 mg, Sodium 165 mg, Total Carb 18 g, Dietary Fiber 5 g, Sugars 5 g, Protein 8 g

Gold Bar Squash Chutney Ⓖ

YIELD: 2 CUPS CHUTNEY

Prep time: 15 minutes, Cook time: 15 minutes, Total time: 30 minutes, Serving size: 1/8 cup, Number of servings: 16

Squash is a nice option to replace higher-calorie vegetables, such as potatoes or corn, adding vibrancy and a sweet mellow flavor. Its yellow hue lets you know of its carotenoid content, which is excellent for immune health. So, eat all you like to accumulate iron, folate, vitamin C, beta-carotene, and lutein! The herbs and other veggies in this chutney nicely flavorize otherwise subtle squash, and the red bell pepper not only gives a lovely color contrast to this dish, but since it's been on the vine longest, adds the most vitamins A and C, folic acid, fiber, and potassium of all peppers. Serve as a topping on Bruschetta (page 163) or as a dip for Jamaican Patties (page 280), chips, or crudités.

2 teaspoons coconut oil
¼ cup diced yellow onion
2 teaspoons seeded and minced jalapeño pepper
1½ teaspoons peeled and minced fresh ginger
3 cups chopped gold bar, crookneck, or pattypan squash (½-inch pieces)
¼ cup seeded and diced red bell pepper
2 tablespoons raw apple cider vinegar
2 tablespoons agave nectar, coconut nectar, organic sugar, or desired sweetener to taste (see page 89)
1 tablespoon freshly squeezed lime juice
½ teaspoon sea salt, or to taste
Pinch of ground cinnamon
Pinch of ground cardamom

Pinch of freshly ground black pepper

1 tablespoon minced fresh cilantro

1. Place the oil in a sauté pan over medium-high heat. Add the onion, jalapeño, and ginger and cook for 3 minutes, stirring frequently.

2. Add the squash and bell pepper and cook for 5 minutes, stirring frequently.

3. Add the vinegar, agave nectar, lime juice, salt, cinnamon, cardamom, and black pepper and cook until the squash is just tender, about 7 minutes, stirring frequently.

4. Add the cilantro, and stir well before serving.

VARIATIONS

♦ For an oil-free version, omit the oil and use the water sauté method (see page 101).

Replace the squash with carrot, beet, or parsnip.

Replace the squash with mango. Be sure the mango is not overripe.

Nutrition Facts per serving (23 g): Calories 220, Fat Calories 5, Total Fat 1 g, Saturated Fat 1 g, Cholesterol 0 mg, Sodium 73 mg, Total Carb 3 g, Dietary Fiber 0 g, Sugars 2 g, Protein 0 g

QUICKER AND EASIER

Caramelized Onions

Onions are naturally sweet. When you cook onions for a long time, the naturally occurring sugars are released and a deep, rich flavor is created. Add to your wraps and rolls, and as a topping for your veggie burgers, for an elevated culinary experience.

Here's how to do it: Place a small amount of oil or vegetable stock (see page 108) in a heavy-bottomed sauté pan over medium-high heat. Add one large, thinly sliced onion and an optional pinch of organic sugar, if using, and cook for 5 minutes, stirring frequently and adding small amounts of water or vegetable stock, if necessary, to prevent sticking. Lower the heat to medium and cook for 20 to 30 minutes, stirring occasionally and adding small amounts of water or vegetable stock, if necessary, to prevent sticking. Be careful not to burn! You can then add a touch of balsamic vinegar or red wine, if you wish. Store in a glass container in the refrigerator for up to 3 days.

Okra Bruschetta🄖

YIELD: 8 SLICES BRUSCHETTA

Prep time: 10 minutes, Cook time: 10 minutes, Total time: 30 minutes, Serving size: 1 slice, Number of servings: 8

Enjoy this Indian twist on the classic Italian appetizer by using warming curry spices and the uniquely comforting veggie, okra. Okra, a summer crop grown year-round in the South, is also known as lady's fingers, especially in the United Kingdom. The tissue-healing gelatinous seeds on the inside of the okra plant have the bonus health advantage of lowering blood sugar. The vegetable is also superfibrous, low-calorie, and calcium rich. Partake as part of a meal that may include Curry Kale Salad (page 184) and Kitchari (page 257).

4 slices gluten-free or whole-grain bread

2 teaspoons coconut oil

2 teaspoons brown mustard seeds

2 teaspoons cumin seeds, or 1 teaspoon ground

¼ cup diced onion

½ teaspoon seeded and diced jalapeño pepper

2 garlic cloves, pressed or minced

2 cups okra (¼-inch slices)

¼ teaspoon sea salt, or to taste

½ teaspoon curry powder

1 ¼ cups chopped tomato (¼-inch pieces)

1 tablespoon freshly squeezed lime juice

2 teaspoons finely chopped fresh cilantro

1. Place the bread in a toaster oven and toast until just browned.

2. Meanwhile, place the coconut oil in a sauté pan over medium high heat. Add the mustard seeds and cumin seeds and cook for 1 minute, stirring constantly.

3. Add the onion, jalapeño, and garlic and cook for 2 minutes, stirring frequently. Add the okra, salt, and curry powder and cook for 10 minutes, stirring frequently. Add the tomato and cook for 5 minutes, or until the okra is just tender, stirring frequently. Add the lime juice and stir well.

4. Place on top of the toast and top with cilantro. Slice each piece of toast into two or four triangles before serving. Serve warm.

VARIATIONS

◆ For an oil-free version, omit the oil and use the water sauté method (page 101).

Replace the okra with zucchini or gold bar squash.

Nutrition Facts per serving (106 g): Calories 45, Fat Calories 185, Total Fat 2 g, Saturated Fat 1 g, Cholesterol 0 mg, Sodium 90 mg, Total Carb 6 g, Dietary Fiber 2 g, Sugars 2 g, Protein 1 g

Buffalo Cauliflower⊙

YIELD: 5 CUPS CAULIFLOWER

Prep time: 10 minutes, Cook time: 15 minutes, Total time: 25 minutes, Serving size: 1/2 cup, Number of servings: 10

Some like it hot, and this cauliflower is revved up to provide a little fire to further its health-stimulating benefits. Hot chile peppers are low in sugar, carbs, fat, and cholesterol, and high in vitamin C and other vitamins and minerals as well as capsaicin, known for strong analgesic properties. Spicy foods improve circulation, curb the appetite and help with weight loss! The crowd favorite cruciferous cauliflower also has vitamin C and functions as an antioxidant and anti-inflammatory. Serve with Raw Cashew Sour Cream (page 113), Raw Hempseed Ranch Dressing (page 224), Creamy Mexican Dipping Sauce (page 234), or Easy Cheezy Sauce (page 233).

1 bunch cauliflower, cut into large florets (5 cups)

½ cup plus 2 tablespoons low-sodium hot sauce, store-bought or homemade (see Turmeric Hot Sauce, page 109)

1 tablespoon coconut oil

1 teaspoon garlic granules

1 teaspoon onion flakes

½ teaspoon sea salt, or to taste

Oil, for baking sheet

1. Place ½ inch of water in a pot over medium-high heat. Add a steamer basket. Add the cauliflower, cover, and steam until the cauliflower is just tender, about 10 minutes. Be careful not to overcook. Transfer to a bowl.

2. Meanwhile, preheat the oven broiler on HIGH. Place the hot sauce, coconut oil, if using, garlic granules, onion flakes, and salt in a small bowl and whisk well. Add to the cauliflower and gently toss to coat evenly and thoroughly. Transfer to a lightly oiled baking sheet.

3. Place in the oven and broil until just tender, about 5 minutes, being careful not to overbroil. Serve warm.

VARIATIONS

⬥For an oil-free version, omit the oil and use water or vegetable stock (see page 108) when broiling.

Replace the cauliflower with broccoli spears.

Replace the cauliflower with tempeh or tofu, sliced into 2-inch by ½-inch strips.

Nutrition Facts per serving (89 g): Calories 30, Fat Calories 15, Total Fat 2 g, Saturated Fat 1 g, Cholesterol 0 mg, Sodium 138 mg, Total Carb 4 g, Dietary Fiber 1 g, Sugars 1 g, Protein 1 g

Curried Garbanzo Cakes with Poppy Seeds🅖⬥

YIELD: 8 CAKES

Prep time: 15 minutes, Cook time: 15 minutes, Total time: 30 minutes, Serving size: 1/8 cup patty, Number of servings: 8

Did you know it takes about 900,000 poppy seeds (give or take a few) to make a pound of them? Poppy seeds are nutty-flavored oilseeds from the opium poppy plant that date back to ancient Egyptian times. The seeds are especially rich in oleic and linoleic acids, which help lower unhealthy cholesterol levels. They work nicely with the garbanzo flour (sometimes sold as besan flour, chickpea flour, and gram flour) which perfectly complements these flavorful bean creations. Garbanzo bean flour is a stand-out in terms of supply of protein and folate—well above that of wheat flour. Serve with Raw Tamarind Sauce (page 230), Sweet-and-Sour Sauce (page 236), or Cilantro Mint Chutney (page 229).

1 cup garbanzo bean flour
½ cup water
1 ½ tablespoons minced fresh cilantro
1 ½ teaspoons poppy seeds
1 teaspoon garlic flakes
1 teaspoon curry powder
1 ½ teaspoons dehydrated onion flakes
½ teaspoon cumin seeds
½ teaspoon sea salt, or to taste
½ teaspoon ground turmeric (optional)
¼ teaspoon freshly ground black pepper
¼ teaspoon ground coriander
Pinch of cayenne pepper
Oil, for baking sheet (optional)

1. Preheat the oven to 375°F. Place all the ingredients, except the oil, in a bowl and mix well.

2. Scoop out eight equal balls onto a well-oiled or parchment paper–lined baking sheet, and form into small pancakes about ½ inch high.

3. Bake for 12 minutes, or until golden brown. Serve warm.

VARIATIONS

Instead of baking, you can sauté the cakes in coconut oil.

Take this dish in a Mexican direction by replacing the curry powder with chili powder or Mexican Spice Mix (page 106).

Nutrition Facts per serving (38 g): Calories 50, Fat Calories 10, Total Fat 1 g, Saturated Fat 0 g, Cholesterol 0 mg, Sodium 155 mg, Total Carb 8 g, Dietary Fiber 2 g, Sugars 1 g, Protein 3 g

Kentucky Baked Portobello Nuggets^G

YIELD: 2 LARGE MUSHROOMS

Prep time: 10 minutes, Cook time: 30 minutes, Total time: 40 minutes, Serving size: 1/4 mushroom, Number of servings: 8

These tender nuggets are just as cravable as the originals, but with ingredients you can actually feel good about! Portobello mushrooms have a perfect balance of proteins and carbs, while providing a satisfyingly chewy texture and earthiness that serves well as a low-fat base for complimentary herbs. The nutritional yeast, which adds its nice cheesy flavor to the coating, is a helpful source of B vitamins as well as a complete protein, with a bonus: iron. Serve with Sweet-and-Sour Sauce (page 236), Ancho Chile Sauce (page 232), or Smoky BBQ Sauce (page 231).

2 large portobello mushrooms

3 tablespoons water

1 tablespoon olive or melted coconut oil

2 teaspoons wheat-free tamari or other soy sauce

COATING

½ cup nutritional yeast

2 teaspoons garlic flakes

2 teaspoons onion flakes

¾ teaspoon dried oregano

½ teaspoon dried thyme

⅛ teaspoon freshly ground black pepper

Pinch of sea salt, or to taste

Pinch of cayenne pepper

Oil, for baking sheet

1. Preheat the oven to 350°F. Remove and discard the gills from the mushrooms and slice each portobello into four 1-inch-thick strips.

2. Prepare the coating: Place the coating ingredients in a bowl and mix well. Place the olive oil and soy sauce in a small bowl and stir well.

3. Using one hand, dip the mushroom strips, one at a time, into the soy sauce mixture. Using the other hand, remove the mushrooms and place in the coating mixture, coat well, and transfer to a well-oiled baking sheet.

4. Bake until the mushrooms are just tender and the coating begins to slightly brown, about 30 minutes.

VARIATIONS

Replace the portobello mushroom with cubed extra-firm or superfirm tofu, or tempeh.

For an oil-free version, replace the olive oil with water or vegetable stock (see page 108) in the recipe and in the baking pan.

Nutrition Facts per serving (34 g): Calories 45, Fat Calories 15, Total Fat 2 g, Saturated Fat 0 g, Cholesterol 0 mg, Sodium 105 mg, Total Carb 3 g, Dietary Fiber 2 g, Sugars less than 1 g, Protein 3 g

Grilled Plantain Kebabs^G

YIELD: 6 KEBABS

Prep time: 15 minutes, Marinate time: 10 minutes,
Cook time: 10 minutes, Total time: 35 minutes,
Serving size: 1 kebab, Number of servings: 6

Did you know that the plantain has more nutrients, including potassium, than its cousin, the ubiquitous banana? In Mexico, it is called *platano macho* (or masculine banana). Starchier and lower in sugar than a banana, plantain is often treated more like a vegetable than a fruit in cooked dishes. It is especially tasty when grilled, and even more so with this flavorsome marinade and colorful accompaniments on the skewer. Serve with Almond Dipping Sauce (page 233), Smoky BBQ Sauce (page 231), or Zesty Chimichurri Sauce (page 231).

KEBAB MARINADE

1 ½ tablespoons melted coconut oil
   (optional)
2 teaspoons rice vinegar or mirin
1 tablespoon freshly squeezed lime juice
¼ teaspoon sea salt, or to taste
⅛ teaspoon freshly ground black pepper
Pinch of chipotle chile powder

1 large ripe plantain, cut into 12 (½-inch)
   slices
1 small yellow bell pepper, halved
1 small zucchini, cut into 6 (¾-inch) rounds
12 cherry tomatoes
6 cremini mushrooms

1. Prepare the kebab marinade: Place the marinade ingredients in a shallow baking dish and whisk well.

2. Add the plantain slices and bell pepper, and toss well. Allow to sit for 10 minutes, or up to overnight.

3. When ready to cook, preheat a grill. Preheat the oven to 400°F. Soak six small bamboo skewers in water while the grill and oven heat.

4. Remove the plantain and pepper from the marinade, reserving the liquid in its baking dish. Grill the plantain and pepper until char marks appear and the plantain is just tender, about 4 minutes on each side, depending upon the heat of the grill. Remove from the heat. When cooled enough to handle, slice the bell pepper into six 1-inch squares.

5. Meanwhile, place the zucchini, cherry tomatoes, and mushrooms in the reserved marinade and coat well. Place in the oven and bake for 7 minutes.

6. To assemble the kebabs, place the plantain and vegetables on the skewers in the following order: yellow bell pepper, cherry tomato, plantain, zucchini, mushroom, plantain, cherry tomato.

VARIATIONS

◆ For an oil-free version, replace the oil with water or vegetable stock (page 108).

Add additional vegetables, such as red bell pepper, roasted Brussels sprouts, turnips, or portobello mushroom.

Add cubed and marinated tofu or tempeh (see page 100).

Nutrition Facts per serving (108 g): Calories 90,
Fat Calories 30, Total Fat 4 g, Saturated Fat 3 g,

Cholesterol 0 mg, Sodium 160 mg, Total Carb 15 g, Dietary Fiber 1 g, Sugars 8 g, Protein 1 g

Black Bean Tostones ⊙ ◗

YIELD: 8 TOSTONES

Prep time: 15 minutes, Cook time: 15 minutes, Total time: 30 minutes, Serving size: 1 tostone (1/8 cup), Number of servings: 8

Traditionally, tostones (from the Spanish "to toast"), are twice-fried plantains. You can't go wrong with this healthier, baked version that includes two Latin American staples: black beans and plantains. What a savory treat they become when baked into a low-fat patty with herbs, spices, and versatile green onions or scallions—known for their rich abundance of vitamin K. Serve with Vegan Sour Cream (page 112), Creamy Mexican Dipping Sauce (page 234) or Roasted Red Pepper Sauce (page 235).

2 very ripe plantains (see Chef's Tips and Tricks) (1 cup mashed)

¼ cup flour (try with gluten-free, such as brown rice or garbanzo)

2 tablespoons diced green onion

2 teaspoons minced fresh cilantro

2 garlic cloves, minced

½ teaspoon sea salt, or to taste

¼ teaspoon chili powder or chipotle chile powder

¼ cup cooked black beans (see page 98)

1. Preheat the oven to 400°F. Place the mashed plantains, flour, green onion, cilantro, garlic, salt, and chili powder in a bowl and mix well. Add the black beans and stir well.

Chef's Tips and Tricks

Working with Plantains

Plantains are often referred to as *cooking bananas*. They are common in the cuisines of the tropics, including Africa, South and Central America, and the Caribbean. They are much larger and starchier than the common banana and are not eaten raw. The unripe plantains are hard and green. As the plantain ripens, it is easier to peel. It will become softer, and yellow. As it continues to ripen, black spots will appear. A fully ripe plantain is black. This recipe works best with slightly ripe plantains. To peel them, cut off the very bottom and top, and carefully make a slit with a knife along the side. Peel off the skin completely. You can then slice the fruit.

2. Form into eight equal-size patties with a small ice-cream scoop, and place on a parchment paper–lined baking sheet. Bake for 7 minutes. Carefully flip and bake for an additional 7 minutes. Serve warm.

VARIATIONS

Replace the black beans with adzuki beans, black-eyed peas, or pinto beans.

Alternatively, lightly oil the baking sheet instead of lining with parchment paper.

Replace the plantains with just-ripe bananas.

Add 2 teaspoons of curry powder and ½ teaspoon of cumin seeds, for an Indian treat.

Replace the cilantro with fresh dill.

Add 2 teaspoons of an ethnic spice blend, such as Moroccan (page 106) or Ethiopian (page 106).

Instead of baking, you can sauté the tostones in coconut oil over medium-high heat until just crispy on each side, about 3 minutes on each side.

Nutrition Facts per serving (58 g): Calories 50, Fat Calories 0, Total Fat 0 g, Saturated Fat 0 g, Cholesterol 0 mg, Sodium 180 mg, Total Carb 11 g, Dietary Fiber 1 g, Sugars 3 g, Protein 1 g

Quinoa Amaranth Cakes 🅖 ◖

YIELD: 8 CAKES

Prep time: 10 minutes, Cook time: 45 minutes, Total time: 55 minutes, Serving size: 1 cake (1/4 cup), Number of servings: 8

Impress your friends at your next cocktail party with these savory, certified seafood-free cakes made with ancient grains, hearts of palm, and artichoke hearts. The secret bonus is that this recipe also may stimulate cell growth and repair, reduce inflammation, and provide a large dose of protein, calcium, and iron, courtesy of the hearty gluten-free grain amaranth, as well as the high-protein quinoa. Top with Avocado Mousse (page 152) and serve with Raw Cashew Sour Cream (page 113), Vegan Sour Cream (page 112), or Creamy Mexican Dipping Sauce (page 234).

2 tablespoons ground flaxseeds plus ¼ cup water
2 cups water or vegetable stock (see page 108)
½ cup uncooked quinoa, rinsed and drained well (see pages 95, 144)

¼ cup uncooked amaranth
¼ cup diced shallot
2 large garlic cloves, pressed or minced
½ teaspoon sea salt, or to taste
¼ cup flour (try gluten-free, such as oat)
½ cup chopped hearts of palm (go for sustainably harvested; see page 169)
½ cup chopped artichoke hearts
2 tablespoons finely chopped fresh parsley, or 2 teaspoons minced fresh dill
1 tablespoon freshly squeezed lemon juice
1 teaspoon Dijon mustard (optional)
½ teaspoon celery seeds (optional)
¼ teaspoon freshly ground black pepper
¼ teaspoon crushed red pepper flakes
1 cup bread crumbs (see page 112, try gluten-free)
Oil, for baking sheet (optional)

1. Preheat the oven to 375°F. Place the flaxseeds and ¼ cup of water in a small bowl. Allow to sit for 10 minutes, stirring occasionally, until gelled.

2. Meanwhile, place the 2 cups of water or stock, quinoa, amaranth, shallot, garlic, and ¼ teaspoon of the sea salt in a pot over medium-high heat. Bring to a boil. Cover, lower the heat to a simmer, and cook until all the liquid is absorbed, about 25 minutes.

3. Meanwhile, place the flour, hearts of palm, artichoke hearts, parsley, lemon juice, Dijon mustard, if using, remaining ¼ teaspoon of salt, celery seeds, if using, black pepper, and crushed red pepper flakes in a bowl and mix well. Add the flaxseed mixture and the cooked grain, and mix well. Taste and add additional salt, if necessary, to taste.

4. Place the bread crumbs in a separate bowl. Form eight equal-size cakes. Coat well with bread crumbs and place on a well-oiled or parchment paper–lined baking sheet. Bake for 10 minutes. Carefully flip and bake for an additional 10 minutes.

VARIATIONS

Reduce the salt, and add 2 teaspoons of Old Bay Seasoning, or to taste.

Replace the hearts of palm with ¼ cup of chopped sun-dried tomato and ¼ cup diced kalamata olives. Add 1 tablespoon of chiffonaded fresh basil, ½ teaspoon of fresh oregano, and ¼ teaspoon of minced fresh rosemary.

For an Indian direction, replace the parsley with fresh cilantro and add 1 tablespoon of curry powder.

For a Mexican direction, replace the parsley with fresh cilantro and add 2 teaspoons of chili powder and 1 teaspoon of cumin seeds.

Nutrition Facts per serving (112 g): Calories 165, Fat Calories 25, Total Fat 3 g, Saturated Fat 0 g, Cholesterol 0 mg, Sodium 260 mg, Total Carb 30 g, Dietary Fiber 3 g, Sugars 5g, Protein 6 g

Pecan Veggie Pâté ♥◉◆▱

YIELD: 2 ½ CUPS PÂTÉ

Prep time: 10 minutes, Soak time: 20 minutes, Total time: 30 minutes, Serving size: 1/8 cup, Number of servings: 22

This rich and dense pâté is part nut, part seed, and part root vegetables, making for a hearty, healthful item in which to dip crackers or chips, or fill a collard leaf. Both pecans and sunflower seeds are energy donors, and have you covered for protein and vitamin E. Colorful carrots and beets are cool-season roots that greatly complement this dish with their color and sweetness and have several combined health preserving benefits, which include cancer prevention, heart health, and even brain enhancement. Spread on celery sticks, stuff in tomatoes or bell pepper slices, or enjoy as a filling for Nori Rolls (see page 263) or Raw Collard Veggie Rolls (page 260).

½ cup raw pecans
½ cup raw sunflower seeds
1 cup diced carrot
1 cup diced beet

2 tablespoons freshly squeezed lemon juice

1 teaspoon curry powder

½ teaspoon ground cumin

1 ½ tablespoons minced fresh cilantro

¾ teaspoon sea salt, or to taste

¼ teaspoon freshly ground black pepper

Pinch of cayenne pepper

¼ teaspoon ground coriander (optional)

Water or vegetable juice (optional)

1. Place the pecans and sunflower seeds in a bowl with ample room-temperature water to cover. Allow to sit for 20 minutes, or up to a few hours. Rinse and drain well.

2. Transfer to a food processor along with the remaining ingredients and process until smooth. Add small amounts of water or vegetable juice to reach your desired consistency.

Nutrition Facts per serving (31 g): Calories 30, Fat Calories 20, Total Fat 2.5 g, Saturated Fat 0 g, Cholesterol 0 mg, Sodium 90 mg, Total Carb 2 g, Dietary Fiber less than 1 g, Sugars less than 1 g, Protein less than 1 g

TEMPLATE RECIPE
Raw Pâté

- -

Seed or nut component: Replace the pecans and sunflower seeds with other nuts or seeds, such as walnuts, almonds, cashews, pumpkin seeds, or hemp seeds.

Veggie component: Replace the beets and carrots with such vegetables as parsnip, bell peppers, mushrooms, cabbage, or zucchini.

Herb component: Replace the cilantro with other fresh herbs to taste (start with small amounts and work your way up). Try dill, basil, parsley, sorrel, rosemary, or marjoram.

Spice component: Replace the curry and cumin with a different ethnic spice blend to taste (see pages 105–107).

Creamy Herbed Polenta ⓖ

YIELD: 3 ½ CUPS POLENTA

Prep time: 10 minutes, Cook time: 20 minutes, Cooling time: 10 minutes, Total time: 40 minutes, Serving size: 1/4 cup, Number of servings: 14

Polenta, a course cornmeal used frequently in Italian cooking, is one of my favorite ingredients to work with because of its naturally buttery and rich flavor and its amazing versatility. There is no end to the number of ingredients you can add to polenta to create different flavor profiles. It is also a great source for the fibrous benefits of corn, not to mention its phytochemicals that help promote healthy vision and skin. Cooked into the mix are the immunity-boosting and healing properties of potent garlic and mixed herbs. Have your cookie cutter handy and have fun creating small decorative portions. Top with Pesto (page 215), or Sun-Dried Tomato Tapenade (page 156).

2 cups unsweetened soy, rice, or almond milk (for homemade, see Plant-Based Milk, page 104)

1 ½ cups water

4 garlic cloves, pressed or minced

¾ teaspoon sea salt, or to taste

⅛ teaspoon freshly ground black pepper

¼ teaspoon crushed red pepper flakes

1 cup polenta

¼ cup chiffonaded fresh basil

3 tablespoons finely chopped fresh parsley

¾ teaspoon minced fresh rosemary

2 tablespoons nutritional yeast (optional)

½ cup grated vegan mozzarella-style cheese (optional)

Oil, for casserole dish

1. Place the soy milk and water in a large pot over high heat. Add the garlic, salt, black pepper, and crushed red pepper flakes and bring to a boil.

2. Lower the heat to low. Slowly whisk in the polenta. Whisk constantly for 5 minutes. Cover, and cook for 15 minutes, whisking occasionally.

3. Add the remaining ingredients, except the oil, and stir well. Taste and add additional salt if necessary.

4. Transfer to a well-oiled 8 by 8-inch casserole dish, and allow to cool until it is firm enough to cut, about 10 minutes. Cut into your desired shapes with cookie cutters or a knife. Serve warm.

VARIATIONS

Give it a Mexican twist by replacing the herbs with 3 tablespoons of minced fresh cilantro, 1 ½ tablespoons of chili powder, 1 teaspoon of ground cumin, and ¼ teaspoon of chipotle chile powder.

Add 1 ½ cups of thinly sliced spinach, kale, chard, leek, or arugula along with the basil.

You can also blend the herbs with ½ cup of water and add after the polenta has cooked for 10 minutes.

Add ½ cup of thinly sliced sun-dried tomatoes and/or ½ cup of pitted and diced olives.

Replace the soy milk with water or vegetable stock (see page 108).

Add 1 to 2 tablespoons of coconut oil or vegan butter along with the polenta.

◗ For an oil-free version, use a parchment paper–lined pan with a small amount of water.

Nutrition Facts per serving (75 g): Calories 75, Fat Calories 15, Total Fat 2 g, Saturated Fat 0 g, Cholesterol 0 mg, Sodium 140 mg, Total Carb 13 g, Dietary Fiber 2 g, Sugars 0 g, Protein 3 g

CHAPTER 12

Salads and Sides

To start eating in a more healthy way, my recommendation can be summed up in three words: eat more salads! It takes very little effort to begin to get more creative with your salads, and they are the perfect way to meet your daily requirements for fresh veggies. When it comes to salads, think color! There is wisdom in the "eat a rainbow" advice. The more colorful your selection of veggies, the wider the range of phytonutrients you will be ingesting.

Salads often get lumped into the "boring side dish" category, so this chapter shares many ways to take your salads to the next level—that's why this is the longest chapter in the book. You can add raw or toasted nuts and seeds and cooked grains. Add sprouts, such as sunflower, buckwheat, broccoli, or pea. Add vegetables—lots of them—be they chopped, grated, roasted, grilled, or steamed. Add legumes or roasted and cubed tofu or tempeh (see page 100). Try experimenting with a new veggie each week. Soon you will have a vast culinary repertoire. Combine this creativity with the dressings in Chapter 13 and you are ready to rock your salad world!

This chapter provides a bountiful selection of dishes to choose from, including a variety of salads and an assortment of side dishes to complement every meal. As you go through the recipes, consider combining a few to create the ultimate plant-based meal.

These salads and sides range from lighter options to more hearty dishes. Some light salads include the Super Sprout Salad (page 173), Simple Chop Salad (page 174), and Asian Cucumber Salad (page 175). For heartier fare, try the Curry Kale Salad (page 184), Three Greens with Tomato Sauce (page 197), or Pearled Barley with Mushrooms and Corn (page 210). There are many raw food selections in this chapter, including Walnut Taco Salad (page 187), Green Papaya Salad (page 175), and Provençal Salad (page 183). Cultured food recipes include Quick Kimchi (page 178) and Simple Sauerkraut (page 176). For pickling aficionados, be sure to check out Pickled Okra (page 181).

With the suggestions in this chapter and your newfound knowledge of template recipes, the range of salads and sides available to you is as limitless as your imagination. Go for it!

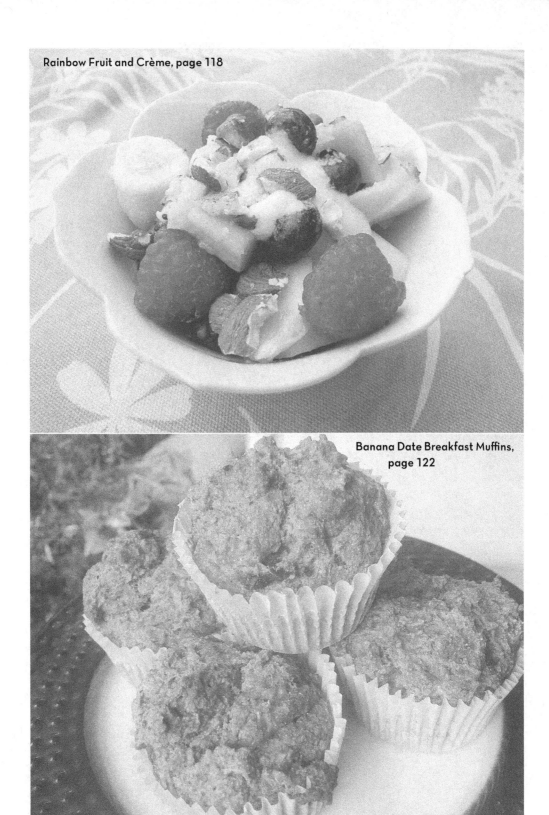

Rainbow Fruit and Crème, page 118

Banana Date Breakfast Muffins, page 122

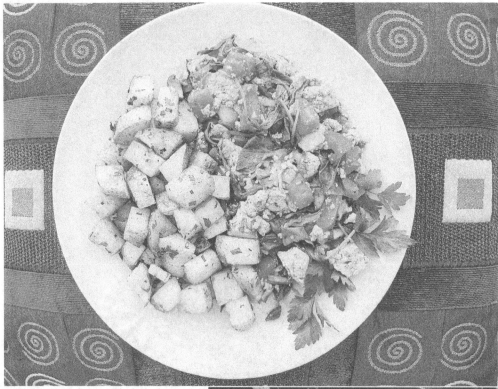

ABOVE:
Garden Veggie Scramble, page 128,
Herb-Roasted Potatoes, page 214

RIGHT:
Purple Potato Tempeh Hash, page 130

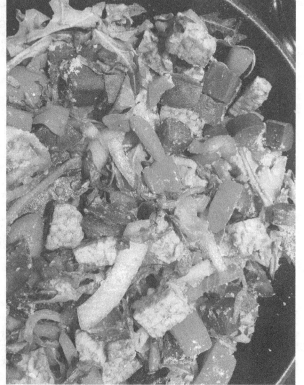

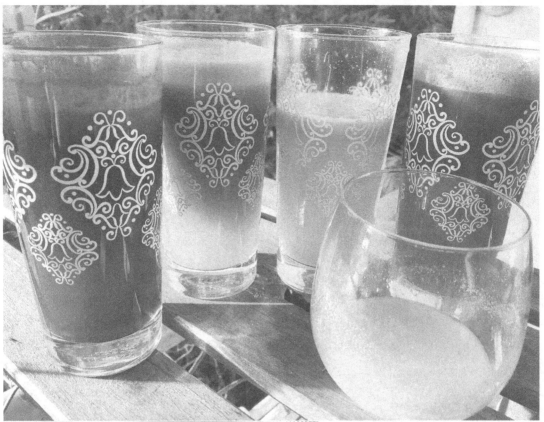

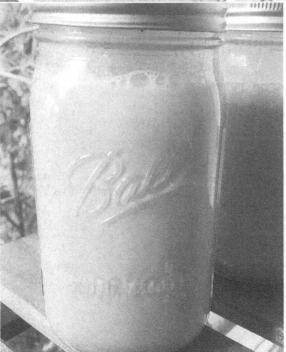

Various teas, juices, elixirs, and smoothies. See chapter 10.

LEFT:
Gold Milk, page 144

Avocado Mousse-Stuffed Tomatoes, page 152

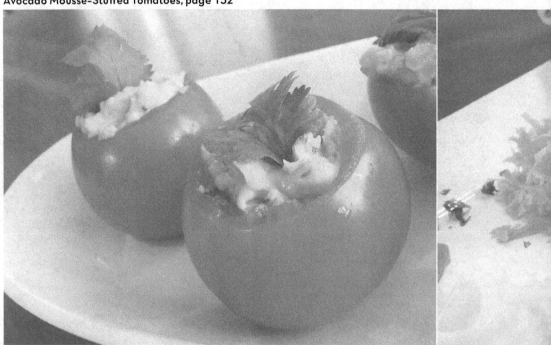

Grilled Plantain Kebabs, page 166

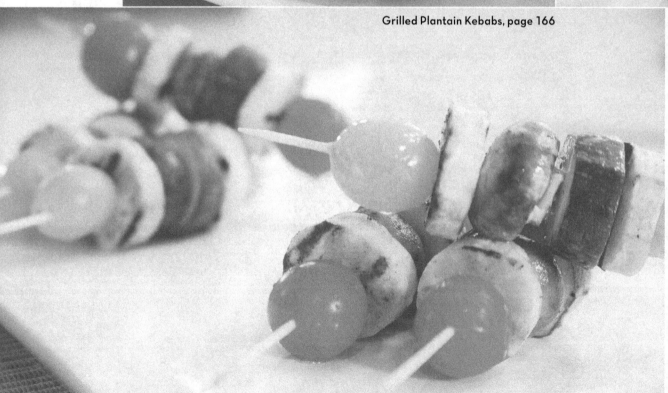

Veggie Lettuce Boats, page 160

Curried Garbanzo Cakes with
Poppy Seeds, page 164

Black Bean Tostones, page 167

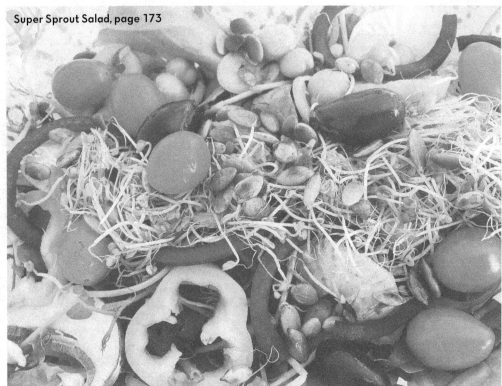

Super Sprout Salad, page 173

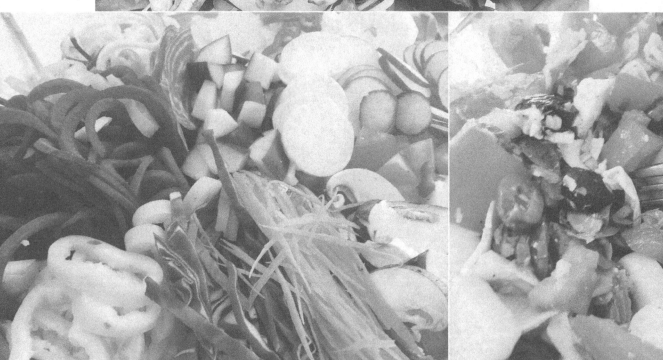

Simple Chop Salad, page 174

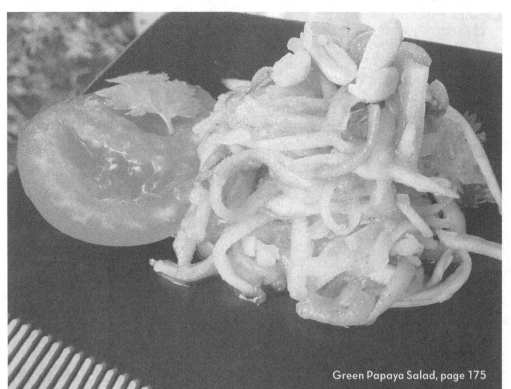

Green Papaya Salad, page 175

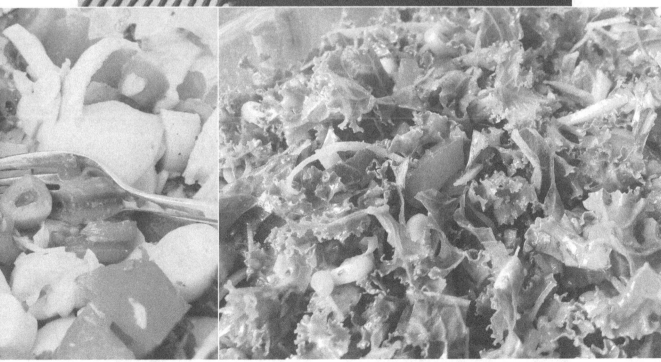

Provençal Salad, page 183

Curry Kale Salad, page 184

Black Bean and Corn Salad, page 189

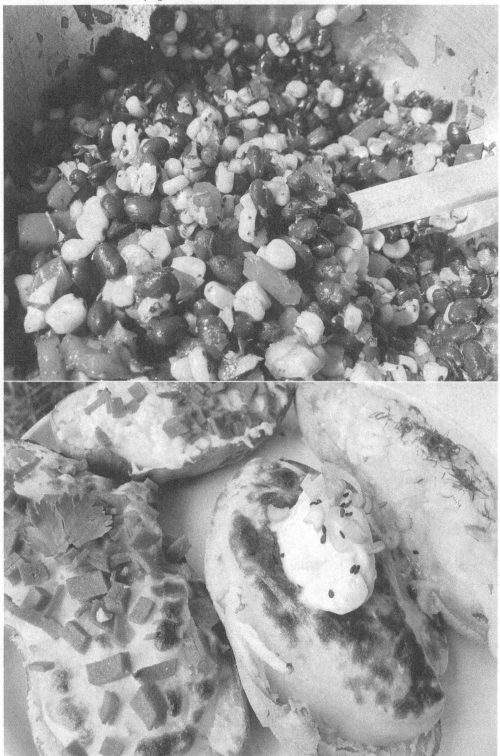

Wasabi Garlic Twice-Baked Potatoes, page 209

Broasted Brussels Sprouts, page 194

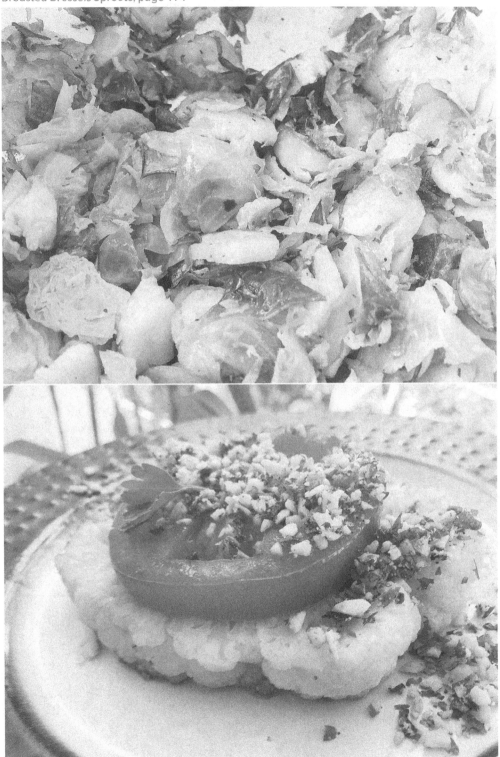

Cauliflower Steaks with Ethiopian-Spiced Almonds, page 200

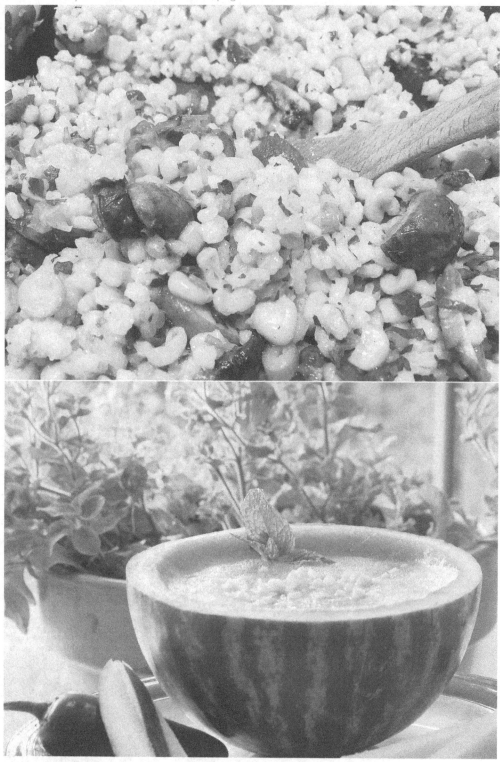

Pearled Barley with Mushrooms and Corn, page 210

Watermelon Gazpacho, page 243

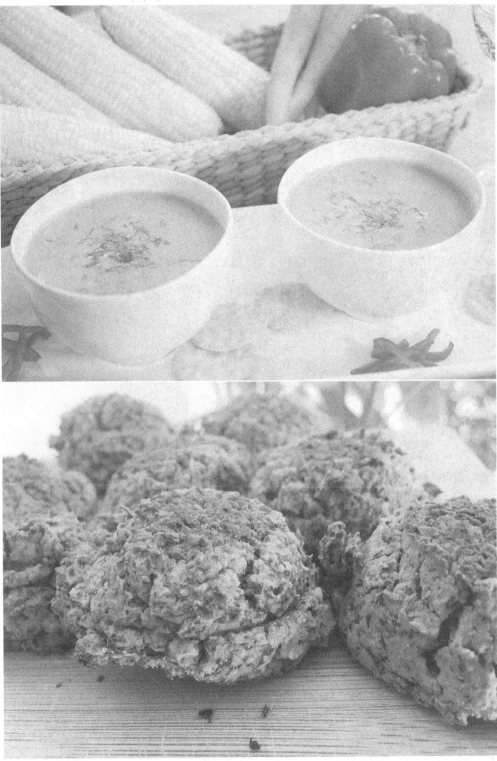

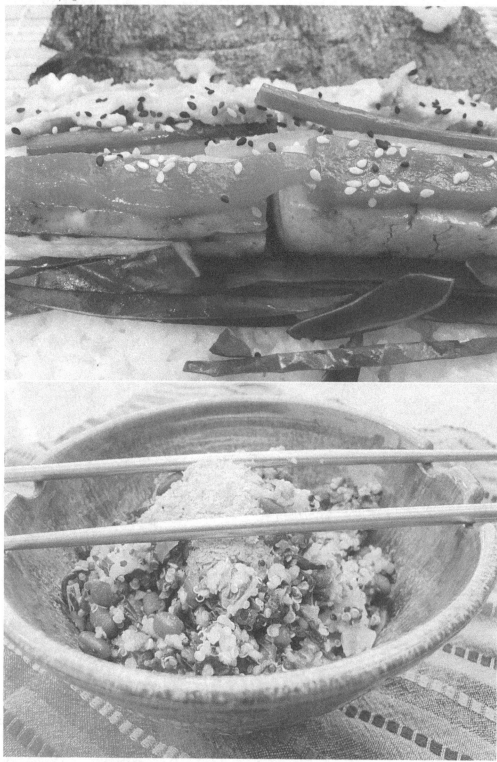

Nori Rolls, page 263

Simple One-Pot Meal, page 266

Raw Coconut Curry Vegetables, page 268

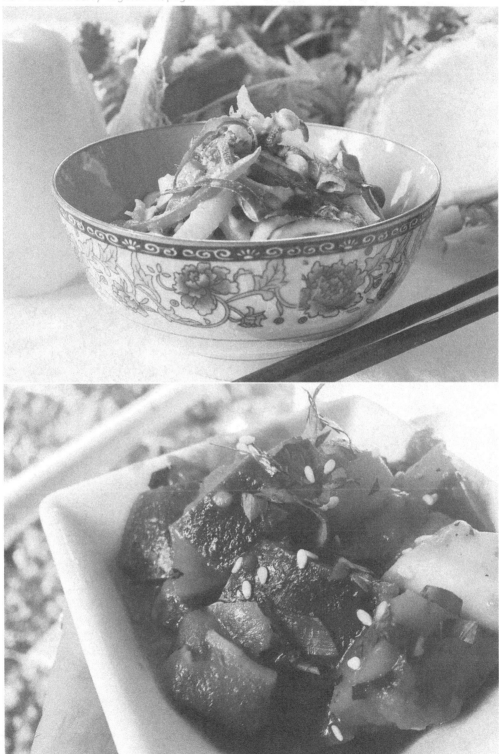

Ratatouille, page 273

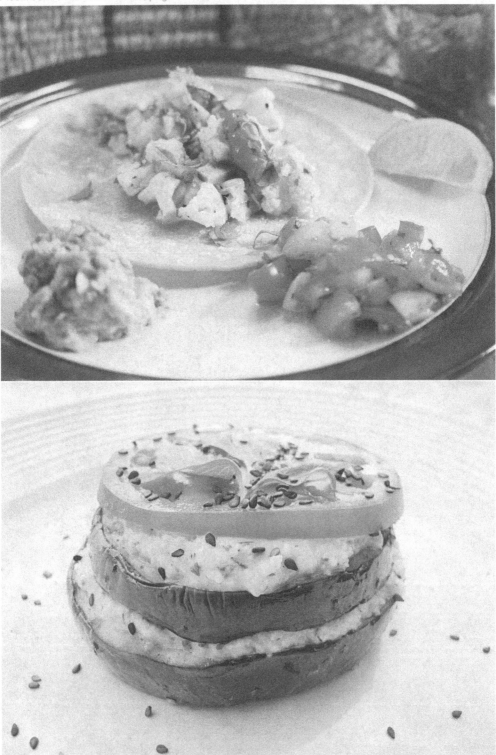

Mushroom Cauliflower Tacos, page 277

Grilled Eggplant Towers with Cashew Ricotta, page 282

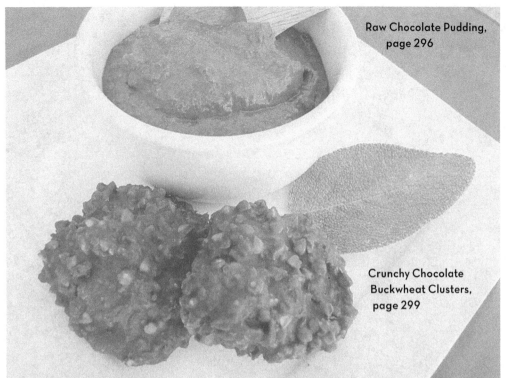

Raw Chocolate Pudding, page 296

Crunchy Chocolate Buckwheat Clusters, page 299

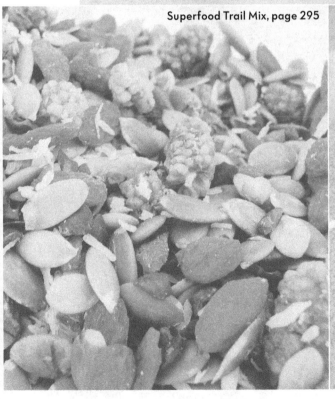

Superfood Trail Mix, page 295

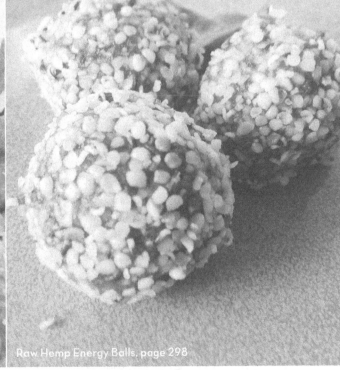

Raw Hemp Energy Balls, page 298

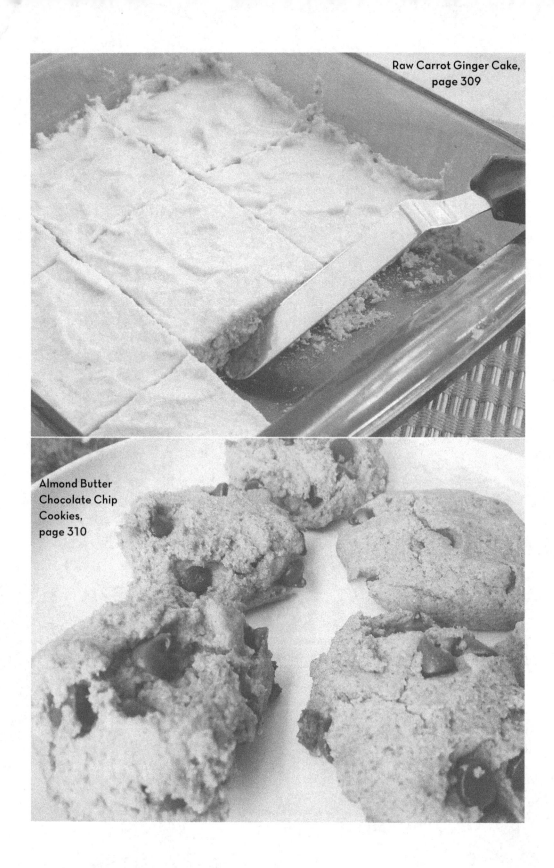

Raw Carrot Ginger Cake, page 309

Almond Butter Chocolate Chip Cookies, page 310

Super Sprout Salad⊙◖◆

YIELD: 7 CUPS SALAD

Prep time: 15 minutes, Total time: 15 minutes, Serving size: 1 3/4 cups, Number of servings 4

Sprouts come in many shapes and sizes, each with their own unique flavor. While this recipe lists a few different types (crunchy sprout mix; smaller sprouts, such as alfalfa; and larger sprouts, such as sunflower), feel free to use just one or two if that is your preference or if that is all that is available. Whatever you decide, this dish includes some of the most beneficial foods you can eat because, as some describe them, they are a "living" food, which goes even a step beyond raw food in terms of high nutrient density and easy absorption by the body. Sprouts are seeds that have received air and water, allowing them to germinate and therefore to retain maximal enzyme activity. Enzymes help you extract more vitamins and minerals, amino acids, and fatty acids from the foods you eat. As such, this salad will enhance the energy-giving properties of the other meals of the day. Serve with your dressing of choice along with Sloppy Joes (page 281) or Designer Seed and Nut Crust Pizzas (page 265).

4 cups loosely packed mixed salad greens
½ cup alfalfa, clover, or broccoli sprouts
½ cup crunchy sprout mix (typically includes lentils, adzuki beans, and peas)
1 cup cooked, drained, and rinsed chickpeas (see page 98)
2 ounces sunflower, buckwheat, or pea sprouts
¾ cup halved cherry tomatoes

2 tablespoons pitted and sliced kalamata olives, or your choice of olives (see page 158)
2 tablespoons hemp seeds (optional)

1. Place the salad greens in a bowl.

2. Top with the alfalfa sprouts and crunchy sprouts. Add the chickpeas and sunflower sprouts.

3. Top with the cherry tomatoes and olives, sprinkle with hemp seeds, if using, drizzle with your dressing of choice, and feel the power!

VARIATIONS

Replace the chickpeas with your favorite beans, such as kidney, navy, or great northern.

Add chopped vegetables of your choosing, such as red cabbage, cucumber, tomato, broccoli, or cauliflower.

Add sliced avocado.

Replace the hemp seeds with other raw or toasted seeds and/or nuts (page 101), such as sesame, pumpkin, walnuts, or pecans.

Top with pomegranate seeds.

Nutrition Facts per serving (157 g): Calories 110, Fat Calories 20, Total Fat 2.5 g, Saturated Fat 0 g, Cholesterol 0 mg, Sodium 150 mg, Total Carb 18 g, Dietary Fiber 5 g, Sugars 4 g, Protein 6 g

Greens component: Rotate through different types of lettuce, such as buttercup, romaine, or mixed salad greens. Try arugula, baby spinach, or baby kale.

Sprouts component: Rotate through alfalfa, clover, broccoli, sunflower, buckwheat, pea, mung bean, lentil, and mixed sprouts,

Raw veggie component: Rotate through carrot, beet, daikon, cabbage, avocado, celery, bell pepper, zucchini, broccoli, cauliflower, cabbage, tomato, Simple Sauerkraut (page 176), Quick Kimchi (page 178), cucumber, kohlrabi, corn, red, white, or green onion, or your favorites. Rotate through different cuts: slice, dice, chop, and grate.

Cooked veggies components: Add steamed, grilled, roasted, or sautéed veggies.

Seed and nut component: Add a sprinkle of raw or toasted (page 101) sunflower seeds, pumpkin seeds, almonds, pecans, walnuts, hemp seeds, sesame seeds, and more.

Legume component: Add cooked chickpeas, black beans, fava beans, kidney, green lentils, black lentils, edamame, or roasted tofu cubes or tempeh cubes (see page 100).

Dressing component: Use simple freshly squeezed lemon juice, or any dressing in Chapter 13.

Other optional components: Add a scoop of Pecan Veggie Pâté (page 169) or Truffled Cashew Cheese (page 159).

Simple Chop Salad♥ⓖ♦

YIELD: 6 CUPS SALAD

Prep time: 20 minutes, Total time: 20 minutes, Serving size: 1 cup, Number of servings: 6

For a salad that breaks free from the lettuce-based model, try this mix and match of chopped-up superpowers. The radish brings a peppery crunch while incorporating an antiviral, antifungal, and blood-purifying element, and like the cabbage and broccoli here, is another member of the health-supportive cruciferous family. Serve with Golden Turmeric Dressing (page 223) or your dressing of choice along with Smoky Split Pea Soup (page 254), or Sloppy Joes (page 281).

1 cup chopped zucchini (½-inch pieces)
1 cup gold bar or crookneck squash (½-inch pieces)
1 cup chopped broccoli (½-inch pieces)
½ cup thinly sliced radish
1 cup chopped cabbage (1-inch pieces)
¼ cup thinly sliced red onion
½ cup cherry tomatoes
2 tablespoons minced fresh cilantro

1. Combine all the ingredients in a bowl and mix well.

2. Toss with your dressing of choice.

VARIATIONS

Add a handful of mixed organic salad greens or arugula.

Top with raw or toasted (page 101) nuts or seeds, such as sunflower, pumpkin, or hazelnuts.

Replace the cilantro with fresh basil, tarragon, parsley, or dill.

Add sliced avocado.

Nutrition Facts per serving (88 g): Calories 25, Fat Calories 0, Total Fat 0 g, Saturated Fat 0 g, Cholesterol 0 mg, Sodium 15 mg, Total Carb 5 g, Dietary Fiber 2 g, Sugars 2 g, Protein 1 g

Asian Cucumber Salad♥ⓖ♦

YIELD: 4 CUPS SALAD

Prep time: 15 minutes, Total time: 15 minutes, Serving size: 1/2 cup, Number of servings: 8

Offering a palate-pleasing way to hydrate the body, and especially helpful for skin and hair, cucumbers make a delightful base for this tangy salad. In concert here with vitamin C and antioxidant lycopene-rich tomatoes and energy- and protein-packed peanuts are the cleansing and immunity-strengthening bold flavors of cilantro and green onion. No need to peel the cucumbers if they are organic. If not, I would definitely recommend peeling them. Serve as a light side dish for heavier mains, such as Thai Curry Vegetables (page 289) or Lemon Tempeh with Kale and Rice Noodles (page 276).

2 cups quartered, seeded, and sliced
   cucumber (¼-inch pieces)
2 cups chopped tomato (½-inch pieces)
1 ½ tablespoons finely chopped fresh cilantro
¼ cup raw peanuts
3 tablespoons thinly sliced green onion

OIL-FREE ASIAN DRESSING
1 ½ tablespoons rice vinegar
1 tablespoon freshly squeezed lime juice
1 teaspoon peeled and minced fresh ginger
1 garlic clove, pressed or minced
½ teaspoon seeded and diced jalapeño pepper
¼ teaspoon sea salt, or to taste
⅛ teaspoon Chinese five-spice powder
   (optional)

1. Place the cucumber, tomato, and cilantro in a bowl and toss well.

2. Prepare the dressing: Place the dressing ingredients in a small bowl and whisk well.

3. Add to the cucumber mixture and toss to coat. Top with the peanuts and green onion before serving.

VARIATIONS

Add 1 tablespoon of sesame oil and ¼ teaspoon of toasted sesame oil to the dressing.

Add two kaffir lime leaves and 2 inches of lemongrass to the dressing ingredients and blend.

Add 1 ½ cups of additional vegetables, such as chopped cabbage, bell pepper, and/or grated carrot.

Top with 1 cup of mung bean sprouts.

Nutrition Facts per serving (107 g): Fat Calories 50, Total Fat 5 g, Saturated Fat 0 g, Cholesterol 0 mg, Sodium 195 mg, Total Carb 6 g, Dietary Fiber 2 g, Sugars 4 g, Protein 2 g

Green Papaya Salad♥ⓖ♦

YIELD: 3 CUPS SALAD

Prep time: 20 minutes, Total time: 20 minutes, Serving size: 1/2 cup, Number of servings: 6

Popular in Thailand and pretty much anywhere papayas are grown, green papaya salad is a flavorful way to get your digestive juices flowing before your meal. Green papayas are underripe papayas that are firmer, less sweet, and contain a larger enzyme content than the ripened fruit. This makes for excellent digestive properties, and promotes overall healthy cell metabolism. When selecting green papaya at the market, be sure to select one that is firm, without any blotches or soft spots. If there is some ripeness in the papaya, don't fret. As long as there is enough firmness to grate the papaya, it will work in this tart, crunchy, and refreshing salad combo. Try serving in a stuffed tomato (see page 152), or on its own along with Raw Coconut Curry Sauce (page 237) or Thai Curry Vegetables (page 289).

3 cups seeded, peeled, and grated green papaya

¼ cup thinly sliced green onion

2 tablespoons finely chopped fresh cilantro

¼ cup mung bean sprouts (optional)

¼ cup raw peanuts (optional)

OIL-FREE PAPAYA SALAD DRESSING

2 tablespoons rice vinegar

2 tablespoons freshly squeezed lime juice

¾ teaspoon wheat-free tamari or other soy sauce, or to taste

1 to 2 teaspoons coconut nectar, agave nectar, or sweetener of choice (optional)

½ teaspoon seeded and diced hot chile pepper (see page 179), or ¼ teaspoon crushed red pepper flakes

¼ teaspoon chili powder

Pinch of sea salt, or to taste

⅛ teaspoon freshly ground black pepper

Pinch of ancho chile powder (optional)

1. Place the papaya, green onion, and cilantro in a bowl and gently mix well.

2. Prepare the dressing: Combine all the dressing ingredients in a small bowl and whisk well.

3. Transfer the dressing to the papaya mixture and gently toss well.

VARIATIONS

Top with ½ cup of roasted unsalted peanuts or chopped cashews.

Add 1 tablespoon of chiffonaded fresh mint.

Add 1 cup of chopped tomato and/or green beans, cut into 1-inch pieces.

Top with mung bean sprouts before serving.

Depending on the sweetness of the papaya, add 1 tablespoon of pure maple syrup, Date Syrup (page 88), or other sweetener to taste (see page 89).

Add 1½ tablespoons of sesame oil, flax oil, or hemp oil to the dressing.

Nutrition Facts per serving (91 g): Calories 40, Fat Calories 0, Total Fat 0 g, Saturated Fat 0 g, Cholesterol 0 mg, Sodium 245 mg, Total Carb 9 g, Dietary Fiber 0 g, Sugars 2 g, Protein 0 g

Simple Sauerkraut ♥ⓖ♦

YIELD: 4 CUPS SAUERKRAUT

Prep time: 15 minutes, Fermenting time: 4–5 days, Total time: 4–5 days, Serving size: 1/4 cup, Number of servings: 16

Although it's an established staple in German cuisine, sauerkraut actually originated in China. The fermented cabbage dish is well known in the healthy eating community for supplying probiotics that rebuild friendly flora in the digestive system. The cabbage in sauerkraut contains anti-inflammatory iso-thiocyanates and the amino acid glutamine, which can actually repair and replenish digestive tissues, including healing stomach ulcers. It is a good source of vitamin C and, as a cruciferous vegetable, may be considered an anticancer food. Be sure to save the outer leaves of the cabbage when prepping. Serious sauerkraut connoisseurs will want to purchase a fermenting crock, available online or at a kitchen supply store. Serve as part of a large mixed salad, or on top of veggie dogs or Magnificent Mushroom Burgers (page 270).

1 large green cabbage (5 cups grated or chopped)

¾ cup water

1 teaspoon sea salt, or to taste

2 teaspoons minced fresh ginger

2 teaspoons minced fresh dill

1 teaspoon caraway seeds (optional)

1. Peel off the outer layers of the cabbage and set aside. Coarsely grate or finely chop the cabbage and place in a large bowl. Remove ¾ cup of the cabbage and place in a blender with the water and salt. Blend for a minute or so and return to the bowl. Mix well.

2. Place the cabbage mixture in a half-gallon glass jar. Cover with the outer layer cabbage leaves and press down firmly. You can place a smaller glass jar filled with water on top of the cabbage to weigh the contents down. All the cabbage should be covered with liquid. If not, add additional water. Cover with plastic wrap and secure with a rubber band.

3. Allow this mixture to sit for 4 or 5 days in a dark, warm place. Check every day and press the outer layers down firmly to make sure cabbage is always covered with water. It should have a slightly fermented taste but should not be gray or moldy.

4. Transfer the cabbage to a bowl and add the ginger, dill, and caraway seeds, if using. Add additional salt to taste, if necessary. Will last for several days or longer if stored in a glass container in the refrigerator.

VARIATIONS

Alter the type of cabbage used.

Add 2 cups of shredded vegetables, such as carrot, celery, daikon radish, burdock root, or beet before culturing.

You can even add small amounts of soaked sea vegetables, such as arame or dulse.

Try replacing the dill with your favorite fresh herbs, such as cilantro, parsley, chives, marjoram, or basil.

Replace the ginger with minced fresh garlic.

Spice it up by adding 2 teaspoons of seeded and diced hot chile pepper (see the Scoville scale on page 179).

Nutrition Facts per serving (29 g): Calories 10, Fat Calories 0, Total Fat 0 g, Saturated Fat 0 g, Cholesterol 0 mg, Sodium 150 mg, Total Carb 2 g, Dietary Fiber 1 g, Sugars 0 g, Protein 0 g

Quick Kimchi ⊙ ◗

YIELD: 3 CUPS KIMCHI

Prep time: 30 minutes, Fermenting time: 3-4 days, Total time: 3-4 days, Serving size: 1/4 cup, Number of servings: 12

Kimchi is a traditional spicy and fermented food of Korea, and is Korea's national dish, which makes sense when you learn that it is served at almost every Korean meal. The fermentation of kimchi, and its abundance of lactic acid bacteria, is key to a healthy digestive system and for building immune system strength. Pungent daikon radish further supports digestive and immunity balance, promotes energy circulation, and increases the metabolic rate. Daikon also contains natural diuretics, decongestants, and digestive enzymes, which help prevent the common cold, flu, and respiratory infections. Be sure to save the outer leaves of the cabbage when prepping so you can use them to top off the shredded leaves. Serve on top of your salad or as part of a Nori Roll (page 263), a Monk Bowl (see pages 100, 267), or Simple One-Pot Meal (page 266).

6 cups tightly packed chopped napa cabbage (1- to 2-inch pieces), whole outer leaves reserved

1 teaspoon sea salt, or to taste

1 cup chopped green onion (½-inch pieces)

1 cup peeled and julienned daikon radish (1 ½-inch pieces)

2 tablespoons minced fresh garlic

½ to 1 teaspoon crushed red pepper flakes

½ to ¾ cup water

1. Place the chopped cabbage in a large bowl with the salt and mix well.

Massage the salt into the cabbage and allow to sit for 20 minutes.

2. Add the green onion, daikon, garlic, and crushed red pepper flakes and mix well.

3. Transfer to a 1-quart mason jar and press down tightly. Top with the outer cabbage leaves and press down tightly. Add water to cover completely. Seal the jar and leave out at room temperature for 2 to 3 days, opening the jar once or twice a day to allow the cabbage to breathe. It should have a slightly fermented taste but should not be gray or moldy.

4. Place in the refrigerator. The flavors will continue to mature the longer it is kept in the fridge.

VARIATIONS

Add 1 cup of thinly sliced carrot or cucumber.

Replace the garlic with fresh ginger.

Add 2 tablespoons of chopped fresh cilantro.

Nutrition Facts per serving (96 g): Calories 15, Fat Calories 0, Total Fat 0 g, Saturated Fat 0 g, Cholesterol 0 mg, Sodium 210 mg, Total Carb 4 g, Dietary Fiber 2 g, Sugars 2 g, Protein 1 g

Chef's Tips and Tricks

Fermentation will be faster if a small amount of already-made sauerkraut is added to fresh shredded cabbage as a starter.

Chef's Tips and Tricks

Scoville Scale

Some like it hot. Some like it hotter! There are many flavorful chile peppers to sample—ranging from mild to inferno. The heat of the peppers is determined by the amount of capsaicin they contain. They are rated using Scoville units, a method developed by Wilbur Scoville in 1912. The scale is from 0 (being the mildest) to 10 (having the highest heat). Try them all and see how hot you can take it. To avoid burning your fingers while chopping, wear rubber gloves and be sure not to touch your eyes!

From cool to hot: Sweet Bells/Pimiento, Cherry, Ancho, Jalapeño/Chipotle/Poblano, Serrano, Cayenne, Habanero, Scotch Bonnet, and Red Savina Habanero.

Watercress with Pistachios and Currants ♥ Ⓖ

YIELD: 6 CUPS SALAD

Prep time: 15 minutes, Total time: 15 minutes, Serving size: 1 cup, Number of servings: 6

Peppery watercress ranks amongst the lowest-calorie and most nutrient-dense foods available, and it's no wonder with all its isothiocyanates, which help remove impurities from the body. Tossed with sweet currants and pistachio nuts, a lower-calorie nut that lowers cholesterol and supplies hefty quantities of vitamin B$_6$, thiamine, and phosphorus, this salad delivers plenty of concentrated nutrition in every bite. Top with the following Simple Balsamic Dressing or with any dressing from Chapter 13.

2 cups loosely packed chopped watercress
2 cups loosely packed arugula
½ cup raw or roasted pistachio nuts
¼ cup dried currants
¼ cup thinly sliced green onion
1 cup halved cherry tomatoes

1. Place the watercress and arugula in a large bowl and gently toss well.

2. Decoratively top with pistachio nuts, currants, green onion, and cherry tomatoes.

3. Drizzle with your dressing of choice and enjoy.

VARIATIONS

Replace the watercress and arugula with mixed salad greens.

Replace the pistachios with nuts or seeds, such as pumpkin, walnuts, or hazelnuts.

Replace the currants with dried cranberries or raisins.

Add additional vegetables, such as seeded and thinly sliced bell pepper or cabbage, grated carrot or beet, or chopped cucumber.

Nutrition Facts per serving (63 g): Calories 85, Fat Calories 40, Total Fat 5 g, Saturated Fat 1 g, Cholesterol 0 mg, Sodium 9 mg, Total Carb 9 g, Dietary Fiber 2 g, Sugars 6 g, Protein 3 g

QUICKER AND EASIER

Simple Balsamic Dressing

Combine the following in a bowl and whisk well: 1/4 cup of olive oil, 1 1/2 tablespoons of balsamic vinegar, 2 teaspoons of pure maple syrup, 1 1/2 teaspoons of Dijon mustard, a pinch of sea salt, a pinch of freshly ground black pepper, and a pinch of crushed red pepper flakes.

Nutrition Facts per serving (178 g): Calories 210, Fat Calories 140, Total Fat 16 g, Saturated Fat 2 g, Cholesterol 0 mg, Sodium 185 mg, Total Carb 15 g, Dietary Fiber 4 g, Sugars 7 g, Protein 6 g

Waldorf Salad ⓖ◆

YIELD: 4 CUPS SALAD

Prep time: 15 minutes, Total time: 15 minutes, Serving size: 1 cup, Number of servings: 4

This hearty salad is famous for its perfect combination of a rich, creamy dressing with a delightful balance of fiber-filled crunchable veggies and fruit and just the right amount of grounding protein to call it a meal. The Waldorf salad was created in the late nineteenth century at the Waldorf-Astoria hotel in midtown Manhattan, where it was an instant smash sensation. With this plant-based version of the dressing, which leaves out the mayonnaise, you can savor the same distinctive flavor and texture combo while preserving your heart, brain, and circulatory health and giving your immune system an energetic boost. Toss with Waldorf dressing (recipe follows) or your dressing of choice, and serve with the Corn Casserole (page 286) or Cauliflower Casserole (page 285).

1 small head lettuce, whole leaves
½ cup Waldorf Dressing (recipe follows)
½ cup walnuts, raw or toasted (see page 101)
1 small apple, cored and thinly sliced
1 cup sliced celery
½ cup peeled and grated carrot

1. Place the lettuce on a plate. Drizzle with the dressing.

2. Top with the walnuts, apple, celery, and grated carrot before serving.

Waldorf Dressing ⓖ◆

YIELD: 1 CUP DRESSING

Prep time: 20 minutes, Total time: 20 minutes, Serving size: 1/8 cup, Number of servings: 8

½ cup raw cashews
½ cup water
2 tablespoons freshly squeezed lemon juice
½ teaspoon onion flakes
1 ½ teaspoons raw apple cider vinegar
½ teaspoon sea salt, or to taste
⅛ teaspoon freshly ground black pepper

1. Place the cashews in a bowl with ample water to cover. Allow to sit for 15 minutes, or up to 3 hours. Drain and rinse well.

2. Place in a blender with the remaining dressing ingredients, including the ½ cup of fresh water, and blend until creamy.

VARIATIONS

Replace the walnuts with pecans, hazelnuts, almonds, or pumpkin seeds.

Add additional veggies, such as grated beet, julienned red cabbage, or julienned bell pepper.

Replace the lettuce with mixed salad greens, romaine lettuce, or arugula.

Replace the cashews in the dressing with macadamia nuts, Brazil nuts, or hemp seeds.

Nutrition Facts per serving (44 g): Calories 80, Fat Calories 55, Total Fat 6 g, Saturated Fat 1 g, Cholesterol 0 mg, Sodium 150 mg, Total Carb 5 g, Dietary Fiber less than 1 g, Sugars 1 g, Protein 3 g

Caesar Salad🄖

YIELD: 6 CUPS SALAD

Prep time: 10 minutes, Total time: 10 minutes (with dressing and croutons prepared), Serving size: 1 cup, Number of servings: 6

This salad was first served and brought to fame at Caesar's Restaurant in Tijuana in the 1920s by Italian owner Caesar Cardini—although several of his business partners have claimed to have originated it, two of whom allegedly named it the aviator's salad before it was stolen from them. Regardless, its creation was an important moment in culinary history, and it remains a thoroughly delightful way to enjoy romaine's abundant offering of calcium, iron, B vitamins, vitamin K, beta-carotene, omega-3s, and, yes, even protein. Carrot and red onion are perfect nutrient companions, and the Brazil Nut Parmesan (page 111) and homemade croutons add a nutty and crunchy finishing touch. Serve along with Sloppy Joes (page 281), Millet and Butternut Squash with Broccoli (page 284), or Simple One-Pot Meal (page 266).

1 small head romaine lettuce, cut into ½ by 1 ½-inch pieces, rinsed and drained well (5 cups)
¾ cup peeled and grated carrot
3 tablespoons thinly sliced red onion
¾ cup Herb Croutons (page 111)
¾ cup Caesar dressing (page 225)
2 tablespoons Brazil Nut Parmesan (page 111) or nutritional yeast

1. Place the lettuce in a large bowl, or in individual serving bowls.

2. Top with the carrot, onion, and croutons. Drizzle with the dressing and top with the Brazil Nut Parmesan before serving.

VARIATIONS

Replace the lettuce with mixed organic greens, baby spinach, or arugula.

Add additional veggies, such as grated beet or parsnip, or sliced tomato, cucumber, or avocado.

Add sprouts, such as sunflower, buckwheat, pea, broccoli, alfalfa, or clover.

Nutrition Facts per serving (118 g): Calories 170, Fat Calories 80, Total Fat 8 g, Saturated Fat 2 g, Cholesterol 0 mg, Sodium 190 mg, Total Carb 19 g, Dietary Fiber 3 g, Sugars 4 g, Protein 4

Pickled Okra♦🄖🔲

YIELD: 15 OKRA

Prep time: 10 minutes, Cook time: 15 minutes, Pickling time: 7-10 days, Total time: 7-10 days, Serving size: 3 okra, Number of servings: 5

"To know me is to love me" is the official motto of okra—and an invitation to get to know this wonderful plant for those who may be put off by its gelatinous texture. As a verified okra lover, I can say that its earthy flavor and pleasant crunch, as well as its nutritional benefits, make it an important food to include in your culinary repertoire. The gelatinous content is actually what makes it healing and soothing for your digestive tract and throat. Pickling is one of the oldest methods of food preservation and a fabulous way to keep the distinctive flavor and antioxidants of okra around well past its summer and fall season. Okra is high in fiber, vitamin C, folate, calcium, and potassium. Pickling it provides some probiotic benefit, and is also just a fun way to spice up and enjoy this unique vegetable's edible pods and seeds. Serve as a side along with Raw Collard Veggie Rolls (page 260), Millet Black Bean Veggie Burgers (page 269), or BBQ Roasted Tofu with Collards (page 278).

4 cups whole okra (about 15)

½ cup thinly sliced sweet or yellow onion (cut into half-moons)

½ jalapeño pepper, seeded and sliced (optional)

PICKLING SPICE MIX

1 tablespoon brown mustard seeds

1 tablespoon fennel seeds

1 teaspoon coriander seeds

1 teaspoon whole black peppercorns

½ teaspoon whole cloves

1 teaspoon dried rosemary (optional)

½ teaspoon juniper berries (optional)

1 cup raw apple cider vinegar

1 ½ cups water

2 bay leaves

1 tablespoon organic sugar, coconut sugar, or desired sweetener to taste (page 89)

¾ teaspoon sea salt, or to taste

1. Clean, rinse, and dry a 1-quart mason jar with a lid. Place the okra, onion, and jalapeño, if using, in the jar.

2. Prepare the pickling spice mix: Place a pot over medium-high heat. Place the mustard seeds, fennel seeds, coriander seeds, peppercorns, cloves, and juniper berries, if using, in the pot and cook for

3 minutes, stirring constantly. Add the remaining pickling spice ingredients, lower the heat to low, and cook for 10 minutes, stirring occasionally.

3. Pour into the jar that contains the okra. Seal with the lid. Allow to cool at room temperature, then place in the refrigerator. The flavor will improve with time. Enjoy after 7 to 10 days.

Nutrition Facts per serving (151 g) including pickling spice liquid that is not consumed: Calories 50, Fat Calories 10, Total Fat 1 g, Saturated Fat 0 g, Cholesterol 0 mg, Sodium 360 mg, Total Carb 11 g, Dietary Fiber 4 g, Sugars 4 g, Protein 2 g

TEMPLATE RECIPE
Pickled Veggies

Pickling spice component: Experiment with different spice combinations, using the spices listed in the recipe. Add different vinegars, such as coconut, white, sherry, or rice; and different sweeteners (see page 89).

Veggie component: Experiment with different veggies, including carrots, cucumbers, daikon, broccoli, and cauliflower, and ginger. Firmer veggies can be slightly steamed before pickling.

For Pickled Beets and Onion, replace the okra with 2 ½ cups of peeled and chopped beet (¼- to ½-inch pieces), and replace the onion with ½ cup of thinly sliced red onion. You can optionally steam or boil the beets for 10 minutes before adding to the jar.

Provençal Salad ♥ⓖ♦

YIELD: 4 ½ CUPS SALAD

Prep time: 20 minutes, Total time: 20 minutes, Serving size: 1/2 cup, Number of servings: 9

Take a culinary trip to the Mediterranean with this robust tomato-based salad replete with ingredients from the region. Lycopene, a carotenoid found in all tomatoes, well known as an antioxidant said to protect tissues from cancer, is now showing a benefit to bone health. Low-calorie and tasty hearts of palm and artichoke hearts both supply the body with not only carbs and fiber, but also potassium and vitamin B_6. A small dose of healthy-fat olives adds a nice color, texture, and flavor accent. Serve with Broccoli Rabe Penne Pasta with Oil-Free Cream Sauce (page 292) or Corn Casserole (page 286).

2 cups chopped tomato (½-inch pieces)
¼ cup diced assorted pitted and chopped olives
1 cup chopped artichoke hearts
1 cup sliced hearts of palm (½-inch pieces) (see box, page 169)
½ cup thinly sliced fennel bulb (optional)
3 tablespoons thinly sliced green onion

OIL-FREE PROVENÇAL DRESSING
1 tablespoon freshly squeezed lemon juice
2 teaspoons balsamic vinegar
1 garlic clove, pressed or minced
1 tablespoon tightly packed chiffonaded fresh basil
1 teaspoon chopped fresh marjoram
½ teaspoon dried thyme
⅛ teaspoon crushed red pepper flakes
⅛ teaspoon freshly ground black pepper
Pinch of sea salt, or to taste

1. Place the tomato, olives, artichoke hearts, hearts of palm, fennel, if using, and green onion in a bowl and mix well.

2. Prepare the dressing: Place all the dressing ingredients in a small bowl and whisk well.

3. Add the dressing to the vegetables and gently stir well before serving.

VARIATIONS

Add more olives, if it strikes your fancy.

Add 1 cup of fresh or frozen and thawed corn, and/or 1 tablespoon of capers.

Add 1 ½ tablespoons of olive oil to the dressing.

Nutrition Facts per serving (100 g): Calories 60, Fat Calories 7, Total Fat 1 g, Saturated Fat 0 g, Cholesterol 0 mg, Sodium 205 mg, Total Carb 12 g, Dietary Fiber 2 g, Sugars 6 g, Protein 2 g

Tomato Avocado Salad ♥ⓖ♦

YIELD: 4 CUPS SALAD

Prep time: 15 minutes, Total time: 15 minutes, Serving size: 1 cup, Number of servings: 4

With balanced colors, flavors, and nutritional perks, this salad is virtual perfection and easy to prepare with just a little chopping and a simple toss. Cucumbers replenish daily vitamins, especially B vitamins, and tomatoes have an array of goodness beyond their antioxidant prowess, by providing vitamin E, copper, potassium, manganese, beta-carotene, folate, phosphorus, chromium, choline, zinc, and iron. Along with the healthy fats of the beautiful avocado fruit, this is a fiber-rich, health-preserving choice. Top with pine nuts (optionally toasted; see page 101) and serve along with Millet Black Bean Veggie Burgers (page 269) or Mexican Seitan-Stuffed Peppers (page 291).

2 cup chopped tomato (½-inch pieces)
2 cups quartered, seeded, and chopped cucumber (½-inch pieces)
¼ cup thinly sliced green onion
1 tablespoon freshly squeezed lemon juice
1 tablespoon balsamic vinegar
1 tablespoon nutritional yeast (optional)
1 garlic clove, pressed or minced
2 teaspoons minced fresh dill
Pinch of sea salt, or to taste
⅛ teaspoon freshly ground black pepper
⅛ teaspoon crushed red pepper flakes
1 cup chopped avocado (½-inch pieces)

1. Combine all the ingredients, except the avocado, in a bowl and mix well.

2. Add the avocado and gently mix well before serving.

VARIATIONS

Replace all or some of the cucumber and tomato with other chopped veggies, including broccoli, cabbage, celery, or bell pepper.

Add 1 tablespoon of an ethnic spice blend, such as Mexican (page 106), Indian (page 106), or Italian (page 105).

Replace the dill with 2 tablespoons of fresh basil, sorrel, or flat-leaf parsley.

Nutrition Facts per serving (197 g): Calories 90, Fat Calories 50, Total Fat 6 g, Saturated Fat 1 g, Cholesterol 0 mg, Sodium 50 mg, Total Carb 10 g, Dietary Fiber 4 g, Sugars 4 g, Protein 2 g

---

TEMPLATE RECIPE
Kale Salad

- -

Base: Rotate through different varieties of kale, such as curly or dinosaur. Add some other greens, such as chard, arugula, dandelion greens, or spinach.

Dressing or sauce component: Rotate through different dressings and sauces, including Golden Turmeric Dressing (page 223), Zesty Chimichurri Sauce (page 231), Smoky BBQ Sauce (page 231), or Raw Coconut Curry Sauce (page 237).

Veggie component: Rotate through a variety of bite-size, shredded, and diced veggies. Carrots, beets, corn, red cabbage, bell peppers, and green and red onion are some suggestions to start.

Herb and spice component: Use fresh herbs, such as dill, basil, marjoram, tarragon, cilantro, or rosemary; or such spices as poppy seeds, Chinese five-spice powder, curry powder, cumin seeds, or garam masala.

Ethnic spice component: Experiment with the other spice blends (see pages 105–106).

Curry Kale Salad ♥Ⓖ⬙

YIELD: 6 CUPS SALAD

Prep time: 15 minutes, Total time: 15 minutes, Serving size: 1 cup, Number of servings: 6

Bollywood meets kale in this wholesome salad with Indian spices. Curry powder often contains twelve to fifteen different spices, each of which provides its own health benefits. The turmeric in curry powder is an anti-inflammatory and is said to protect against Alzheimer's. Black pepper, cinnamon, bay leaves, cloves, coriander, and cumin all have properties to aid digestion. In this vibrant salad, green, red, yellow, and orange colors are represented several times over! Serve along with Raw Collard Veggie Rolls (page 260), Creamy Lentil Saag (page 290), or a bowl of Kitchari (page 257).

KALE SALAD

4 cups fairly tightly packed stemmed and thinly sliced kale

¾ cup seeded and diced red bell pepper

1 cup fresh or frozen (thawed) corn

½ cup peeled and grated carrot

½ cup pumpkin seeds

½ cup dried currants or raisins (optional)

¼ cup thinly sliced green onion

SIMPLE CURRY DRESSING

3 tablespoons sesame oil

2 tablespoons freshly squeezed lemon juice

1 ½ tablespoons finely chopped fresh cilantro

2 teaspoons wheat-free tamari or other soy sauce to taste

2 teaspoons curry powder

1 teaspoon ground cumin powder (optionally toasted; see page 101)

⅛ teaspoon cayenne pepper

1. Prepare the salad: Combine all the salad ingredients in a large bowl and toss well.

2. Prepare the dressing: Combine the dressing ingredients in a small bowl and whisk well.

3. Add the dressing to the salad and gently massage the dressing into the kale.

VARIATIONS

For Mexican, toss with the Creamy Pepita Dressing (page 227).

For Italian, toss with the Simple Balsamic Dressing (page 179).

For Moroccan, add 2 tablespoons of Moroccan Spice Mix (page 106).

🌢For an oil-free version, replace the sesame oil with ¼ cup of mashed avocado.

Nutrition Facts per serving (130 g): Calories 260, Fat Calories 120, Total Fat 14 g, Saturated Fat 2 g, Cholesterol 0 mg, Sodium 150 mg, Total Carb 29 g, Dietary Fiber 5 g, Sugars 3 g, Protein 8 g

Ranch Kale Salad♥☺🌢

YIELD: 5 CUPS SALAD

Prep time: 25 minutes, Total time: 25 minutes, Serving size: 3/4 cup, Number of servings: 8

"It's all about the sauce" is a well-known phrase in the culinary world. That rings true in this dish, where the rich, creamy, and tangy ranch sauce imparts its magic of the earthiness of kale, affectionately known as the king of the leafy greens. In addition to flavor, the ranch ingredients provide B vitamins, protein, and alkalizing, immunity-boosting, and cleansing benefits. You may feel your vitality increase with every bite. Experiment with the different ways to vary this dish and you will become a kale believer for life! Top with pomegranate seeds and serve along with Broccoli Dill Quiche (page 274) or BBQ Roasted Tofu with Collards (page 278).

RANCH SAUCE

½ cup chopped raw cashew pieces

3 tablespoons freshly squeezed lemon juice

2 to 3 tablespoons water

2 tablespoons nutritional yeast

2 teaspoons coconut vinegar or raw apple cider vinegar

2 garlic cloves

1 teaspoon paprika

¾ teaspoon sea salt, or to taste

¼ teaspoon freshly ground black pepper

1 tablespoon minced fresh dill, or 1 teaspoon dried

¼ teaspoon chipotle chile powder

⅛ teaspoon cayenne pepper

6 cups stemmed, rinsed, drained, and chopped curly kale (½-inch pieces)

½ cup hemp seeds or sesame seeds

1. Prepare the sauce: Place the cashews in a bowl with at least 1 cup of water. Allow to sit for 20 minutes, or up to 3 hours. Drain and rinse well. Place in a blender with the remaining sauce ingredients, including the 2 to 3 tablespoons of fresh water, and blend well.

2. Place the kale in a large bowl.

3. Pour the sauce over the kale and toss well. Garnish with the hemp seeds before serving.

VARIATIONS

♥ For a Raw Kale Ranch Dip, transfer the kale with its sauce to a food processor and process until creamy.

♥ Ranch Kale Chips: Toss the kale with the sauce as above and place in a single layer on three dehydrator sheets. Dehydrate at 115°F for 5 hours.

Cooked Ranch Kale Chips: Preheat the oven to 300°F. Toss the kale with the sauce as above and place in a single layer on a large baking sheet. Bake for 10 minutes. Carefully flip and bake for an additional 15 minutes.

For an out-of-control Ranch Kale Dip, after 10 minutes of baking at 300°F, transfer the kale with its sauce to a food processor and process until creamy.

Nutrition Facts per serving (90 g): Calories 195, Fat Calories 115, Total Fat 13 g, Saturated Fat 2 g, Cholesterol 0 mg, Sodium 245 mg, Total Carb 12 g, Dietary Fiber 3 g, Sugars 2 g, Protein 10 g

Sesame Kale Salad ♥ⓖ

YIELD: 6 CUPS SALAD

Prep time: 15 minutes, Total time: 15 minutes, Serving size: 3/4 cup, Number of servings: 8

This supersatisfying salad is a simple yet powerful blend of flavors and textures. Kale is one of the most nutrient-dense foods available (see page 46); and sesame seeds, appearing in three forms (black, white, and creamed in tahini), are full of calcium and magnesium—though, feel free to stick with just one variety of sesame seeds, if that's all you have on hand! This colorful salad touches a rainbow of different nutrient bases. Serve as a side with Nori Rolls (page 263), Baked Falafel (page 262), or Sloppy Joes (page 281).

5 cups tightly packed stemmed and chopped kale (½-inch pieces)

1 cup seeded and diced red bell pepper

1 cup shredded purple cabbage

1 ½ tablespoons white sesame seeds

1 ½ tablespoons black sesame seeds

¼ cup thinly sliced green onion

TAHINI DIJON DRESSING

¼ cup creamy tahini

¼ cup water

1 tablespoon freshly squeezed lemon juice

1 ½ teaspoons raw apple cider vinegar or coconut vinegar

1 teaspoon wheat-free tamari or other soy sauce, or to taste

1 teaspoon Dijon mustard

1 garlic clove, pressed or minced

Pinch of crushed red pepper flakes

1 tablespoon minced fresh dill

1 tablespoon nutritional yeast (optional)

1. Place the kale, bell pepper, and purple cabbage in a bowl and toss well.

2. Prepare the dressing: Place the dressing ingredients in a small bowl and whisk well.

3. Add to the bowl with the kale and toss well.

4. Top with the sesame seeds and green onion before serving.

VARIATIONS

Add 1 ½ cups of additional veggies, such as grated carrot, beet, parsnip, and/or daikon radish.

Add ½ cup of pitted and diced olives.

Bulk it up with 1 cup of cooked beans, such as chickpeas, or cannellini or black beans.

Add 1 cup of chopped vegetables, such as tomato, cucumber, or radish.

Replace the Tahini Dijon Dressing with any dressing in Chapter 13.

Nutrition Facts per serving (105 g): Calories 100, Fat Calories 55, Total Fat 6 g, Saturated Fat 1 g, Cholesterol 0 mg, Sodium 90 mg, Total Carb 9 g, Dietary Fiber 4 g, Sugars 2 g, Protein 4 g

Walnut Taco Salad ⑥

YIELD: 6 CUPS SALAD

Prep time: 30 minutes, Total time: 30 minutes, Serving size: 1 cup, Number of servings: 6

The walnut crumble is a superb meat alternative in this dish as it provides a nice chewy texture, absorbing the flavors while also maintaining its superfood qualities that promote brain and heart health. Avocado further enhances the healing benefits with wonderful fats, vitamins, and minerals to keep you beautiful and vibrant while indulging in a perfect satisfying meal. completed by herbs and spices that each add both flavor and extra trace minerals. Serve as part of a Mexican feast with Tempeh Fajitas (page 279) and Watermelon Gazpacho (page 243).

4 cups chopped romaine lettuce

1 cup chopped tomato

1 cup chopped avocado

¼ cup plus 2 tablespoons Raw Walnut Crumble (recipe follows)

½ cup Cilantro Lime Vinaigrette (page 221)

Raw Cashew Sour Cream (page 113) (optional)

1. Place the lettuce in a bowl. Top with the tomato and avocado.

2. Sprinkle the Raw Walnut Crumble on top of the salad.

3. Drizzle with the Cilantro Lime Vinaigrette and Raw Cashew Sour Cream, if using, and enjoy!

Nutrition Facts per serving (113 g): Calories 180, Fat Calories 145, Total Fat 16 g, Saturated Fat 2 g, Cholesterol 0 mg, Sodium 60 mg, Total Carb 9 g, Dietary Fiber 4 g, Sugars 3 g, Protein 4 g

Raw Walnut Crumble ♥ⓖ◆

YIELD: 1 CUP CRUMBLE

Prep time: 10 minutes, Total time: 10 minutes, Serving size: 1 tablespoon, Number of servings: 16

2 cups roughly chopped walnuts
1 ½ teaspoons ground cumin
1 teaspoon chili powder
⅛ teaspoon chipotle chile powder or cayenne pepper
1 tablespoon finely chopped fresh cilantro
¼ teaspoon sea salt, or to taste
⅛ teaspoon freshly ground black pepper
1 tablespoon water
2 teaspoons freshly squeezed lime juice

1. Place all the ingredients in a food processor and pulse chop until the walnuts are just ground. Do not overprocess.

VARIATIONS

♥ For a fully raw salad, use the oil-free variation of the Cilantro Lime Vinaigrette (page 221)

Replace the romaine lettuce with mixed salad greens or arugula.

Add your favorite veggies to your salad, including cucumber, radishes, microgreens, sprouts, sliced mushrooms, or bell pepper.

Nutrition Facts per serving (22 g): Calories 100, Fat Calories 85, Total Fat 10 g, Saturated Fat 1 g, Cholesterol 0 mg, Sodium 40 mg, Total Carb 2 g, Dietary Fiber 1 g, Sugars 0 g, Protein 2 g

TEMPLATE RECIPE
Legume and Vegetable Salad

Legume component: Replace the black beans with cannellini or pinto beans, chickpeas, or your favorite.

Vegetable component: Replace the corn and bell pepper with veggies of your choosing, such as peas, chopped cucumber, tomatoes, or celery. Add 1 cup of diced jicama and ½ teaspoon of seeded and diced jalapeño.

Dressing component: Add 1 ½ tablespoons of coconut oil along with the lime juice. Add ½ cup of your dressing of choice, such as Creamy Pepita (page 227), Raw Hempseed Ranch (page 224), or Horseradish Dijon (page 226).

Ethnic spice component: Replace the chile powder, cumin, and oregano with 1 tablespoon of an ethnic spice blend, such as Ethiopian (page 106), Moroccan (page 106), or Indian (page 106).

Herb component: Replace the cilantro with fresh dill, parsley, or basil.

Black Bean and Corn Salad⊕�♦▱

YIELD: 2 ½ CUPS SALAD

Prep time: 20 minutes, Total time: 20 minutes, Serving size: 1/2 cup, Number of servings: 5

A perfect blend of sweet and savory chewiness and crunch, with a Mexican flair, this is a great go-to salad for a party since it is easy to prepare and presents very well. Black beans have a have superior fiber and protein content, which makes this simple salad pack a punch. Strong immunity-boosters, such as garlic and chile; the heart-healthy antioxidants in cumin; and natural cleansing agent cilantro round out this colorful salad. Serve on its own with chips for a light snack, or as a side topped with Glorious Guacamole (page 151).

1 (15-ounce) can black beans, drained and rinsed well, or 1 ½ cups cooked (see page 98)

1 cup fresh or frozen (thawed) corn

¼ cup seeded and diced red bell pepper

¼ cup thinly sliced green onion or diced red onion

3 tablespoons freshly squeezed lime juice

1 ½ tablespoons finely chopped fresh cilantro

1 garlic clove, pressed or minced

½ teaspoon seeded and diced jalapeño pepper (optional)

1 teaspoon chili powder

½ teaspoon ground cumin

½ teaspoon dried oregano (optional)

⅛ teaspoon chipotle chile powder (optional)

½ teaspoon sea salt, or to taste

⅛ teaspoon freshly ground black pepper

1 ½ teaspoons wheat-free tamari or other soy sauce (optional)

1. Combine all the ingredients in a bowl and mix well.

Nutrition Facts per serving (108 g): Calories 200, Fat Calories 20, Total Fat 2 g, Saturated Fat 0 g, Cholesterol 0 mg, Sodium 255 mg, Total Carb 39 g, Dietary Fiber 8 g, Sugars 0 g, Protein 8 g

Ginger Rainbow Chard⊕�♦▱

YIELD: 3 CUPS CHARD

Prep time: 10 minutes, Cook time: 10 minutes, Total time: 20 minutes, Serving size: 3/4 cup, Number of servings: 4

Ginger zests up these greens flavorfully while adding incredible immunity-boosting properties. Upset stomachs and cold and flu are soothed by ginger's antinausea and decongesting benefits. By adding a bunch of chard, you get the extraordinary antioxidant protection of its carotenoid phytonutrients. If that weren't enough, the rainbow chard provides lutein for eye health and calcium for bone health. Serve along with Golden Rice (page 204) and Simple Baked Tofu (page 260) with Zesty Chimichurri Sauce (page 231).

¼ cup water or vegetable stock (see page 108)

1 tablespoon peeled and minced fresh ginger

1 cup thinly sliced carrot

1 large bunch rainbow chard, cut into ½-inch pieces (4 cups tightly packed)

1 tablespoon rice vinegar

½ teaspoon wheat-free tamari or other soy sauce, or to taste

2 tablespoons sesame seeds

1. Place the water or stock in a pot over medium-high heat. Add the ginger and carrot and cook for 3 minutes, stirring frequently and adding a small amount of water, if necessary, to prevent sticking.

2. Add the chard and cook for 5 minutes, stirring frequently with tongs and adding a small amount of water, if necessary, to prevent sticking.

3. Remove the chard with the tongs and place on a serving plate, leaving as much carrot as possible in the pot. Then, use a slotted spoon to place the carrot slices on top of the chard.

4. Drizzle the vinegar and tamari over the vegetables and top with sesame seeds before serving.

VARIATIONS

Add 2 teaspoons of toasted sesame oil along with the tamari.

You can sauté the ginger and carrot in 2 teaspoons of coconut oil, before adding the water.

Replace the ginger with garlic and the rice vinegar with balsamic vinegar.

Toss in 2 cups of raw chopped greens, such as kale, chard, spinach, or arugula.

Nutrition Facts per serving (77 g): Calories 55, Fat Calories 20, Total Fat 2.5 g, Saturated Fat 0 g, Cholesterol 0 mg, Sodium 260 mg, Total Carb 7 g, Dietary Fiber 2 g, Sugars 3 g, Protein 2 g

TEMPLATE RECIPE
Simple Green Sauté

Oil component: Instead of cooking the vegetables in water or stock, use a high-heat oil, such as coconut, sesame, or grapeseed. Small amounts of oils, such as hemp, flax, pumpkin seed, or olive, can be drizzled on after the greens are cooked, to avoid heating.

Green component: Rotate through kale, chard, collards, cabbage, beet greens, dandelion greens, mustard greens, turnip greens, or wild greens.

Veggie add-on component: Rotate through ginger, garlic, onion, mushrooms, or bell peppers.

Dressing component: Simply dress with fresh squeezed lemon or lime juice. Or use a splash of mirin, balsamic vinegar, tamari, rice wine vinegar, or red or white wine.

Heat component: Try cayenne pepper, crushed red pepper flakes, or seeded and diced hot chile peppers (see the Scoville scale on page 179).

Ethnic spice component: Create a world fusion flair by rotating through the various spice blends (see pages 105–106). Always start with a small amount of spices and work your way up until the desired flavor is achieved.

Season with salt and freshly ground black pepper to taste.

Collards and Red Beans

Here is another simple and colorful sauté. Place 1 tablespoon of coconut oil or 3 tablespoons of water in a pot over medium-high heat. Add 1/2 sliced yellow onion and two pressed or minced garlic cloves. Sauté for 3 minutes, stirring frequently. Add one bunch of thinly sliced collards and cook for 5 minutes, stirring frequently. Add one 15-ounce can of kidney beans, drained and rinsed, and cook for 5 minutes, stirring frequently. Season with freshly squeezed lemon juice, a splash of tamari, and 1 tablespoon of an ethnic spice blend, such as Mexican (page 106), Indian (page 106), or Ethiopian (page 106). Add salt, freshly ground black pepper, and crushed red pepper flakes to taste.

Garlicky Greens Ⓖ

YIELD: 2 ½ CUPS GREENS

Prep time: 5 minutes, Cook time: 10 minutes, Total time: 15 minutes, Serving size: 1/2 cup, Number of servings: 5

The name says it all in this simple dish bursting with garlicky goodness. In the onion family, garlic has been imparting its pungent flavor and warding off vampires and sickness for thousands of years. Its healing comes from its role as an immunity booster and an antioxidant source. Greens, such as kale, need little introduction: maximally nutrient dense, low in calories, and plentiful in antioxidant vitamins A, C, and K plus vital phytonutrients. Enjoy along with Maple Baked Tempeh (page 262) topped with Roasted Red Pepper Sauce (page 235) along with Unfried Rice (page 205).

¼ cup water

5 garlic cloves, pressed or minced

1 large bunch kale, stemmed, rinsed well, and chopped into ½-inch pieces (4 cups tightly packed)

2 tablespoons freshly squeezed lemon juice

½ teaspoon sea salt, or to taste

¼ teaspoon freshly ground black pepper

¼ teaspoon crushed red pepper flakes (optional)

1 tablespoon olive, flax, or hemp oil (optional)

1. Place the water in a large sauté pan over medium-high heat. When the water begins to simmer, add the garlic and cook for 2 minutes, stirring frequently.

2. Add the kale, cover, and cook until just tender, about 5 minutes, stirring frequently with tongs. Transfer to a bowl.

3. Add the remaining ingredients, and stir well before serving.

VARIATIONS

Replace the kale with other greens, such as collards, chard, beet greens, dandelion greens, or mustard greens.

You can sauté 1 cup of sliced shiitake mushrooms, and/or 1 cup of seeded diced red bell pepper for 3 minutes before adding the kale.

Add 1 tablespoon of an ethnic spice blend, such as Indian (page 106), Italian (page 105), Mexican (page 106), or Moroccan (page 106).

◆ For an oil-free version, omit the oil.

Nutrition Facts per serving (63 g): Calories 35, Fat Calories 5, Total Fat 0 g, Saturated Fat 0 g,

Cholesterol 0 mg, Sodium 255 mg, Total Carb 7 g,
Dietary Fiber 2 g, Sugars 1 g, Protein 2 g

Roasted Zucchini and Corn G

YIELD: 3 ½ CUPS ZUCCHINI AND CORN

Prep time: 15 minutes, Cook time: 25 minutes,
Total time: 40 minutes, Serving size: 1/2 cup,
Number of servings: 7

Zucchini is part of the gourd family and is a rapid grower, though the smaller ones are the most flavorful. When roasted, zucchini has an almost buttery flavor. It boasts a large vitamin C content, lutein, and zeaxanthin for healthy eye maintenance, folate, vitamin B$_{12}$, and manganese, which protects tissues from harmful free radicals. The red peppers in this summery side dish provide additional vitamin C, eye health benefits from vitamin A, and popping color. The corn adds additional sweetness, fiber, and antioxidant benefits. Toss with cooked rice pasta, top with nutritional yeast, and serve along with Cauliflower Casserole (page 285).

4 cups sliced zucchini (½-inch slices)
½ cup seeded and diced red bell pepper
½ cup thinly sliced yellow onion
4 garlic cloves, pressed or minced
1 ½ tablespoons coconut oil (optional)
¾ teaspoon sea salt, or to taste
¼ teaspoon freshly ground black pepper
¼ teaspoon crushed red pepper flakes
1 cup fresh or frozen (thawed) corn
1 tablespoon minced fresh dill
2 teaspoons freshly squeezed lemon juice
2 teaspoons red wine vinegar or coconut
   vinegar

1. Preheat the oven to 400°F. Place the zucchini, bell pepper, onion, garlic, oil, if using, salt, black pepper, and crushed red pepper in a large bowl and mix well.

2. Transfer to a baking sheet and bake for 15 minutes. Remove from the oven, add the corn, mix well, and cook for an additional 10 minutes.

3. Remove from the oven, add the remaining ingredients, and stir well before serving.

VARIATIONS

Add 1 cup of thinly sliced mushrooms along with the corn.

Replace the dill with 2 tablespoons of fresh cilantro, basil, or flat-leaf parsley.

Go Indian by adding 2 tablespoons of minced fresh cilantro, 1 tablespoon of curry powder, and 2 teaspoons of ground cumin.

Go Mexican by adding 2 tablespoons of minced fresh cilantro, 1 tablespoon of chili powder, 1 teaspoon of ground cumin, and ¼ teaspoon of chipotle chile powder.

♦ For an oil-free version, replace the oil with water or vegetable stock (see page 108).

Nutrition Facts per serving (89 g): Calories 125,
Fat Calories 30, Total Fat 3 g, Saturated Fat 2 g,
Cholesterol 0 mg, Sodium 260 mg, Total Carb 21 g,
Dietary Fiber 3 g, Sugars 1 g, Protein 4 g

Chili Lime Grilled Asparagus with Mushrooms and Bell Pepper ⊙

YIELD: 4 CUPS ASPARAGUS

Prep time: 15 minutes, Cook time: 15 minutes,
Total time: 30 minutes, Serving size: 1 cup,
Number of servings: 4

Hold on to your sombrero as you enjoy the tangy, charred, and Mexican-themed undertones of this grilled veggie dish. Prepare for a double dose of varied health-benefiting properties from this potent combo. Portobello mushrooms deliver quality protein and carbs, plus potassium, phosphorus, and B vitamins. Asparagus's specialties include a detoxifying compound called glutathione, and the amino acid asparagine, a natural diuretic that helps the body eliminate excess salt. Serve as a side with Black Bean Grits (page 272) or Mexican Seitan-Stuffed Peppers (page 291).

MARINADE
¼ cup water
1 ½ tablespoons melted coconut or olive oil
½ teaspoon sea salt, or to taste
¼ teaspoon freshly ground black pepper
¼ teaspoon crushed red pepper flakes
¼ teaspoon chili powder
Pinch of chipotle chile powder (optional)

VEGETABLES
1 bunch asparagus, tough bottoms removed
2 large portobello mushrooms, gills removed
1 red bell pepper, seeded and quartered
1 ½ tablespoons freshly squeezed lime juice
1 tablespoon finely chopped fresh cilantro

1. Preheat a grill to high heat.

2. Prepare the marinade: Place the water, oil, salt, black pepper, crushed red pepper flakes, chili powder, and chipotle chile powder, if using, on a shallow baking sheet and whisk well.

3. Add the asparagus and toss well to evenly coat. Add the mushrooms and bell pepper and flip to coat.

4. Place the asparagus, mushrooms, and bell pepper on the grill, and grill until the vegetables are just tender and char marks appear, about 15 minutes, depending upon the heat of the grill and the thickness of the asparagus and mushrooms. Flip the vegetables with tongs frequently, to prevent burning.

5. Remove the asparagus and place on a serving tray. Remove the mushrooms and bell peppers, and place on a cutting board. Slice into ½-inch pieces. Place on top of the asparagus.

6. Top the vegetables with any remaining marinade. Sprinkle with the lime juice and cilantro before serving.

VARIATIONS
Go Italian by replacing the chili powder in the marinade with 1 tablespoon of Italian Spice Mix (page 105) or 2 teaspoons of dried oregano and 1 teaspoon of dried thyme. Replace the lime juice with freshly squeezed lemon juice and 2 teaspoons of balsamic vinegar, and replace the cilantro with 2 tablespoons chiffonaded fresh basil and 1 tablespoon of finely chopped fresh flat-leaf parsley.

💧 For an oil-free version, replace the oil in the marinade with additional water or vegetable stock (see page 108).

Nutrition Facts per serving (84 g): Calories 65, Fat Calories 50, Total Fat 5.5 g, Saturated Fat 3 g, Cholesterol 0 mg, Sodium 300 mg, Total Carb 4 g, Dietary Fiber 1 g, Sugars 2 g, Protein 1 g

Broasted Brussels Sprouts ⓖ

YIELD: 3 CUPS BRUSSELS SPROUTS

Prep time: 15 minutes, Cook time: 10 minutes, Total time: 25 minutes, Serving size: 1/2 cup, Number of servings: 6

Look no further for a tasty way to feed your children (or anyone you love) Brussels sprouts. Cruciferous Brussels sprouts offer an abundant supply of potassium, iron, protein, vitamin C, fiber, and folate, a B vitamin. Paired with nutritional yeast, a plant-based solution to vitamin B_{12} that also supplies a cheesy flavor, and more vitamin C in the tang of lemon, these sprouts can be enjoyed by kids of all ages. Serve along with Ital Roasted Squash and Sweet Potato Soup (page 251) and Lentil Walnut Loaf (page 288).

¼ cup water
1 ½ tablespoons melted coconut oil (optional)
½ teaspoon sea salt, or to taste
¼ teaspoon freshly ground black pepper
¼ teaspoon crushed red pepper flakes
4 cups thinly sliced Brussels sprouts (⅛-inch slices)
1 ½ tablespoons nutritional yeast
1 tablespoon freshly squeezed lemon juice

1. Preheat the oven broiler on LOW. Place the water, coconut oil, if using, salt, black pepper, and crushed red pepper flakes on a baking sheet and mix well. Add the Brussels sprouts and toss well to coat.

2. Place in the oven and cook for 10 minutes, carefully stirring a few times to ensure even cooking.

3. Remove from the oven and place in a bowl. Add the nutritional yeast and lemon juice, and stir well before serving.

VARIATIONS

Indulge and add ½ cup of grated vegan mozzarella-style cheese after roasting. Replace the coconut oil with olive oil.

Add two pressed or minced garlic cloves and/or 1 cup of seeded and diced red bell pepper along with the Brussels sprouts.

💧 For an oil-free version, replace the oil with vegetable stock (see page 108) or water.

Nutrition Facts per serving (63 g): Calories 30, Fat Calories 0, Total Fat 0g, Saturated Fat 4.5 g, Cholesterol 0 mg, Sodium 210 mg, Total Carb 6 g, Dietary Fiber 3 g, Sugars 1 g, Protein 3 g

Broiled Cauliflower with Sun-Dried Tomatoes ⓖ

YIELD: 3 ½ CUPS CAULIFLOWER

Prep time: 10 minutes, Cook time: 10 minutes, Total time: 20 minutes, Serving size: 1/2 cup, Number of servings: 7

Boasting a host of nutritional benefits, cauliflower may be supplanting kale as the "it" health food! Broiling imparts a smoky flavor and crisps up its outside while leaving the center soft and tender. A member of the cruciferous family, providing vitamin C, potassium, fiber, folic acid, and a sulfur compound called isothiocyanate, cauliflower is versatile in both its raw and cooked forms. Cooked lightly here and enhanced with the protein, fiber, iron, and potassium of nutrient-retaining sun-dried tomatoes and basil, cauliflower shines at its most flavorful. Serve along with Moroccan Chickpea Stew (page 255) and Israeli Couscous Tabouli (page 203).

¼ cup sun-dried tomatoes

¼ cup water

1½ tablespoons coconut oil (optional)

½ teaspoon sea salt, or to taste

⅛ teaspoon freshly ground black pepper

Pinch of crushed red pepper flakes

1 large cauliflower, cut into small florets
　　(5 ½ cups)

1 tablespoon freshly squeezed lemon juice

2 tablespoons chiffonaded fresh basil

Pine nuts, for garnish (optionally toasted;
　　see page 101)

1. Preheat the oven broiler on HIGH. Place the sun-dried tomatoes in a bowl with ample hot water to cover.

2. Place the ¼ cup of water, coconut oil, if using, salt, black pepper, and crushed red pepper flakes on a small baking sheet and mix well. Add the cauliflower and toss well to coat. Place in the oven.

3. Broil for 5 minutes. Carefully remove from the oven and stir well. Return to the oven and broil until the cauliflower is just tender, about 5 minutes. Transfer to a bowl.

4. Meanwhile, when the sun-dried tomatoes are soft, cut into very thin slices. Add to the cauliflower. Add the lemon juice and basil and toss well. Top with the pine nuts before serving.

VARIATIONS

Add additional Italian herbs along with the basil, such as 2 tablespoons of finely chopped fresh flat-leaf parsley, 1 tablespoon of chiffonaded fresh sage, 1 teaspoon of fresh oregano, and ½ teaspoon of fresh thyme.

Go Indian by adding 2 tablespoons of minced fresh cilantro, 1 tablespoon of curry powder, and 2 teaspoons of ground cumin.

Go Mexican by adding 2 tablespoons of minced fresh cilantro, 1 tablespoon of chili powder, 1 teaspoon of ground cumin, and ¼ teaspoon of chipotle chile powder.

◗ For an oil-free version, replace the oil with vegetable stock (see page 108) or water.

Nutrition Facts per serving (90 g): Calories 30, Fat Calories 5, Total Fat 0.5g, Saturated Fat 0 g, Cholesterol 0 mg, Sodium 230 mg, Total Carb 6 g, Dietary Fiber 2 g, Sugars 2 g, Protein 2 g

Steamed Italian Baby Bok Choy⊙

YIELD: 2 BABY BOK CHOY

Prep time: 10 minutes, Cook time: 10 minutes, Total time: 20 minutes, Serving size: 1/2 baby bok choy, Number of servings: 4

What can be better than the merging of Eastern and Western cultures, as found here in this dish uniting bok choy with Italian seasonings. Bok choy, also known as pak choy, is commonly found in Asian produce markets, given its origins in China. A cruciferous vegetable, bok choy is, in one package, low calorie and nutrient dense: high in vitamins, minerals, phytochemicals, antioxidants, as well as water content. This recipe combines it with many other top ingredients, making it a nutritionally complete side. Serve as a side with pasta topped with Fire-Roasted Tomato Sauce (page 239) and cubed and roasted Simple Baked Tofu (page 260).

2 baby bok choy, halved lengthwise
2 teaspoons coconut oil
¾ cup diced shallot or onion
2 garlic cloves, pressed or minced
¼ teaspoon dried oregano
¼ teaspoon dried thyme
½ cup diced shiitake mushrooms
½ cup diced tomato
2 tablespoons freshly squeezed lemon juice
1 ½ tablespoons finely chopped parsley
1 ½ tablespoons chiffonaded fresh basil
1 tablespoon nutritional yeast (optional)
Pinch of sea salt, or to taste
⅛ teaspoon freshly ground black pepper
Pinch of crushed red pepper flakes
2 tablespoons pine nuts (optionally toasted; see page 101)

1. Place water in a pot with a steamer basket over medium-high heat. Add the bok choy. Cover and cook until the bottom of the bok choy is just tender and the leaves are still a darker shade of green, about 5 minutes, depending upon the size of the bok choy. Remove from the heat. Drain well and place on a serving platter.

2. Meanwhile, place the oil in a sauté pan over medium-high heat. Add the shallot, garlic, oregano, and thyme and cook for 2 minutes, stirring frequently. Add the shiitake mushrooms and cook, stirring frequently, for 5 minutes, or until the shiitakes are just tender. Remove from the heat.

3. Add the tomato, lemon juice, parsley, basil, nutritional yeast, if using, salt, black pepper, and crushed red pepper flakes and mix well. Place ¼ cup on top of each baby bok choy, and garnish with pine nuts, if using, before serving.

VARIATIONS

Try grilling the bok choy (see page 101). Replace the baby bok choy with regular-size bok choy, steamed tatsoi, or cabbage.

Replace the bok choy with four romaine lettuce leaves.

Steam the bok choy and replace the topping with Smoky Salsa (page 151), Sloppy Joe filling (page 281) or the filling from Mexican Seitan-Stuffed Peppers (page 291).

You can also chop the bok choy into 1-inch pieces. Steam until just tender, and toss with remaining ingredients.

◆ For an oil-free version, use the water sauté method (see page 101).

Nutrition Facts per serving (579 g): Calories 160, Fat Calories 65, Total Fat 7.5 g, Saturated Fat 3 g, Cholesterol 0 mg, Sodium 100 mg, Total Carb 21 g, Dietary Fiber 7 g, Sugars 10 g, Protein 9 g

Three Greens with Tomato Sauce ⓖ

YIELD: 2 ½ CUPS GREENS

Prep time: 5 minutes, Cook time: 15 minutes, Total time: 20 minutes, Serving size: 1/2 cup, Number of servings: 5

Three greens are better than one, and with collards, kale, and chard, this recipe certainly does the body good. They are all low fat, cholesterol free, and super fibrous, as well as offer vitamins A and C, calcium, and iron. You'll really be able to say you've gone green, and may feel the burst of energy as well. Serve with Green Quinoa (page 203) and Ratatouille (page 273). Also wonderful when served over pasta, rice, or quinoa.

1 tablespoon coconut oil
3 garlic cloves, pressed or minced
2 cups stemmed and thinly sliced collards (⅛ by 1-inch slices)
1 ½ cups vegan tomato sauce, store-bought or homemade (page 239)
1 cup thinly sliced kale (⅛ by 1-inch slices)
1 cup stemmed and thinly sliced Swiss chard (⅛ by 1-inch slices)
1 tablespoon balsamic vinegar

1 tablespoon nutritional yeast (optional)
½ teaspoon sea salt, or to taste
⅛ teaspoon freshly ground black pepper
Pinch of crushed red pepper flakes

1. Place the oil in a pot over medium-high heat. Pour in the oil. Add the garlic and cook for 2 minutes, stirring constantly. Add the collards and cook for 5 minutes, stirring frequently and adding small amounts of water or vegetable stock (page 108), if necessary, to prevent sticking.

2. Add the tomato sauce, kale, and chard, and cook for 5 minutes, stirring frequently.

3. Add the remaining ingredients and stir well before serving.

VARIATIONS

Include additional greens, such as dandelion greens, mustard greens, or beet greens.

Add 1 cup of crumbled tempeh or extra-firm tofu along with the tomato sauce.

Replace the tomato sauce with Oil-Free Cream Sauce (page 235), Roasted Red Pepper Sauce (page 232), or 1 cup of Ancho Chile Sauce (page 232).

◆ For an oil-free version, use the water sauté method (see page 101).

Nutrition Facts per serving (156 g): Calories 70, Fat Calories 30, Total Fat 3 g, Saturated Fat 2.5 g, Cholesterol 0 mg, Sodium 270 mg, Total Carb 10 g, Dietary Fiber 2 g, Sugars 5 g, Protein 2 g

Edamame Arame Salad ⊙◆

YIELD: 6 CUPS SALAD

Prep time: 20 minutes, Cook time: 7 minutes,
Total time: 25 minutes, Serving size: 1 cup,
Number of servings: 6

Edamame is a more exotic name for boiled green soybeans, which are chock-full of fiber and protein as well as vitamins A and C, iron, and calcium. Arame is a nutritious sea vegetable that boasts a slew of nutrients including vitamin A, calcium, iron, zinc, manganese, folate, and iodine, helpful for healthy thyroid function. The base of this salad is napa cabbage, a Beijing area–originating Chinese cabbage that may have emanated from a cross between bok choy and turnips. It features a springlike light green color, a sweet and celery-like crunch, and is loaded with antioxidants and fiber, alongside folates and vitamins C and K. Toss with the following dressing or the Oil-Free Asian Umeboshi Dressing (page 220), and serve with Nori Rolls (page 263) and Miso Vegetable Soup (page 246).

3 tablespoons arame sea vegetable (see page 86)
1 ¼ cups shelled edamame
3 cups thinly sliced napa cabbage
1 cup thinly sliced purple cabbage
1 cup fresh or frozen (thawed) corn
¾ cup seeded and diced red bell pepper
1 ½ tablespoons finely chopped fresh cilantro
¼ cup thinly sliced green onion

ARAME SALAD DRESSING
1 ½ tablespoons umeboshi vinegar (see page 220)
1 tablespoon water
¼ teaspoon wheat-free tamari or other soy sauce, or to taste
1 tablespoon apple juice (optional)
2 teaspoons peeled and minced fresh ginger
1 teaspoon Dijon or Chinese mustard
Pinch of crushed red pepper flakes

1. Place the arame in a small cup or bowl.

2. Bring a pot of water to boil over high heat. Remove about 1 cup of the water and add to the arame. Lower the heat to medium, add the edamame to the pot, and cook until just soft, about 8 minutes.

3. Meanwhile, combine the napa cabbage, purple cabbage, corn, bell pepper, cilantro, and green onion in a large bowl and toss well.

4. Prepare the dressing: Combine the dressing ingredients in a small bowl and whisk well.

5. When the edamame are done cooking, drain well, and rinse under cold water until cool. Add to the vegetables.

6. Drain the arame, add to the vegetables, and toss to combine. Discard the soak water or use to water your plants.

7. Add the dressing and gently toss well.

VARIATIONS

Top with sesame seeds (optionally toasted; see page 101).

Add 1 tablespoon of melted coconut oil or toasted sesame oil to the dressing.

Replace all or some of the red cabbage, corn, and bell pepper with assorted chopped vegetables, including cucumber, jicama, or zucchini.

Add 1 cup of grated carrot, beet, parsnip, or daikon.

Top with mung bean sprouts before serving.

Nutrition Facts per serving (158 g): Calories 170, Fat Calories 25, Total Fat 3 g, Saturated Fat 0 g, Cholesterol 0 mg, Sodium 310 mg, Total Carb 32 g, Dietary Fiber 6 g, Sugars 4 g, Protein 7 g

Parsnip Fries [Ⓖ]

YIELD: 4 CUPS FRIES

Prep time: 10 minutes, Cook time: 35 minutes, Total time: 45 minutes, Serving size: 1 cup, Number of servings: 4

Do you fancy some fries with a side of folate and potassium? Try this parsnippy version. A root vegetable native to Eurasia, parsnips have a close relation with the more commonly used carrot, including the similarity of raw edibility and hint of sweetness. One of my favorite veggies, they are creamy when roasted. Serve with Magnificent Mushroom Burger (page 270) or Millet Black Bean Veggie Burgers (page 269) and Waldorf Salad (page 180) or Caesar Salad (page 181).

4 medium-size parsnips
1 tablespoon coconut oil
1 ½ tablespoons nutritional yeast (optional)
¼ teaspoon sea salt, or to taste
¼ teaspoon paprika
⅛ teaspoon freshly ground black pepper
Pinch of cayenne pepper
Oil, for baking sheet
1 tablespoon freshly squeezed lime juice

1. Preheat the oven to 400°F. Slice the parsnips into matchsticks about 3 inches long and ½ inch thick. Measure out 4 cups for this recipe.

2. Place in a bowl with the oil, nutritional yeast, if using, salt, paprika, black pepper, and cayenne and toss well.

3. Transfer to a well-oiled baking sheet and bake until just crispy, about 35 minutes, stirring occasionally with a spatula to prevent sticking.

4. Drizzle with the lime juice before serving.

VARIATIONS

Replace the parsnip with sweet potato, russet potato, carrot, turnip, or rutabega.

Add 1 tablespoon of an ethnic spice blend, such as Mexican (page 106), Indian (page 106), or Ethiopian (page 106), along with the salt and pepper.

🍴 Replace the oil in the recipe with 3 tablespoons of water or vegetable stock (see page 108). Replace the oil on the baking sheet with additional water or vegetable stock.

Nutrition Facts per serving (190 g): Calories 130, Fat Calories 35, Total Fat 4 g, Saturated Fat 3 g, Cholesterol 0 mg, Sodium 160 mg, Total Carb 24 g, Dietary Fiber 7 g, Sugars 6 g, Protein 2 g

Cauliflower Steak with Ethiopian-Spiced Almonds⊙

YIELD: 4 PORTIONS

Prep time: 10 minutes, if spice mix is already made,
Cook time: 30 minutes, Total time: 40 minutes,
Serving size: 1 steak, Number of servings: 4

Cut flat and thick and then roasted, our friendly neighborhood cauliflower offers a new way to enjoy a perfectly cooked "steak," as well as the health benefits of a tasty crucifer. The exotically flavored almonds, used as a "steak" topping, also bring protein, fiber, vitamin E, manganese, and magnesium. Serve with Cream of Kale (page 201) and Unfried Rice (page 205).

¼ cup water or vegetable stock (see page 108)
2 teaspoons melted coconut or olive oil
½ teaspoon sea salt, or to taste
⅛ teaspoon freshly ground black pepper
1 medium-size cauliflower
1 large tomato, cut into ½-inch slices
1 ½ tablespoons freshly squeezed lemon juice
1 ½ tablespoons nutritional yeast (optional)

ETHIOPIAN-SPICED ALMONDS
½ cup raw almonds
½ teaspoon Ethiopian (Berbere) spice mix, store-bought or homemade (page 106)
Pinch of sea salt, or to taste
Pinch of freshly ground black pepper

1. Preheat the oven to 400°F. Place the water or stock, oil, salt, and pepper in a baking dish and whisk well.

2. Cut off the very bottom of the cauliflower and remove the outer leaves. Carefully slice the cauliflower vertically into ½-inch-thick slices. Place in the baking dish along with any loose florets. Coat well.

3. Place in the oven and roast for 15 minutes. Carefully flip and roast for an additional 5 minutes. Remove from the oven, top each cutlet with a slice of tomato, and return to the oven. Bake for 10 minutes. Remove from the oven, and top with the lemon juice and nutritional yeast, if using.

4. Meanwhile, prepare the spiced almonds: Place the spiced almond ingredients in a small food processor and process until just ground.

5. Top each cauliflower steak with the Ethiopian-Spiced Almonds before serving.

VARIATIONS

Top with chopped olives and diced green onion.

Replace the cauliflower with tempeh or tofu cutlets.

Replace the Berbere spice mix with 1 teaspoon of Mexican Spice Mix (page 106) or Indian Spice Mix (page 106), or 1 tablespoon of Italian Spice Mix (page 105).

Replace the almonds with seeds or nuts of your choosing, such as hazelnuts, pecans, pistachios, hemp seeds, or pumpkin seeds.

♦For an oil-free version, omit the oil.

Nutrition Facts per serving (268 g): Calories 170, Fat Calories 100, Total Fat 11.5 g, Saturated Fat 3 g, Cholesterol 0 mg, Sodium 340 mg, Total Carb 13 g, Dietary Fiber 6 g, Sugars 5 g, Protein 7 g

Cream of Kale⊙

YIELD: 3 CUPS CREAM OF KALE

Prep time: 15 minutes, Cook time: 10 minutes, Total time: 25 minutes, Serving size: 1/2 cup, Number of servings: 6

Convert any kale-doubters by this modern-day, plant-based version of the old favorite cream of spinach, no heavy cream needed. The outside flavors allow anyone to reap the benefits of a hearty kale portion: fiber; vitamins A, B_6, C, and K; and the minerals calcium, potassium, copper, and manganese. Serve along with Maple Baked Tempeh (page 262), Unfried Rice (page 205), and Broiled Cauliflower with Sun-Dried Tomatoes (page 194).

2 teaspoons coconut oil

1 cup diced yellow onion

2 tablespoons minced garlic

1 teaspoon fennel seeds

½ cup thinly sliced shiitake mushrooms

4 cups finely chopped kale

¾ cup soy, almond, coconut, or rice milk (for homemade, see Plant-Based Milk, page 104)

¼ cup raw cashews

½ teaspoon sea salt, or to taste

⅛ teaspoon freshly ground black pepper

1 tablespoon freshly squeezed lemon juice

1 ½ tablespoons nutritional yeast (optional)

1. Place the oil in a sauté pan over medium-high heat. Add the onion, garlic, and fennel seeds and cook for 3 minutes, stirring frequently. Add the mushrooms and cook for 3 minutes, stirring frequently and adding small amounts of water, if necessary, to prevent sticking.

2. Add the kale and cook for 5 minutes, stirring frequently.

3. Transfer to a food processor with the remaining ingredients and process until just pureed. Serve warm.

VARIATIONS

Add 1 teaspoon of seeded and diced jalapeño pepper along with the shiitake mushrooms.

Replace the soy milk with soy yogurt.

Replace the kale with spinach, broccoli, cauliflower, corn, or Romanesco.

Top with toasted pumpkin seeds or sunflower seeds (see page 101).

For a taste of India, add 2 teaspoons of curry powder, 1 teaspoon of ground cumin, and 1 ½ tablespoons of minced fresh cilantro.

⬥For an oil-free version, use the water sauté method (see page 101).

Nutrition Facts per serving (169 g): Calories 120, Fat Calories 60, Total Fat 7 g, Saturated Fat 2 g, Cholesterol 0 mg, Sodium 230 mg, Total Carb 12 g, Dietary Fiber 3 g, Sugars 3 g, Protein 5 g

Smashed Roasted Cauliflower and Parsnip◉

YIELD: 3 CUPS CAULIFLOWER AND PARSNIP

Prep time: 20 minutes, Cook time: 40 minutes,
Total time: 60 minutes, Serving size: 1/2 cup,
Number of servings: 6

Anytime you crave that starch-heavy old standby, mashed potatoes, try this super-comforting (and lighter) alternative, made from cauliflower and parsnip, instead! Cruciferous cauliflower gets its name from the Latin root *caulis*, meaning "cabbage," which makes it fitting that its ancestry goes back to the wild cabbage of Asia Minor. You may find cauliflower in other colors, such as purple, orange, or green—the hue is dependent on the amount of chlorophyll received during growth. White cauliflower is easy to find and preserves that mashed potato look. Here, it teams up with parsnips (cousin to the carrot) to offer much vitamin C, fiber, folic acid, and potassium. If you wish, you can garnish with smoked paprika and minced chives, and serve with a salad along with Simple Baked Tofu (page 206) or Maple Baked Tempeh (page 262) and Oil-Free Mushroom Gravy (page 240).

4 cups small cauliflower florets
3 cups chopped parsnip (½-inch pieces)
5 large garlic cloves
2 teaspoons coconut oil
½ teaspoon sea salt, or to taste
¼ teaspoon freshly ground black pepper
½ teaspoon crushed red pepper flakes
½ cup water or vegetable stock (page 108)
Oil, for baking sheet
¼ cup light or full-fat coconut milk

1. Preheat the oven to 400°F. Place the cauliflower, parsnip, garlic, coconut oil, salt, black pepper, crushed red pepper flakes, and water or stock on a well-oiled baking sheet, and toss well.

2. Roast until the vegetables are thoroughly cooked through, about 45 minutes, stirring occasionally.

3. Transfer to a food processor along with the coconut milk and pulse chop five or six times, until well mashed.

VARIATIONS

◆For an oil-free version, replace the oil with ¼ to ½ cup of water or vegetable stock (see page 108), as needed to prevent sticking.

Replace the coconut milk with other plant-based milks, such as soy, rice, almond, or quinoa (see pages 104 and 143).

Add ½ cup of grated vegan mozzarella-style cheese when pulse chopping.

Add 2 teaspoons of minced fresh dill, or 1 tablespoon of minced fresh cilantro, basil, sorrel, or parsley when mashing.

Top with fresh, minced chives.

Nutrition Facts per serving (192 g): Calories 90, Fat Calories 25, Total Fat 2.5 g, Saturated Fat 2 g, Cholesterol 0 mg, Sodium 225 mg, Total Carb 17 g, Dietary Fiber 5 g, Sugars 5 g, Protein 2 g

Israeli Couscous Tabouli

YIELD: 5 CUPS TABOULI

Prep time: 20 minutes, Cook time: 15 minutes, Total time: 35 minutes, Serving size: 1 cup, Number of servings: 5

Discover the benefits of chewy and tender Israeli couscous, also known as pearled couscous—larger and sturdier than its North African counterpart. Made of semolina and wheat flour, its most helpful nutrient is selenium, otherwise found in Brazil nuts, required in trace amounts for normal health but not available in many foods. One cup of Israeli couscous offers more than 60 percent of your daily requirement for selenium. Serve along with Baked Falafel (page 262) and Provençal Salad (page 183).

2 cups water or vegetable stock (see page 108)
1 cup uncooked Israeli couscous
1 cup finely chopped fresh flat-leaf parsley
3 tablespoons finely chopped fresh mint
2 tablespoons freshly squeezed lemon juice
1 ½ tablespoons olive oil
¼ cup diced red onion
2 cups seeded and chopped tomato (½-inch pieces)
½ teaspoon sea salt, or to taste
⅛ teaspoon freshly ground black pepper
¼ teaspoon crushed red pepper flakes
1 garlic clove, pressed or minced
2 teaspoons balsamic vinegar
2 tablespoons capers (optional)

1. Place the water or stock in a pot over medium-high heat. You can optionally add a small amount of salt to the water to enhance the flavor. Bring to a boil. Add the couscous and lower the heat to simmer. Cook until the couscous is just tender, about 8 minutes. Drain and rinse well.

2. Meanwhile place the remaining ingredients in a bowl and mix well.

3. Add the couscous and toss well. Enjoy warm or cold.

VARIATIONS

Replace the couscous with bulgur wheat and cook according to the instructions on page 97.

Add 1 cup of seeded and diced cucumber.

Add ¼ cup of thinly sliced olives and ½ cup of chopped artichoke hearts.

🄖 For a gluten-free version, replace the couscous with rice or quinoa.

🄗 For an oil-free version, omit the olive oil.

Nutrition Facts per serving (175 g): Calories 155, Fat Calories 5, Total Fat 0.5 g, Saturated Fat 0 g, Cholesterol 0 mg, Sodium 250 mg, Total Carb 32 g, Dietary Fiber 3 g, Sugars 3 g, Protein 6 g

Green Quinoa 🄖 ●

YIELD: 3 CUPS QUINOA

Prep time: 10 minutes, Cook time: 20 minutes, Total time: 30 minutes, Serving size: 3/4 cup, Number of servings: 4

Instead of green beer on St. Patrick's Day, try this quinoa special, gone green. With three different shades of green from the darker oregano to vibrant parsley to spring-green onion, quinoa gets not only a dash of color, but vitamins A, C, and K, among other nutrients.

Serve with Roasted Veggies and Beans (page 267), Three Greens with Tomato Sauce (page 197), or Grilled Eggplant Towers (page 282).

1 cup uncooked quinoa, rinsed and drained well (see pages 95, 144)

1 ¾ cups water or vegetable stock (see page 108)

2 teaspoons dried marjoram or oregano

½ teaspoon sea salt, or to taste

¼ teaspoon freshly ground black pepper

¼ cup minced fresh flat-leaf parsley

¼ cup diced green onion

1. Place the quinoa, water or stock, marjoram, salt, and pepper in a pot over medium-high heat. Bring to a boil. Cover, lower the heat to simmer, and cook until all the liquid is absorbed, about 15 minutes.

2. Allow to sit for 5 minutes. Fluff with a fork, then transfer to a bowl.

3. Add the parsley and green onion and gently stir well.

VARIATIONS

Replace the quinoa with rice, millet, or farro. See the cooking chart on page 96 for their liquid-to-grain ratio.

Add some sautéed veggies: In a separate pan, sauté 1 cup of diced onion, ½ cup of diced shiitake mushrooms, and 1 cup of julienned kale or spinach. Gently stir into the cooked quinoa. Use as filling for stuffed peppers (pages 206 or 291) or zucchini.

Nutrition Facts per serving (103 g): Calories 160, Fat Calories 25, Total Fat 2.6 g, Saturated Fat 0, Cholesterol 0 mg, Sodium 300 mg, Total Carb 28 g, Dietary Fiber 4 g, Sugars 0 g, Protein 6 g

Golden Rice Ⓖ ◐

YIELD: 3 CUPS RICE

Prep time: 10 minutes, Cook time: 50 minutes, Total time: 60 minutes, Serving size: 3/4 cup, Number of servings: 4

Make brown rice golden with the addition of yellow and orange ingredients, such as carrots or gold beets, ginger, and turmeric, the vivid yellow of the spice world. Golden beets are slightly sweeter and oftentimes have a less earthy flavor than red beets, though their nutritional benefits are the same: Beets are a good source of fiber, potassium, and calcium, making them a great food for weight loss, heart health, and even bone strength. Serve as a side along with Ratatouille (page 273), Thai Curry Vegetables (page 289), or Creamy Lentil Saag (page 290).

1 cup uncooked brown basmati rice

2 cups water or vegetable stock (see page 108)

¼ teaspoon sea salt, or to taste

¼ cup peeled and diced gold beets or carrots

1 ½ teaspoons peeled and minced fresh turmeric, or ½ teaspoon ground

2 teaspoons peeled and minced fresh ginger

1. Place all the ingredients in a pot over medium-high heat. Bring to a boil.

2. Lower the heat to simmer, cover, and cook until all the liquid is absorbed, about 50 minutes. Remove from the heat.

3. Allow to sit for 5 minutes. Fluff with a fork before serving.

Replace the basmati rice with other varieties, such as short- or long-grain, or sushi rice; or replace the rice with quinoa, farro, or millet. Just be sure to alter your liquid amount and cooking time accordingly—see the chart on page 96.

Top with slivered almonds (optionally toasted; see page 101).

Nutrition Facts per serving (82 g): Calories 180, Fat Calories 15, Total Fat 1.5 g, Saturated Fat 0 g, Cholesterol 0 mg, Sodium 160 mg, Total Carb 37 g, Dietary Fiber 2 g, Sugars 1 g, Protein 4 g

Unfried Rice ⊙⬦

YIELD: 4 CUPS RICE

Prep time: 10 minutes, Cook time: 50 minutes, Total time: 60 minutes, Serving size: 1 cup, Number of servings: 4

Using ingredients typically associated with the fried version, this recipe takes your health into consideration without compromising on flavor. Brown rice is the better-for-you, nonstripped version of its more frequently found counterpart, white rice. Selenium, manganese, antioxidants, and fiber can all shine in brown rice's whole-grain form. Cooking it in nourishing, tasty, alkalizing vegetable broth, and adding your favorite veggies, ensures this unfried rice is a powerhouse of minerals. The liquid smoke here is optional, though it contributes to the sense of enjoying fried rice. Serve as a side along with Thai Curry Vegetables (page 289) and Super Sprout Salad (page 173).

2 cups water or vegetable stock (see page 108)
1 cup uncooked long-grain brown rice

½ teaspoon sea salt, or to taste
2 cups carrot, pea, and corn frozen vegetable mixture
½ cup diced green onion
1 ¼ teaspoons Chinese five-spice powder
¼ teaspoon wheat-free tamari or other soy sauce, or to taste
¼ teaspoon liquid smoke (optional, see page 85)
¼ teaspoon freshly ground black pepper
⅛ teaspoon cayenne pepper

1. Place the water or stock, rice, and salt in a pot over high heat. Bring to a boil. Cover, lower the heat to low, and cook until all the liquid is absorbed, about 40 minutes. Remove from the heat and allow to sit for 5 minutes. Fluff with a fork.

2. Meanwhile, place the remaining ingredients in a large bowl and mix well. Add the rice and gently toss well. Transfer to a large baking sheet.

3. Heat the oven broiler on HIGH. Place the rice mixture in the oven and cook for 5 minutes. Carefully toss well and return to the oven. Cook for 3 minutes. Serve warm.

VARIATIONS

Add 1 ½ cups of cooked or canned chickpeas along with the green onion.

Replace the frozen corn, pea, and carrot mixture with fresh corn, peas, and diced carrot. Steam until just tender before using in this recipe.

You can sauté the rice in 3 tablespoons of oil once cooked. Add the remaining ingredients and cook for 5 minutes, stirring frequently.

Replace the rice with farro, millet, or quinoa. See the cooking chart on page 96.

Change up the vegetables with chopped broccoli, asparagus, and Romanesco.

For Unfried Rice–Stuffed Peppers, preheat the oven to 375°F. Slice four peppers in half and remove the seeds. Place ½ cup of the rice mixture (prepared through step 3) in each pepper, top with grated vegan cheese, place on a well-oiled casserole dish, and cook until the peppers are just soft and the cheese melts, about 20 minutes.

Nutrition Facts per serving (130 g): Calories 220, Fat Calories 15, Total Fat 1.5g, Saturated Fat 0 g, Cholesterol 0 mg, Sodium 340 mg, Total Carb 46 g, Dietary Fiber 5 g, Sugars 3 g, Protein 6 g

Spicy Pinto Beans⊙◖

YIELD: 2 CUPS BEANS

Prep time: 10 minutes, Cook time: 15 minutes, Total time: 25 minutes, Serving size: 1/2 cup, Number of servings: 4

Jalapeño pepper, chili powder, and chipotle chile powder provide ample flavorful spice to this recipe while simultaneously revving up the body's metabolism. The capsicum in all three is also efficient as a digestive aid and circulation booster, not to mention a means of heating up the body up on a cold day. Similarly warming pinto beans are a perennial favorite for cholesterol-lowering dietary fiber, iron, and antioxidants. Serve along with rice and Walnut Taco Salad (page 187).

½ cup water
¼ cup diced yellow onion
3 garlic cloves, pressed or minced
½ teaspoon seeded and diced jalapeño pepper
1 (15-ounce) can pinto beans, drained and rinsed well, or 1 ½ cups cooked (see page 98)
1 teaspoon chili powder
¾ teaspoon ground cumin
¼ teaspoon sea salt, or to taste
⅛ teaspoon freshly ground black pepper
⅛ teaspoon chipotle chile powder (optional)
1 teaspoon wheat-free tamari or other soy sauce (optional)
1 tablespoon finely chopped fresh cilantro

1. Place the water in a small pot over medium-high heat. Add the onion, garlic, and jalapeño and cook for 3 minutes, stirring frequently and adding a small amount of additional water, if necessary, to prevent sticking.

2. Lower the heat to low, add the pinto beans, and mix well. Add the chili powder, cumin, salt, black pepper, and chipotle chile powder, if using, and cook for 7 minutes, stirring occasionally.

3. Add the tamari, if using, and cilantro and stir well before serving.

VARIATIONS

Sauté the onion and garlic in 1 tablespoon of coconut oil for 2 minutes, stirring constantly, before adding the water.

Add ¼ cup of seeded and diced red bell pepper along with the onion.

Feel free to replace the pinto beans with kidney, black, fava, great northern, or navy beans.

Add ½ cup of grated vegan cheese just before adding the cilantro.

Nutrition Facts per serving (80 g): Calories 100, Fat Calories 10, Total Fat 1 g, Saturated Fat 0 g, Cholesterol 0 mg, Sodium 160 mg, Total Carb 19 g, Dietary Fiber 6 g, Sugars 1 g, Protein 6 g

Spaghetti Squash with Broccoli ◉

YIELD: 5 CUPS SQUASH AND BROCCOLI

Prep time: 10 minutes, Cook time: 35 minutes, Total time: 45 minutes, Serving size: 1 cup, Number of servings: 5

Spaghetti squash is from the cucurbit family, along with the likes of cucumbers, watermelons, and pumpkins. As its name suggests, kids may mistake its noodlelike strands for a yellow/orange spaghetti in a boat of its own skin. There are many ways to vary the colorful veggie sauté that is mixed in with the squash. See the variations for some ideas and discover your (and your kids'!) favorite. Both spaghetti squash and the broccoli in this recipe have digestive benefits in the form of their fiber content. Serve with Golden Rice (page 204) and Maple Baked Tempeh (page 262) with Roasted Red Pepper Sauce (page 235).

1 medium-size spaghetti squash (3 cups cooked and shredded)
½ cup water or vegetable stock (see page 108)
2 teaspoons coconut oil
¾ cup diced shiitake mushrooms
¼ cup finely chopped fennel bulb
2 cups finely chopped broccoli
½ cup seeded and diced red bell pepper
½ cup soy, rice, almond, or coconut milk (optional; for homemade, see Plant-Based Milk, page 104)
2 tablespoons freshly squeezed lime juice
2 tablespoons nutritional yeast (optional)
1 ½ tablespoons finely chopped fresh parsley or cilantro
½ teaspoon sea salt, or to taste
⅛ teaspoon freshly ground black pepper
¼ teaspoon chipotle chile powder
Pinch of cayenne pepper
¼ cup thinly sliced green onion

1. Preheat the oven to 375°F. Slice the squash lengthwise. Use a spoon to scoop out and discard the seeds. Place the water or stock in a 9 by 13-inch casserole dish. Add the squash, cut side down, and bake until the flesh is just tender, about 30 minutes.

2. Using a fork, carefully scrape the flesh out of the skin lengthwise to form spaghetti-like strands and transfer to a bowl. Save the hard outer skins.

3. Meanwhile, place the oil in a sauté pan over medium-high heat. Add the shiitakes and fennel and cook for 5 minutes, stirring frequently. Add the broccoli and cook for 7 minutes, stirring frequently and adding small amounts of water or vegetable stock, as necessary, to prevent sticking. Add the bell pepper and cook for 5 minutes, stirring frequently. Add all the remaining ingredients, except the green onion and squash skins, and mix well.

4. Transfer to the shredded spaghetti squash and mix well. To serve, scoop into the squash skins, and top with green onion.

VARIATIONS

Replace the broccoli with other veggies, such as cauliflower, chopped zucchini or parsnip, shredded kale, or Brussels sprouts.

Replace the shiitake with other mushrooms, such as oyster, cremini, or button.

Add 2 teaspoons of chili powder and 1 teaspoon of ground cumin, for a taste of Mexico.

◖ For an oil-free version, use the water sauté method (see page 101) to cook the vegetable mixture.

Nutrition Facts per serving (204 g): Calories 70, Fat Calories 25, Total Fat 2.5 g, Saturated Fat 2 g, Cholesterol 0 mg, Sodium 270 mg, Total Carb 11 g, Dietary Fiber 3 g, Sugars 4 g, Protein 3 g

Date Glazed Sweet Potatoes Ⓖ ◖

YIELD: 5 CUPS SWEET POTATOES

Prep time: 10 minutes, Cook time: 40 minutes, Total time: 50 minutes, Serving size: 1 cup, Number of servings: 5

Aside from being candy-sweet, dates are loaded with dietary fiber, iron, and potassium. The sweet potatoes provide even more sweetness, fiber and potassium, and their additional vitamins B_6, C, and E, beta-carotene, and manganese make this dessertlike dish also nutrition smart. Serve as part of a holiday feast along with Lentil Walnut Loaf (page 288) and Oil-Free Mushroom Gravy (page 240).

5 cups peeled and sliced sweet potato (1-inch pieces)
¼ cup water
¾ cup freshly squeezed orange juice
¼ cup tightly packed pitted Medjool dates
1 teaspoon pure vanilla extract
½ teaspoon ground cinnamon
⅛ teaspoon ground nutmeg
Pinch of sea salt
1 tablespoon finely chopped fresh mint (optional)

1. Preheat the oven to 400°F. Place the potato slices in a 9 by 13-inch casserole dish.

2. Place the water, orange juice, dates, vanilla, cinnamon, nutmeg, and salt in a blender and blend well. Pour over the potato and toss well.

3. Place in the oven and bake until the potato is just soft and the sauce begins to caramelize, about 30 minutes. Garnish with the fresh mint, if using, before serving.

VARIATIONS

Drizzle 1 ½ tablespoons of coconut oil or melted vegan butter over the sweet potato before roasting.

For additional sweetness, add pure maple syrup, coconut nectar, or desired sweetener of choice to taste (see page 89).

Experiment with different varieties of sweet potato or winter squash, such as butternut, acorn, or buttercup.

Nutrition Facts per serving (183 g): Calories 165, Fat Calories 0, Total Fat 0 g, Saturated Fat 0 g, Cholesterol 0 mg, Sodium 130 mg, Total Carb 40 g, Dietary Fiber 5 g, Sugars 16 g, Protein 3 g

Wasabi Garlic Twice-Baked Potatoes ☉ ◆

YIELD: 2 LARGE POTATOES

Prep time: 15 minutes, Cook time: 55 minutes, Total time: 70 minutes, Serving size: 1/2 potato, Number of servings: 4

Wasabi is famous for its pungent sinus-clearing effects, which are attributed to its unique biochemically available isothiocyanates (the anticancer phytochemicals that all cruciferous veggies are known for). Besides being fun to eat, it also has potent antibiotic and anti-inflammatory properties. With fiber powerhouse potatoes and immunity-boosting garlic, this comforting side is a flavorful way to get some important nutrients. Top with grated vegan cheese, store-bought bacon-analogue bits or Coco Bacon (page 112), Vegan Sour Cream (page 112), and chopped chives, dill, or green onion.

2 large russet potatoes (about 2 pounds)

½ cup unsweetened soy, rice, coconut, or almond milk (for homemade, see Plant-Based Milk, page 104)

4 large garlic cloves, pressed or minced

1 tablespoon nutritional yeast (optional)

2 to 3 teaspoons wasabi powder (see page 85)

¼ teaspoon sea salt, or to taste

¼ teaspoon freshly ground black pepper

Paprika

1. Preheat the oven to 450°F. Poke several holes in the potatoes, using a fork, and place on a small baking sheet. Bake until a knife can pass easily through the potatoes, about 50 minutes, depending upon the size of the potatoes.

2. Slice the potatoes in half. Using a baking mitt or clean towel to hold each potato, carefully scoop out the inside of the potatoes into a large bowl. Taste and add additional salt, if necessary. Return the skins to the baking sheet.

3. Preheat the oven broiler on LOW. Mash the potatoes with a potato masher or strong whisk. Add all the remaining ingredients, except the paprika and potato skins, and mix well. Portion out the mixture evenly into the potato skins on the baking sheet. Sprinkle with paprika and return to the top rack of the oven. Cook until the potato starts to brown, about 5 minutes.

VARIATIONS

Feel free to omit the wasabi.

Replace the soy milk with Vegan Mayonnaise (page 113) or Vegenaise.

Experiment with different types of potatoes, or replace the potatoes with acorn or delicata squash.

Nutrition Facts per serving (222 g): Calories 160, Fat Calories 10, Total Fat 1 g, Saturated Fat 0 g, Cholesterol 0 mg, Sodium 170 mg, Total Carb 35 g, Dietary Fiber 5 g, Sugars 2 g, Protein 5 g

Pearled Barley with Mushrooms and Corn

YIELD: 3 CUPS BARLEY, MUSHROOMS, AND CORN

Prep time: 15 minutes, Cook time: 55 minutes, Total time: 70 minutes, Serving size: 1/2 cup, Number of servings: 6

Pearled barley is faster cooking than regular barley and easier to eat because it has had the bran removed along with the hull (which is removed on all varieties of barley). Always the superb antidote to a chilly day, chewy tender and slightly nutty barley is a respectable source of protein and fiber, with portions of your daily dose of copper, manganese, thiamine, niacin, magnesium, and selenium. Serve along with Simple Chop Salad (page 174) and Simple Baked Tofu (page 260) topped with Tahini Oat Sauce (page 238).

1 cup uncooked pearled barley
2 ½ cups water or vegetable stock (see page 108)
½ teaspoon sea salt, or to taste
1 teaspoon dried thyme
2 teaspoons coconut oil
2 cups sliced mushrooms (try cremini or shiitake)
¼ teaspoon ground nutmeg
1 ½ cups fresh or frozen (thawed) corn
3 tablespoons finely chopped fresh flat-leaf parsley
3 tablespoons thinly sliced green onion
¼ teaspoon freshly ground black pepper
Pinch of crushed red pepper flakes

1. Place the barley, water or stock, salt, and thyme in a pot over medium-high heat. Bring to a boil. Cover, lower the heat to simmer, and cook until the barley is tender and all the liquid is absorbed, 55 to 60 minutes. (If the barley is tender and there is still liquid after 55 minutes, you can drain the excess liquid). Transfer to a bowl.

2. Meanwhile, after 30 minutes while the barley is still cooking, place the coconut oil in a pan over medium-high heat. Add the mushrooms and nutmeg and cook for 4 minutes, stirring frequently. Add the corn and cook for 3 minutes, stirring frequently. Add the parsley, green onion, black pepper, and crushed red pepper flakes and mix well.

3. Add to the cooked barley and gently mix well before serving. Serve warm or cool.

VARIATIONS

Add three minced or pressed garlic cloves along with the mushrooms.

G Replace the barley with rice or quinoa. See the grain-cooking chart on page 96 for the liquid-to-grain ratio.

For an oil-free version, use the water sauté method (see page 101).

Nutrition Facts per serving (191 g): Calories 310, Fat Calories 40, Total Fat 4.5 g, Saturated Fat 2 g, Cholesterol 0 mg, Sodium 223 mg, Total Carb 62 g, Dietary Fiber 10 g, Sugars 3 g, Protein 9 g

Quinoa Chickpea Pilaf⊙♦

YIELD: 5 CUPS PILAF

Prep time: 15 minutes, Cook time: 15 minutes,
Total time: 25 minutes, Serving size: 1 cup,
Number of servings: 5

Coming at you from the Andes mountains, quick-cooking quinoa imparts its slightly nutty flavor and abundance of nutritional benefits to this Mediterranean-themed pilaf. Botanically a seed, this ancient food of the Incas is a complete protein while also offering iron, magnesium, manganese, folate, and lysine, which aid tissue growth and repair. Chickpeas, from the legume family, provide more protein, more fiber, and more manganese and folate in this hardy pilaf. Enjoy as a stuffing in stuffed bell peppers (page 262), or along with Baked Falafel (page 262) and Watercress with Pistachios and Currants (page 179).

1 ½ cups uncooked quinoa, rinsed and
   drained well (see pages 95, 144)
2 ¼ cups water or vegetable stock (see page
   108)
½ teaspoon sea salt, or to taste
1 garlic clove, pressed or minced
1 (15-ounce) can chickpeas, drained and
   rinsed well, or 1 ½ cups cooked (see page
   98)
1 cup fresh or frozen (thawed) corn
   (optional)
½ cup seeded and diced red bell pepper
2 tablespoons minced kalamata olives
2 tablespoons freshly squeezed lemon juice
2 tablespoons diced green onion
1 ½ tablespoons finely chopped fresh dill
2 teaspoons balsamic vinegar

¼ teaspoon freshly ground black pepper
¼ teaspoon crushed red pepper flakes

1. Place the quinoa, water or stock, salt, and garlic in a pot on high heat and bring to a boil. Cover, lower the heat to low, and cook until all the liquid is absorbed, about 15 minutes. Remove from the heat. Allow to sit for 5 minutes, then fluff with a fork.

2. Meanwhile, place the remaining ingredients in a bowl and mix well.

3. Add the cooked quinoa and gently toss to combine evenly before serving.

VARIATIONS

Replace the quinoa with rice, millet, farro, or rice pasta.

Omit the chickpeas or replace with pinto, adzuki, kidney, or black beans. Add 1 ½ tablespoons of olive oil along with balsamic vinegar.

Replace the kalamatas with olives of your choosing (see page 158).

Add ½ cup of grated carrot and/or thinly sliced fennel.

Add ½ cup of thinly sliced sun-dried tomatoes.

Replace the dill with minced fresh cilantro, basil, sorrel, or flat-leaf parsley.

Nutrition Facts per serving (129 g): Calories 280, Fat Calories 40, Total Fat 5 g, Saturated Fat 0.5 g, Cholesterol 0 mg, Sodium 275 mg, Total Carb 48 g, Dietary Fiber 8 g, Sugars 4 g, Protein 12 g

Grilled Mediterranean Vegetables and Quinoa 🅖 ▱

YIELD: 4 ½ CUPS VEGETABLES AND QUINOA

Prep time: 20 minutes, Cook time: 10 minutes, Total time: 30 minutes, Serving size: 3/4 cup, Number of servings: 6

Nothing beats the smoky and rich flavor of grilling. When vegetables are grilled, they cook quickly and have the highest likelihood of retaining maximal nutrients. This is wonderful, since they tend to always be a hit at barbecue gatherings, and may be a nice way to introduce more nutrients to someone with a less veggie-heavy diet. Mixed in with protein-abundant quinoa, this dish is sure to be a favorite at your next pot luck. Seek out sustainably harvested hearts of palm! (See page 169 for more information about hearts of palm.)

Serve with Baked Falafel (page 262) and Ratatouille (page 273) or with a Super Sprout Salad (page 173) with Creamy Lemon Tahini Dressing (page 228).

1 cup uncooked quinoa, rinsed and drained well (see pages 95, 144)

2 cups water or vegetable stock (see page 108)

½ teaspoon sea salt, or to taste

2 tablespoons plus 1 teaspoon freshly squeezed lemon juice

1 tablespoon olive oil

1 teaspoon dried oregano

⅛ teaspoon dried thyme

¼ teaspoon freshly ground black pepper

1 red bell pepper, quartered

1 large portobello mushroom, gills removed

1 red bell pepper, quartered

4 hearts of palm

½ cup chopped artichoke hearts

3 tablespoons diced kalamata olives

1 garlic clove, pressed or minced

2 tablespoons chiffonaded fresh basil

2 tablespoons finely chopped fresh flat-leaf parsley

3 tablespoons thinly sliced green onion

2 teaspoons balsamic vinegar

¼ teaspoon crushed red pepper flakes

1. Preheat a grill. Place the quinoa, 1 ¾ cups of the water or stock, and ¼ teaspoon of the sea salt in a pot over medium-high heat. Bring to a boil. Cover, lower the heat to low, and cook until all liquid is absorbed, about 15 minutes. Remove from heat. Allow to sit for 10 minutes.

2. Meanwhile, place the remaining ¼ cup of water or stock, 2 tablespoons of the lemon juice, the olive oil, if using, oregano, and thyme, the remaining ¼ teaspoon of salt, and the black pepper in a shallow baking dish and whisk well. Add the portobello, red bell pepper, hearts of palm, and artichoke hearts and coat well.

3. Grill the marinated vegetables until tender and char marks appear, 3 to 5 minutes on each side, depending upon the heat of the grill. Chop into ½-inch pieces, and place in a large bowl.

4. Add the cooked quinoa and all the remaining ingredients, including the remaining teaspoon of lemon juice, and gently mix well. Serve warm or cold.

💧 For an oil-free version, omit the oil and add 3 tablespoons of additional water to the marinade.

Add ¼ cup of diced sun-dried tomatoes.

Nutrition Facts per serving (170 g): Calories 185, Fat Calories 50, Total Fat 6 g, Saturated Fat 1 g, Cholesterol 0 mg, Sodium 340 mg, Total Carb 28 g, Dietary Fiber 4 g, Sugars 7 g, Protein 6 g

---

TEMPLATE RECIPE
Grain Vegetable Dish

- -

Grain component: Replace the quinoa with rice, millet, or rice pasta.

Vegetable component: Replace the grilled vegetables with your favorites, such as corn, asparagus, carrots, or eggplant. Instead of grilling, you can add steamed, roasted, or sautéed vegetables. Replace the raw veggies with tomatoes, cucumbers, chopped broccoli, spinach, or sun-dried tomato.

Herb component: Replace the basil and parsley with fresh cilantro, dill, or sorrel. Add additional fresh herbs, such as minced rosemary, oregano, sage, and thyme.

Ethnic component: Add 1 tablespoon of an ethnic spice blend, such as Moroccan (page 106), Ethiopian (page 106) or Herbes de Provence (page 106).

Optional legume component: Add 1 cup of cooked and drained chickpeas, kidney beans, black-eyed peas, black beans, pinto beans, or your favorites.

Mushroom Kasha 🄖

YIELD: 4 CUPS MUSHROOM KASHA

Prep time: 15 minutes, Cook time: 20 minutes, Total time: 35 minutes, Serving size: 1 cup, Number of servings: 4

Popular in Russian and Eastern European cuisine, kasha (pretoasted buckwheat groats) is a blood-friendly grain because it contains elevated levels of rutin, which gives strength to capillaries and helps prevent blood clotting. It is also an excellent source of magnesium, which helps lower blood pressure. Complemented with the earthiness of cremini or shiitake mushrooms, this flavorful grain dish contributes to full nutritional satisfaction. Top with cubed and roasted tofu (see page 100) and serve with Simple Chop Salad (page 174).

1 ½ cups water or vegetable stock (see page 108)

1 cup uncooked kasha

½ teaspoon sea salt, or to taste

2 teaspoons coconut oil

½ cup diced yellow onion

3 garlic cloves, pressed or minced

1 ½ cups diced cremini or shiitake mushrooms

¼ teaspoon dried thyme

Pinch ground nutmeg

⅛ teaspoon freshly ground black pepper

2 tablespoons finely chopped fresh flat-leaf parsley

1. Place the water or stock in a small pot over high heat and bring to a boil. Add the kasha and salt. Lower the heat to low, cover, and cook until all liquid is absorbed, about 10 minutes. Allow to sit for 5 minutes, then fluff with a fork.

2. Meanwhile, place the coconut oil in a sauté pan over medium-high heat. Add the onion and garlic and cook for 3 minutes, stirring frequently. Add the mushrooms, thyme, nutmeg, and black pepper and cook for 7 minutes, stirring frequently and adding a small amount of water, if necessary, to prevent sticking. Add the parsley and mix well.

3. When the kasha is done cooking, add to the mushrooms and gently stir to combine. Serve warm or cool.

VARIATIONS

Add 1 cup of thinly sliced celery and/or ¾ cup of seeded and diced bell pepper along with the mushrooms.

Replace the parsley with 1 tablespoon of minced fresh dill.

♦ For an oil-free version, use the water sauté method (see page 101).

For **Kasha-Stuffed Tomatoes,** preheat the oven to 400°F. Scoop out the center of six to eight tomatoes. Place in an oiled baking dish and cook for 10 minutes. Fill with the Mushroom Kasha and top with grated vegan mozzarella-style cheese. Place in the oven broiler on HIGH and cook for 3 minutes, or until the cheese melts.

For **Kasha Varnishkes,** gently toss the Mushroom Kasha with 14 ounces of cooked and optionally lightly oiled bow-tie pasta.

Nutrition Facts per serving (96 g): Calories 185, Fat Calories 35, Total Fat 4 g, Saturated Fat 2 g, Cholesterol 0 mg, Sodium 295 mg, Total Carb 34 g, Dietary Fiber 5 g, Sugars 1 g, Protein 7 g

Herb-Roasted Potatoes ⒢

YIELD: 4 CUPS POTATOES

Prep time: 10 minutes, Cook time: 25 minutes, Total time: 35 minutes, Serving size: 3/4 cup, Number of servings: 4

Nothing says "filling and down-home comfort food" as much as roasted potatoes. Garlic's nutritional benefits make up a lengthy list; chief among them are its immune system strengthening. With some of its strong flavor and that of such herbs as rosemary and parsley, this recipe is a dream come true when served as part of a breakfast feast with Garden Veggie Scramble (page 128) and Lemon Blueberry Pancakes (page 123).

5 cups chopped potatoes (½-inch pieces)
3 garlic cloves, pressed or minced
1 tablespoon melted coconut oil
¼ teaspoon sea salt, or to taste
¾ teaspoon paprika
⅛ teaspoon freshly ground black pepper
¼ teaspoon crushed red pepper flakes
Oil, for baking sheet
2 tablespoons finely chopped fresh flat-leaf parsley
1 teaspoon finely chopped fresh rosemary
½ teaspoon balsamic vinegar
½ teaspoon wheat-free tamari or other soy sauce (optional)

1. Preheat the oven to 400°F. Place the potatoes, garlic, coconut oil, salt, paprika, black pepper, and crushed red pepper flakes in a bowl and toss well. Transfer to an oiled baking sheet, place in the oven, and bake for 15 minutes.

2. Gently toss the potatoes and add a small amount of water, if necessary, to

prevent sticking. Cook until the potatoes are just soft and golden brown, about 10 minutes.

3. Transfer to a bowl along with the remaining ingredients and gently toss well before serving.

VARIATIONS

♦ For an oil-free version, replace the oil with ¾ cup of water or vegetable stock (see page 108).

Add ½ cup of chopped fennel bulb and/ or seeded and diced red bell pepper along with the potatoes.

Add ¼ teaspoon of smoked paprika along with the paprika.

Replace the potatoes with sweet potatoes, turnips, rutabagas, or parsnips.

Replace the parsley and rosemary with 1 ½ tablespoons of minced fresh dill.

For an Indian dish, replace the parsley and rosemary with 2 tablespoons of minced fresh cilantro and add 1 ½ tablespoons of curry powder or Indian Spice Mix (page 106).

For a Mexican dish, replace the parsley and rosemary with 2 tablespoons of minced fresh cilantro, 1 tablespoon of chili powder, 1 teaspoon of ground cumin, and ¼ teaspoon of chipotle chile powder.

For a Moroccan dish, add 2 tablespoons of Moroccan Spice Mix (page 106).

Nutrition Facts per serving (197 g): Calories 180, Fat Calories 30, Total Fat 4 g, Saturated Fat 3 g, Cholesterol 0 mg, Sodium 160 mg, Total Carb 34 g, Dietary Fiber 4 g, Sugars 2 g, Protein 4 g

Fingerling Potatoes with Pesto🄶

YIELD: 4 CUPS POTATOES

Prep time: 15 minutes, Cook time: 15 minutes, Total time: 30 minutes, Serving size: 1/2 cup, Number of servings: 8

Originating in Genoa in northern Italy, pesto is one of my all-time favorite foods to prepare. So many variations are possible! This cashew-based version brings out the best of the enticingly fragrant basil plant, which is also a source of cell-protecting nutrients. Simply divine on its own, here we are enjoying this Italian gift from the gods over low-fat, fiber-rich potatoes. The nutritional yeast adds not only the important cheesy component but a concentrated dose of B vitamins. The pesto can last for a few days when stored in a glass jar in the refrigerator, so make a double batch and keep some extra on hand. Serve with Ranch Kale Salad (page 185) and BBQ Roasted Tofu with Collards (page 278).

1 ½ pounds fingerling or new potatoes, chopped into ½-inch pieces (4 cups)
Sea salt and freshly ground black pepper (optional)

PESTO SAUCE
½ cup tightly packed fresh basil
2 tablespoons raw cashew pieces
2 tablespoons olive oil
2 tablespoons water
1 tablespoon freshly squeezed lemon juice
1 tablespoon diced green onion
1 garlic clove
½ teaspoon seeded and diced jalapeño pepper
2 teaspoons nutritional yeast

Potato Madness

Cultivated since 8,000 BC by Peruvian Incas, potatoes are now the leading vegetable crop in the United States and the fourth largest crop in the world. They are mostly commonly consumed in French fry form, but also in chips, baked, boiled, mashed, and in stews.

Potatoes are on the "Dirty Dozen" list (see page 61) so securing organic is recommended. Over one hundred varieties of potatoes are available, in the following categories:

White potatoes are most often medium-size and dense with a thin, no-need-to-peel skin and white interior, and are appropriate for mashing, baking, frying, and boiling.

Yellow potatoes are larger and yield a golden interior that lends a buttery quality. Ideal for roasting, mashing, or potato salads, they also have a mild sweetness, enhancing the buttery essence.

Creamy and sweet, red (or "new") potatoes tend to size out at small or medium. The red is the skin, not the white interior, and they tend to maintain a firmness despite any cooking procedure, which makes red potatoes good for salads and stews alike.

Smaller and purple or dark blue on both the outside and inside, purple potatoes are small and shape-maintaining. They are eye-catching in salads and also do well grilled and baked.

Russet potatoes are on the large end and cook up light and fluffy despite a thicker, chewier skin. They make terrific oven fries or light mashed potatoes as well as being the classic baked potato.

Finger-size fingerling potatoes and petite mini-potatoes both come in a variety of colors and have an earthiness alongside a buttery flavor, making them a versatile addition to any stew, salad, or side dish.

~~~~~~

½ **teaspoon sea salt, or to taste**

⅛ **teaspoon freshly ground black pepper**

1. Place a steamer basket in a pot filled with about ½ inch of water over high heat. Bring to a boil. Lower the heat to low. Add the potatoes and cook until just tender, about 15 minutes. Transfer to a bowl.

2. Meanwhile, prepare the pesto: Place all the sauce ingredients in a blender or food processor and blend until smooth.

3. Add to the potatoes and gently mix well. Add additional salt and pepper to taste, if necessary, before serving. Serve warm or cooled.

VARIATIONS

Add ¾ cup of thinly sliced celery and ¼ cup of diced red onion to the bowl along with the potatoes.

Add ½ cup of seeded and diced red bell pepper and 1 teaspoon of lemon zest.

Add ¼ cup of thinly sliced olives.

Replace the water with an additional 2 tablespoons of olive oil.

◆ For an oil-free version, replace the oil and water with ¼ cup of mashed avocado.

Top with 1 cup of Coco Bacon (page 112).

Nutrition Facts per serving (66 g): Calories 75, Fat Calories 45, Total Fat 5 g, Saturated Fat 1 g, Cholesterol 0 mg, Sodium 150 mg, Total Carb 7 g, Dietary Fiber 1 g, Sugars 0 g, Protein 2 g

Green Beans with White Bean Fennel Sauce⊙

YIELD: 3 CUPS GREEN BEANS

Prep time: 15 minutes, Cook time: 10 minutes, Total time: 25 minutes, Serving size: 3/4 cup, Number of servings: 4

Two beans are present in this dish, but one is considered a vegetable and the other a legume. White beans work well as the base for this delicious creamy protein-rich sauce, accented by a slight sweetness from fennel. These legumes have a trace mineral called molybdenum, which makes detoxifying enzymes for the body, as well as potent quantities of magnesium. Green or string beans are a nutrient-rich vegetable, containing vitamins A, C, and K, and the mineral manganese. Serve as a side along with Golden Rice (page 204) and Ratatouille (page 273). The sauce is also amazing over steamed vegetables or tossed in with your favorite pasta.

WHITE BEAN FENNEL SAUCE

2 teaspoons coconut oil

½ cup diced yellow onion

4 garlic cloves, pressed or minced

½ cup thinly sliced fennel bulb

1 (15-ounce) can cannellini beans, drained and rinsed, or 1 ½ cups cooked (see page 98)

½ cup water or vegetable stock (see page 108)

¼ teaspoon sea salt, or to taste

⅛ teaspoon freshly ground black pepper

⅛ teaspoon crushed red pepper flakes

1 tablespoon chiffonaded fresh basil

3 cups green beans (¾ pound)

¼ cup thinly sliced green onion

¼ cup seeded and diced red bell pepper

1 tablespoon finely chopped fresh summer savory (optional)

1. Make the sauce: Place the coconut oil in a sauté pan over medium-high heat. Add the onion and cook for 1 minute, stirring frequently. Add the garlic and cook for 1 minute, stirring frequently. Add the fennel and cook for 5 minutes, stirring frequently, adding small amounts of water, if necessary, to prevent sticking.

2. Transfer to a food processor, along with the cannellini beans, water or stock, salt, black pepper, and crushed red pepper flakes, and process until smooth. Return to the pan over low heat. Add the basil and mix well.

3. Meanwhile, place a steamer basket in a pot with 1 inch of water over high heat and bring to a boil. Add the green beans, cover, and cook until the beans are just tender, about 5 minutes. Place in a serving dish.

4. Top with the White Bean Fennel Sauce, and garnish with green onion, red bell pepper, and summer savory, if using, before serving.

VARIATIONS

Replace the cannellini beans with chickpeas, kidney beans, or white navy beans.

Replace the water with soy, rice, coconut, or almond milk (for homemade, see Plant-Based Milk, page 104) or coconut beverage.

Add 1 tablespoon of finely chopped fresh flat-leaf parsley and 1 teaspoon of fresh marjoram to the sauce.

Replace the basil with fresh dill or cilantro.

◆ For an oil-free version, use the water sauté method (see page 101).

Nutrition Facts per serving (244 g): Calories 140, Fat Calories 25, Total Fat 3 g, Saturated Fat 2 g, Cholesterol 0 mg, Sodium 160 mg, Total Carb 24 g, Dietary Fiber 8 g, Sugars 4 g, Protein 8 g

CHAPTER 13

Dressings and Sauces

This chapter will equip you with all of the tools you need to create an infinite array of flavorful and innovative dressings and sauces, which can add just the right note to take a dish from satisfying to sensational.

When it comes to salads, the dressing is the pièce de résistance. The most simple and healthful dressing is freshly squeezed lemon juice. If you're looking for oil-free dressings, you can take comfort in the selection ranging from the lightest Orange Tarragon Dressing (page 220) and Asian Umeboshi Dressing (page 220) to the more decadent and creamier Raw Hempseed Ranch Dressing (page 224) and Oil-Free Macadamia Wasabi Dressing (page 226). As with other sections, the classic template recipe format can be applied to the Creamy Pepita Dressing (page 227) and Strawberry Vinaigrette (page 222) to create hundreds of variations.

In the realm of sauces, you will enjoy the light Cilantro Mint Chutney (page 229) and Raw Tamarind Sauce (page 230), and the richer Creamy Mexican Dipping Sauce (page 234) and Almond Dipping Sauce (page 233). The Oil-Free Mushroom Gravy (page 240) is perfect for all your holiday feasts and when you are looking for a down-home comfort food.

A range of ethnic sauces can complement your Vegan Fusion meals, whether you are seeking Italian (Fire-Roasted Tomato Sauce, page 239), South American (Zesty Chimichurri Sauce, page 231), Mexican (Ancho Chile Sauce, page 232), Indian (Raw Coconut Curry Sauce, page 237) or Asian (Sweet-and-Sour Sauce, page 236). With a sauce on hand, you are bound to enjoy your culinary tour de force!

Oil-Free Orange Tarragon Dressing ♥Ⓖ◊

YIELD: 1 CUP DRESSING

Prep time: 10 minutes, Total time: 10 minutes, Serving size: 2 tablespoons, Number of servings: 8

This fresh orange juice-based dressing is excellent for salads and steamed veggies alike—try blood orange juice for a slight difference in color and flavor. Popular in French cuisine, tarragon is a lesser-known herb with a potent, unique flavor best described as similar to that of anise and pepper. It has an impressive quantity of potassium, and also has built a reputation for easing digestive problems and water retention, as well as having sleep-inducing effects. Almost universally known is the vitamin C content of oranges (40 percent more in blood oranges), which aids in repairing tissues and ensuring gum health.

1 cup freshly squeezed orange juice
1 ¼ teaspoons raw apple cider vinegar or coconut vinegar
¾ teaspoon Dijon mustard
1 tablespoon finely chopped fresh tarragon
¼ teaspoon sea salt, or to taste
Pinch of freshly ground black pepper
Pinch of cayenne pepper
¾ teaspoon wheat-free tamari or other soy sauce (optional)
1 ½ teaspoons raw agave nectar, coconut nectar, or pure maple syrup (optional)

1. Place all the ingredients in a bowl and whisk well.

VARIATIONS

Add 3 tablespoons of olive, grapeseed, safflower, or sunflower oil.

Replace the agave nectar with one large, pitted date, and blend well with all the ingredients.

Replace the tarragon with minced fresh mint, dill, cilantro, or basil.

Nutrition Facts per serving (33 g): Calories 15, Fat Calories 0, Total Fat 0 g, Saturated Fat 0 g, Cholesterol 0 mg, Sodium 85 mg, Total Carb 3 g, Dietary Fiber 0 g, Sugars 3 g, Protein 0 g

Oil-Free Asian Umeboshi Dressing ♥Ⓖ◊

YIELD: ¾ CUP DRESSING

Prep time: 10 minutes, Total time: 10 minutes, Serving size: 2 tablespoons, Number of servings: 6

Umeboshi (also known as pickled plums or Japanese salt plums) have been used widely in Asia for hundreds of years, appearing in a medical text some thousand years ago, where it is said to help with fatigue, escort toxins out of the body, and even remedy typhoid and food poisoning. Umeboshi vinegar is salty, fruity, and sour, contributing a nirvana-like flavor that makes this dressing stand out. Enjoy on salads and as a dipping sauce for Nori Rolls (page 263).

½ cup pineapple juice
2 tablespoons water
1 tablespoon plus 1 teaspoon umeboshi vinegar
1 tablespoon freshly squeezed lime juice
1 tablespoon diced green onion

1 teaspoon peeled and minced fresh ginger

1 small garlic clove, pressed

½ teaspoon seeded and diced jalapeño or other hot chile pepper (see Scoville scale, page 179)

Pinch of sea salt, or to taste

⅛ teaspoon Chinese five-spice powder

1. Place all the ingredients in a bowl and whisk well.

VARIATIONS

For a creamier dressing, soak ½ cup of raw cashew pieces for 30 minutes. Drain well and add to a blender with the remaining ingredients.

Nutrition Facts per serving (33 g): Calories 20, Fat Calories 0, Total Fat 0 g, Saturated Fat 0 g, Cholesterol 0 mg, Sodium 145 mg, Total Carb 5 g, Dietary Fiber 0 g, Sugars 4 g, Protein 0 g

Simple Flax or Hemp Oil Dressing♥ⓖ

YIELD: ½ CUP DRESSING

Prep time: 5 minutes, Total time: 5 minutes, Serving size: 2 tablespoons, Number of servings: 4

Hippocrates, the father of modern medicine, would be proud of this recipe, which makes use of flaxseeds, one of the foods he recommended to his patients. Flaxseed oil is one of the richest sources of alpha-linoleic acid in a plant-based diet. Hemp seed oil is a complete protein, and also contains essential fatty acids, such as DHA, required for brain development and ongoing sharpness. Both have been studied for their benefits of regulating cholesterol levels and calming inflammation.

The oil in both seeds is more than 75 percent polyunsaturated fats—the most unsaturated oils in the plant kingdom. It contributes a wonderful nutty flavor when poured over salads, steamed veggies, and Monk Bowls (see pages 100, 267).

¼ cup plus 1 tablespoon flax oil or hemp oil

2 tablespoons freshly squeezed lemon juice

1 tablespoon raw apple cider vinegar

1 teaspoon minced fresh dill

Pinch of sea salt

Pinch of freshly ground black pepper

Pinch of cayenne pepper

1. Place all the ingredients in a bowl and whisk well.

VARIATIONS

Replace the dill with fresh cilantro, basil, or oregano.

Add ¼ teaspoon of dried thyme and a pinch of dried summer savory.

Add 2 teaspoons of nutritional yeast.

Nutrition Facts per serving (36 g): Calories 155, Fat Calories 150, Total Fat 17 g, Saturated Fat 2 g, Cholesterol 0 mg, Sodium 40 mg, Total Carb less than 1 g, Dietary Fiber 0 g, Sugars 0 g, Protein 0 g

Cilantro Lime Vinaigretteⓖ

YIELD: ¾ CUP VINAIGRETTE

Prep time: 20 minutes, Total time: 20 minutes, Serving size: 2 tablespoons, Number of servings: 6

Cleansing and *refreshing* are good descriptions of this tasty vinaigrette with its addition of cilantro, a natural detoxifier, and hydrating limes, which appear in many cleansing regimens. Ginger is also widely recommended as one of the best detoxifying herbs. Toss with mixed salads that include jicama, tomatoes, and corn and enjoy with Mushroom Cauliflower Tacos (page 277) or Mexican Seitan-Stuffed Peppers (page 291).

½ cup sunflower or safflower oil

¼ cup freshly squeezed lime juice

2 tablespoons water

1 small garlic clove

1 tablespoon agave nectar

1 teaspoon balsamic vinegar

¼ teaspoon peeled and minced fresh ginger

¼ teaspoon ground coriander

¼ teaspoon sea salt, or to taste

⅛ teaspoon freshly ground black pepper

⅛ teaspoon chile powder

⅛ teaspoon chipotle chile powder

¼ cup finely chopped fresh cilantro

1. Place all the ingredients, except the cilantro, in a blender and blend well.

2. Add the cilantro and blend for a few seconds.

VARIATIONS

Replace the cilantro with fresh basil or parsley, or 1 ½ tablespoons of fresh dill.

Replace the chili powder and chipotle with 1 teaspoon of curry powder, for an Indian touch.

For a richer dressing, replace the water with additional safflower or sunflower oil.

⬧ For an oil-free version, replace the oil with mashed avocado and add additional water, if necessary, to reach your desired consistency.

Nutrition Facts per serving (51 g): Calories 180, Fat Calories 160, Total Fat 18 g, Saturated Fat 2 g, Cholesterol 0 mg, Sodium 100 mg, Total Carb 4 g, Dietary Fiber 0 g, Sugars 3 g, Protein 0 g

Strawberry Vinaigrette Ⓖ🖐

YIELD: 1 ½ CUPS VINAIGRETTE

Prep time: 10 minutes, Total time: 10 minutes, Serving size: 2 tablespoons, Number of servings: 12

This tangy and slightly sweet vinaigrette provides a delicious way to ingest fine quantities of vitamin C, manganese, iodine, folate, and fiber from the delightfully colorful strawberry. Aromatic and spicy ginger is a great accent not only for its bold flavor but for its boost to blood circulation and the immune system. Lime, mint, and cardamom add extra dashes of both flavor and nutrition. Enjoy over salad as part of a romantic summer meal that includes Broccoli Dill Quiche (page 274) and a glass of Basil Rose Lemonade (page 141).

½ cup safflower or sunflower oil

½ cup water

½ cup strawberries

1 tablespoon plus 2 teaspoons balsamic vinegar

2 teaspoons freshly squeezed lime juice

1 teaspoon peeled and minced fresh ginger

½ teaspoon sea salt, or taste

¼ teaspoon Dijon mustard

Pinch of cayenne

Pinch of ground cardamom

Pinch of freshly ground black pepper

1 teaspoon finely chopped fresh mint

1. Place all the ingredients, except the mint, in a blender and blend well.

2. Pour into a bowl. Add the mint and gently mix well.

VARIATION

◆For an oil-free version, replace the oil with soaked and drained raw cashew pieces.

Nutrition Facts per serving (37 g): Calories 85, Fat Calories 80, Total Fat 9 g, Saturated Fat 1 g, Cholesterol 0 mg, Sodium 100 mg, Total Carb 1 g, Dietary Fiber 0 g, Sugars 0 g, Protein 0 g

TEMPLATE RECIPE
Vinaigrette

Oil component: Replace with grapeseed or olive oil. For an oil-free version, replace the oil with mashed avocado.

Vinegar component: Replace with raspberry vinegar, champagne vinegar, raw apple cider vinegar, sherry vinegar, or coconut vinegar.

Fruit component: Replace with kiwi, pineapple, or mango. Omit the fruit and replace with vegetables, such as carrot, beet, sautéed shiitake mushrooms, or roasted red bell pepper.

Salt component: Replace with tamari or coconut aminos (see page xv).

Seasoning component: Replace the ginger with garlic. Replace the cayenne and cardamom with 1 teaspoon of an ethnic spice blend, such as Indian (page 106) or Mexican (page 106).

Herb component: Replace the mint with fresh dill, cilantro, or basil.

Sweetener component: Add 1 tablespoon of your sweetener of choice, such as pure maple syrup, coconut nectar, or two pitted dates.

Golden Turmeric Dressing ⓖ

YIELD: ¾ CUP DRESSING

Prep time: 10 minutes, Total time: 10 minutes, Serving size: 2 tablespoons, Number of servings: 6

Want in on the secret to the endurance of builders of the Taj Mahal? It's all about the turmeric! If you have any inflammatory issues, run, don't walk, to make this rich and tangy dressing. Anti-inflammatory agents are found in turmeric, in the form of its yellow pigment called curcumin, and in ginger, in the form of compounds called gingerol. This dressing, with its bright visual effect and supercharged health benefits, is indeed like pouring liquid gold over a salad. Pairs very well with the Simple Chop Salad (page 174).

¼ **cup olive oil**
¼ **cup water**
1 **teaspoon peeled and minced fresh turmeric**
1 **teaspoon peeled and minced fresh ginger**
1 **tablespoon freshly squeezed lemon juice**
2 **teaspoons raw apple cider vinegar**
½ **teaspoon Dijon mustard**
½ **teaspoon agave nectar, coconut nectar, pure maple syrup, or desired sweetener to taste (optional, see page 89)**
Pinch of ground turmeric

¼ teaspoon sea salt, or to taste

Pinch of cayenne pepper

1. Place all the ingredients in a blender and blend until creamy.

VARIATION

⬥ For an oil-free version, replace the oil with soaked and drained raw cashew pieces.

Nutrition Facts per serving (32 g): Calories 85, Fat Calories 80, Total Fat 9 g, Saturated Fat 1.5 g, Cholesterol 0 mg, Sodium 110 mg, Total Carb 1 g, Dietary Fiber 0 g, Sugars 0 g, Protein 0 g

Raw Hempseed Ranch Dressing ♥ⓖ⬥

YIELD: 1 CUP DRESSING

Prep time: 20 minutes, Total time: 20 minutes, Serving size: 2 tablespoons, Number of servings: 8

A creamy ranch dressing for healthy brain, skin, and heart! Hemp seeds are a true gift of nature. Many consider them the most nutritious seed in the world, qualifying as a super superfood for all of their life-sustaining benefits. They feature a huge quantity of readily bioavailable protein (almost 4 grams in 1 tablespoon) including all ten amino acids and no phytic acid, so they don't need to be soaked like many other nuts and seeds for proper digestion. They also contain both omega-6 and omega-3 fatty acids, which are important to have in balance for optimal health. Heart-healthy cashews also provide the base for this low-fat and delicious version of the classic creamy dressing. Toss with the Super Sprout Salad (page 173) and serve with Jamaican Patties (page 280).

¼ cup raw cashew pieces

¾ cup plus 2 tablespoons water

½ cup hulled hemp seeds

2 tablespoons nutritional yeast

2 tablespoons freshly squeezed lemon juice

2 teaspoons raw apple cider vinegar

1 peeled garlic clove, peeled

½ teaspoon Dijon mustard

½ teaspoon sea salt, or to taste

¼ teaspoon onion flakes

¼ teaspoon wheat-free tamari or coconut aminos (page xv, optional)

Pinch of crushed red pepper flakes

Pinch of freshly ground black pepper

1 teaspoon minced fresh flat-leaf parsley

1 teaspoon minced fresh dill

Pinch of paprika

1. Soak the cashews in a bowl with water to cover for 15 minutes, up to 3 hours. Drain and rinse well.

2. Transfer the cashews to a blender with the ¾ cup plus 2 tablespoons of fresh water and the hemp seeds, nutritional yeast, lemon juice, vinegar, garlic, mustard, salt, onion flakes, tamari, if using, crushed red pepper flakes, and black pepper and blend until creamy.

3. Place in a bowl along with the parsley, dill, and paprika and whisk well before serving.

VARIATIONS

Replace the cashews with macadamia, pine, or Brazil nuts.

Try smoked paprika instead of regular, for an extra-savory flair.

Nutrition Facts per serving (29 g): Calories 130, Fat Calories 85, Total Fat 10 g, Saturated Fat 1 g, Cholesterol 0 mg, Sodium 150 mg, Total Carb 4 g, Dietary Fiber 1 g, Sugars 0 g, Protein 7 g

QUICKER AND EASIER

Oil-Free Avocado Dressing

For a supersimple oil-free dressing, combine 1/2 cup of mashed avocado, 1 1/2 tablespoons of freshly squeezed lemon or lime juice, water to your desired consistency (start with 1/4 cup), and salt and freshly ground black pepper to taste. Add a pinch of cayenne, crushed red pepper flakes, or chipotle chile powder for some heat. Enjoy!

Caesar Dressing ◉ ◆

YIELD: 1 ½ CUPS DRESSING

Prep time: 25 minutes, Total time: 25 minutes, Serving size: 2 tablespoons, Number of servings: 12

The key to the flavor in this vegan version of a classic dressing comes from nutritional yeast. Nutritional yeast is derived from a long-named organism, *Saccharomyces cerevisiae*, which is grown on molasses and subsequently harvested, washed, and dried, providing iron, protein, folic acid, and selenium. Capers, another flavor enhancer in this dressing, may have surprising benefits. Being flower buds, capers are very low in calories, 23 calories per 100 grams, and contain many phytonutrients, including well-known antioxidants rutin and quercetin. The spicy caper pickles were traditionally added to recipes as an appetite stimulant, and therefore help to prevent indigestion. Serve it on . . . you got it, the Caesar Salad (page 181), and even over steamed veggies.

½ cup raw cashew pieces
½ cup water
3 tablespoons nutritional yeast
2 tablespoons freshly squeezed lemon juice
1 tablespoon miso paste (see page 248)
2 teaspoons Dijon mustard
2 tablespoons sherry vinegar
1 tablespoon minced garlic
1 tablespoon capers
2 teaspoons vegan Worcestershire sauce (optional)
2 teaspoons wheat-free tamari or other soy sauce (optional)
¼ teaspoon sea salt, or to taste
Pinch of freshly ground black pepper

1. Place the cashews in a bowl with ample water to cover. Allow to sit for 20 minutes, up to overnight. Drain and rinse well.

2. Transfer to a strong blender with the remaining ingredients, including the ½ cup of fresh water, and blend until creamy.

VARIATION

Replace the cashews with macadamia nuts or Brazil nuts.

Nutrition Facts per serving (26 g): Calories 60, Fat Calories 35, Total Fat 4 g, Saturated Fat 1 g, Cholesterol 0 mg, Sodium 90 mg, Total Carb 4 g, Dietary Fiber 1 g, Sugars 1 g, Protein 2 g

Horseradish Dijon Dressing⊙

YIELD: ¾ CUP DRESSING

Prep time: 15 minutes, Total time: 15 minutes, Serving size: 2 tablespoons, Number of servings: 6

Horseradish is a spicy root that has a dramatic flavor profile. It comes from the mustard family, and thereby keeps company with the greats: kale, radish, mustard, and cabbage, for example. (The popular wasabi served at Japanese restaurants is a derivative of horseradish.) It has medicinal qualities, thanks to its mustard oil, which impedes bacterial growth and, as you may have experienced, can have a wonderful immediate effect on clearing sinus congestion.

May be enjoyed tossed in salads or as a sauce for Simple Baked Tofu (page 250) or Grilled Plantain Kebabs (page 166).

¼ cup plus 2 tablespoons grapeseed, safflower, or sunflower oil

3 tablespoons water

3 tablespoons prepared horseradish

1 tablespoon sherry vinegar, raw apple cider vinegar, coconut vinegar, or your favorite

2 tablespoons diced green onion or shallot

2 teaspoons Dijon mustard

⅛ teaspoon freshly ground black pepper

Pinch of sea salt, or to taste

Pinch of cayenne pepper or crushed red pepper flakes

1. Place all the ingredients in a bowl and whisk well.

VARIATIONS

Add 1 tablespoon of minced pickled ginger.

🜄 For an oil-free version, replace the oil with soaked raw cashew pieces, raw macadamia nuts, or pine nuts (see page 105), and blend.

Nutrition Facts per serving (32 g): Calories 130, Fat Calories 120, Total Fat 14 g, Saturated Fat 1.5 g, Cholesterol 0 mg, Sodium 90 mg, Total Carb 1 g, Dietary Fiber 0 g, Sugars 0 g, Protein 0 g

Oil-Free Macadamia Wasabi Dressing♥⊙🜄

YIELD: 1 CUP DRESSING

Prep time: 25 minutes, Total time: 25 minutes, Serving size: 2 tablespoons, Number of servings: 8

With a burst of heat, courtesy of wasabi powder, and a touch of creamy decadence, thanks to exotic macadamia nuts, this dressing will add an element of elegance to any salad or side veggie. Macadamia nuts are native to Australia and are cultivated nowadays also in Hawaii, where they were introduced in the late nineteenth century. Known as the fattiest of all nuts, and somewhat caloric, macadamias are a worthwhile indulgence every once in a while because the fat is monounsaturated—beneficial to cardiovascular health. Be sure to use a strong blender to produce the creamiest dressing. Enjoy tossed with salads or as a dipping sauce for Grilled Plantain Kebabs (page 166) or Veggie Lettuce Boats (page 160).

½ cup raw macadamia nuts

¾ cup water

2 teaspoons rice vinegar

1 ¼ to 1 ½ teaspoons wasabi powder (see page 85)

1 tablespoon freshly squeezed lemon juice

1 small garlic clove

1 teaspoon pickled ginger

½ teaspoon onion powder

¼ teaspoon sea salt, or to taste

Pinch of freshly ground black pepper

Pinch of crushed red pepper flakes

1 tablespoon minced fresh flat-leaf parsley

1. Place the macadamia nuts in a bowl with ample water to cover. Allow to sit for 20 minutes, or up to overnight. Rinse and drain well.

2. Transfer to a strong blender with all the remaining ingredients, including the ½ cup of fresh water and except the parsley, and blend well.

3. Pour into a bowl, add the parsley, and mix well before serving.

VARIATIONS

To turn this dressing into a sauce, simply leave out the vinegar.

Replace the macadamia nuts with raw cashew pieces or Brazil nuts.

Replace the parsley with fresh basil or cilantro, or 1 teaspoon of minced fresh dill.

Nutrition Facts per serving (26 g): Calories 65, Fat Calories 55, Total Fat 6.5 g, Saturated Fat 1 g, Cholesterol 0 mg, Sodium 120 mg, Total Carb 2 g, Dietary Fiber less than 1 g, Sugars 0 g, Protein 0 g

Creamy Pepita Dressing ⊙⬭

YIELD: 1 CUP DRESSING

Prep time: 10 minutes, Total time: 10 minutes, Serving size: 2 tablespoons, Number of servings: 8

Pumpkin seeds, also known as pepitas, are remarkable for their stunning nutritional content contained in their petite size. Most renowned for their magnesium dosage, which contributes to heart, bone, and blood vessel function, pepitas also contain plant-based omega-3 fats, phytosterols, antioxidants, and an abundance of the mineral zinc—important for prostate health. Enjoy at your next Cinco de Mayo celebration tossed with a watercress salad and served with Mexican Seitan-Stuffed Peppers (page 291).

½ cup water

¼ cup pumpkin seeds (pepitas)

¼ cup safflower or grapeseed oil

1 ½ tablespoons freshly squeezed lime juice

1 tablespoon finely chopped fresh cilantro (optional)

1 tablespoon raw apple cider vinegar or coconut vinegar

1 teaspoon wheat-free tamari or other soy sauce

1 teaspoon pure maple syrup, coconut nectar, agave nectar, or sweetener of choice

¾ teaspoon chili powder

½ teaspoon ground cumin (optionally toasted; see page 101)

¼ teaspoon sea salt, or to taste

⅛ teaspoon freshly ground black pepper

Pinch of cayenne pepper or chipotle chile powder

1. Place all the ingredients in a blender and blend well.

VARIATION

⬧ For an oil-free version, replace the oil with avocado or soaked raw cashews and add additional water to attain your desired consistency.

Nutrition Facts per serving (18 g): Calories 90, Fat Calories 80, Total Fat 9 g, Saturated Fat 1 g, Cholesterol 0 mg, Sodium 120 mg, Total Carb 1 g, Dietary Fiber 0 g, Sugars 0 g, Protein 1 g

---

TEMPLATE RECIPE
Creamy Dressings

- -

Liquid component: Replace the water with plant-based milk, such as soy, rice, almond, or coconut (for homemade, see page 104).

Oil component: Replace with grapeseed or olive oil.

♦ For an oil-free version, use mashed avocado, or soaked and drained raw cashews, Brazil nuts, or macadamia nuts.

Sweetener component: Replace the maple syrup with your sweetener of choice, such as coconut nectar, agave nectar, or two pitted dates (see page 89).

Creamy component: Replace the pepitas with sunflower seeds, walnuts, pecans, or macadamia nuts.

Vinegar component: Replace with champagne vinegar, rice vinegar, balsamic vinegar, or sherry vinegar.

Herb component: Replace the cilantro with fresh basil or dill.

Ethnic spice component: Add 2 teaspoons of an ethnic spice blend, such as Ethiopian (page 106), Herbes de Provence (page 106), or Indian (page 106).

Creamy Lemon Tahini Dressing ♥ Ⓖ

YIELD: 1 ½ CUPS DRESSING

Prep time: 10 minutes, Total time: 10 minutes, Serving size: 2 tablespoons, Number of servings: 12

The quintessential house dressing of many a natural foods restaurant, creamy tahini showcases all the benefits of the sesame seed, which is packed with calcium, magnesium, and amino acid building proteins. This dressing enlivens the palate with the unique flavor mix of miso, a great probiotic food, as well as enzyme-stimulating lemon, vinegar, and tamari. You may need to add slightly more water, depending upon the consistency of the tahini and the desired consistency of your dressing. A go-to dressing for Monk Bowls (see pages 100, 267) and simple salads.

½ cup plus 2 tablespoons water
1 tablespoon unpasteurized miso paste (see page 248)
½ cup creamy tahini
2 teaspoons wheat-free tamari or other soy sauce, or to taste
2 tablespoons freshly squeezed lemon juice
2 teaspoons raw apple cider vinegar or coconut vinegar
2 teaspoons nutritional yeast (optional)
Pinch of cayenne pepper
1 tablespoon minced green onion (optional)
1 garlic clove, pressed, or 1 teaspoon peeled and minced fresh ginger (optional)

1. Combine the water and miso in a small bowl and whisk well.

2. Add the remaining ingredients and whisk well.

Add 1 tablespoon of finely chopped fresh flat-leaf parsley or 1 teaspoon of minced fresh dill.

Replace the lemon juice with freshly squeezed lime juice and add 1 tablespoon of minced fresh cilantro, 1 teaspoon of chili powder, and a pinch of chipotle chile powder, for a Mexican twist.

Experiment with different types of miso paste and see how the flavor of the dressing is affected.

Nutrition Facts per serving (14 g): Calories 60, Fat Calories 50, Total Fat 5.5 g, Saturated Fat 1 g, Cholesterol 0 mg, Sodium 70 mg, Total Carb 2 g, Dietary Fiber 1 g, Sugars 0 g, Protein 2 g

Oil-Free Creamy Sweet Potato Dressing 🅖◆

YIELD: 1¼ CUPS DRESSING

Prep time: 10 minutes, Cook time: 10 minutes, Total time: 20 minutes, Serving size: 2 tablespoons, Number of servings: 10

Try this velvety dressing, which capitalizes not only on sweet potato's creamy texture but on its substantial provision of vitamins A, B_6, and C, as well as potassium and manganese, helping to strengthen our immune system and eyesight, among many other virtues. Add additional liquid to reach your desired consistency. Serve on salads alongside Lentil Walnut Loaf (page 288) or Corn Casserole (page 286).

½ cup peeled, cooked, and mashed sweet potato (see Purple Potato Hash recipe, page 130, for cooking method)

¾ cup unsweetened soy, rice, or almond milk (for homemade, see Plant-Based Milk, page 104)

2 tablespoons raw apple cider vinegar

1 teaspoon Dijon or stone-ground mustard

1½ tablespoons finely chopped fresh flat-leaf parsley, basil, or cilantro

¼ teaspoon sea salt, or to taste

⅛ teaspoon freshly ground black pepper

Pinch of cayenne pepper

Pinch of smoked paprika or chipotle chile powder

1. Place all the ingredients in a blender and blend well.

VARIATIONS

Experiment with different varieties of sweet potato, such as purple, garnet, or jewel.

Replace the raw apple cider vinegar with coconut vinegar, sherry vinegar, or raspberry vinegar.

Nutrition Facts per serving (45 g): Calories 20, Fat Calories 5, Total Fat 0 g, Saturated Fat 0 g, Cholesterol 0 mg, Sodium 90 mg, Total Carb 3 g, Dietary Fiber 0 g, Sugars 0 g, Protein 1 g

Cilantro Mint Chutney ♥🅖◆

YIELD: 1 CUP CHUTNEY

Prep time: 15 minutes, Total time: 15 minutes, Serving size: 2 tablespoons, Number of servings: 8

Cilantro (or coriander, for those across the pond) boasts a wide array of phytonutrients, antioxidants, and essential oils and has been used in traditional medicine for ages as an antiseptic, analgesic, pick-me-up, and digestive aid. Mint, its counterpart in this chutney, is not only a terrific palate cleanser but also is a boost for digestion—just its aroma activates the salivary glands, which kicks off the digestive process. Enjoy as a dipping sauce with Curried Garbanzo Cakes with Poppy Seeds (page 164), Buffalo Cauliflower (page 163), or Broiled Artichoke Fritters (page 155).

2 cups loosely packed chopped fresh cilantro

¼ cup chopped fresh mint

¼ cup dried shredded unsweetened coconut (optionally toasted; see page 101)

¼ cup plus 1 tablespoon water

1 tablespoon peeled and minced fresh ginger

2 tablespoons plus 1 teaspoon freshly squeezed lime juice

¾ teaspoon seeded and diced jalapeño or other hot pepper (see Scoville scale, page 179)

½ teaspoon raw apple cider vinegar or coconut vinegar

1 teaspoon ground cumin

½ teaspoon ground coriander

¼ teaspoon sea salt, or to taste

1. Place all the ingredients in a blender and blend until smooth.

VARIATIONS

Add 1 tablespoon of olive oil.

Add 2 tablespoons of shredded and optionally toasted (page 101) coconut.

Replace the ginger with garlic.

Add 1 teaspoon each of cumin seeds, coriander seeds, and fennel seeds.

Nutrition Facts per serving (20 g): Calories 50, Fat Calories 40, Total Fat 5 g, Saturated Fat 4 g, Choles-

sterol 0 mg, Sodium 80 mg, Total Carb 2 g, Dietary Fiber 1 g, Sugars 0 g, Protein 0 g

Raw Tamarind Sauce ♥ⓖ◆

YIELD: ¾ CUP SAUCE

Prep time: 10 minutes, Total time: 10 minutes, Serving size: 2 tablespoons, Number of servings: 6

Tamarind is an ancient native of Africa and Southeast Asia, where it continues to be popularly used in regional cuisine. Both sweet and sour, tamarind is a fruit that, unusually, contains calcium. It is a surefire go-to for digestive issues, and has been used for centuries for fevers, scratchy throats, and relief of inflammation. Serve with Veggie Lettuce Boats (page 160), Jamaican Patties (page 280), or Curried Garbanzo Cakes with Poppy Seeds (page 164).

½ cup plus 3 tablespoons water

¼ cup tightly packed pitted dates

1 tablespoon tamarind paste

½ teaspoon ground ginger

½ teaspoon garam masala

¼ teaspoon sea salt, or to taste

⅛ teaspoon cayenne pepper

Pinch of ground cinnamon

1. Place all the ingredients in a blender and blend well.

VARIATIONS

Replace the dates with your desired sweetener to taste (see page 89). Try pure maple syrup or coconut sugar.

Nutrition Facts per serving (29 g): Calories 35, Fat Calories 0, Total Fat 0 g, Saturated Fat 0 g, Cholesterol 0 mg, Sodium 100 mg, Total Carb 9 g, Dietary Fiber less than 1 g, Sugars 8 g, Protein 0 g

Zesty Chimichurri Sauce🅖

YIELD: 1 ½ CUPS SAUCE

Prep time: 30 minutes, Total time: 30 minutes, Serving size: 2 tablespoons, Number of servings: 12

Chimichurri originates in Argentina and Uruguay. Argentinian cowboys, or gauchos, who herded the cattle, came up with this flavorful, super-easy-to-mix-together, rustic blend of herbs, spices, and oil to top their cowboy-cooked meals. The name *chimichurri* evolved from the Basque word *tximitxurri*, which means "a mixture of a lot of things"! There are some variations in its ingredients, but most often parsley provides the base, which supplies varied key vitamins that boost immunity, flush out toxins, and tone bones. This flavor blend gives a little zest to any meal. Awesome on top of Simple Baked Tofu (page 260), Maple Baked Tempeh (page 262), or Millet and Butternut Squash with Broccoli (page 284).

¾ cup olive oil
1 cup finely chopped fresh flat-leaf parsley
¼ cup finely chopped fresh cilantro
3 tablespoons freshly squeezed lemon juice
3 tablespoons diced shallot
2 tablespoons minced garlic
1 ½ tablespoons sherry vinegar
1 ½ tablespoons red wine vinegar
1 ½ teaspoons dried oregano
½ teaspoon sea salt, or to taste
⅛ teaspoon freshly ground black pepper
¼ teaspoon crushed red pepper flakes

1. Place all the ingredients in a small bowl and whisk well. Alternatively, you can place all the ingredients in a food processor and pulse chop until just pureed.

VARIATION

💧For an oil-free version, replace the oil with ½ cup mashed avocado. Add water to reach your desired consistency.

Nutrition Facts per serving (45 g): Calories 130, Fat Calories 120, Total Fat 14 g, Saturated Fat 2 g, Cholesterol 0 mg, Sodium 100 mg, Total Carb 2 g, Dietary Fiber 0 g, Sugars 0 g, Protein 0 g

Smoky BBQ Sauce🅖💧

YIELD: 2 CUPS SAUCE

Prep time: 20 minutes, Total time: 20 minutes, Serving size: 1/4 cup, Number of servings: 8

The obsession with barbecue in American culture is in many cases all about the sauce, and with several regional varieties of the ubiquitous condiment, we had to get in on the action. This BBQ sauce, lower in sugar than store-bought brands, richly enhances a dish with its smoky, sweet sultriness, topping it off with tomato's vitamin C and lycopene, and the notable iron content of molasses (especially blackstrap). A touch of smoke and accent of warm, stimulating cloves and chili complete the full sensory experience. Serve with BBQ Roasted Tofu with Collards (page 278), Simple One-Pot Meal (page 266), or as a dipping sauce for Grilled Plantain Kebabs (page 166).

1 (6-ounce) can tomato paste
½ cup filtered water

¼ cup molasses

1 tablespoon pure maple syrup (optional)

1 tablespoon raw unfiltered apple cider vinegar

1 ½ teaspoons chili powder

¼ teaspoon sea salt, or to taste

1 teaspoon wheat-free tamari or other soy sauce, or to taste

¼ teaspoon freshly ground black pepper

¼ teaspoon liquid smoke (see page 85)

⅛ teaspoon ground cloves

⅛ teaspoon chipotle chile powder (optional)

1. Place all the ingredients in a bowl and whisk well.

Nutrition Facts per serving (48 g): Calories 50, Fat Calories 0, Total Fat 0 g, Saturated Fat 0 g, Cholesterol 0 mg, Sodium 150 mg, Total Carb 12 g, Dietary Fiber 1 g, Sugars 9 g, Protein 1 g

Ancho Chile Sauce ♥ⓖ◐

YIELD: 2 CUPS SAUCE

Prep time: 25 minutes, Cook time: 5 minutes, Total time: 30 minutes, Serving size: 1/4 cup, Number of servings: 8

Originating in Mexico, where it is known as the poblano pepper, the ancho chile has a color range from green to a very dark red. The dark red phase is the one where the pepper takes on its flavorful spice, and on the hot pepper scale it is known for mild heat with sweet. Like most hot peppers, ancho chiles contain capsaicin, a pain relieving anti-inflammatory chemical that may also have potent cardiovascular benefits, such as increasing nitric oxide. This powerful substance can sometimes irritate the skin and eyes, so just be sure to wash your hands or wear food han-

dler gloves when handling the soaked chile pepper. You can also open the dried chiles and shake the seeds out while they're still dry. Serve over Creamy Herbed Polenta (page 170), as a sauce for Millet Black Bean Veggie Burgers (page 269), or with your Simple One-Pot Meal (page 266).

½ cup chopped raw cashews

1 to 2 dried ancho chiles

1 ¼ cups water

½ cup seeded and chopped tomato

1 tablespoon plus 2 teaspoons freshly squeezed lime juice

2 large or 4 medium-size pitted dates (2 tablespoons)

½ teaspoon sea salt, or to taste

½ teaspoon ground cumin

½ teaspoon dried oregano

¼ teaspoon chipotle chile powder

⅛ teaspoon freshly ground black pepper

Pinch of ground cinnamon

1. Place the cashews in a bowl with ample water to cover. Allow to sit for 20 minutes, or up to an hour.

2. Place the ancho pepper in a separate bowl with ample hot water to cover. Allow to sit for 20 minutes.

3. Meanwhile, place the remaining ingredients, including the 1 ¼ cups of fresh water, in a blender.

4. Remove the seeds from the ancho chile. Discard the soak water. Measure out ⅓ cup of the chile and place in the blender.

5. Drain and rinse the cashews well. Discard the soak water. Place the cashews in the blender and blend until creamy.

Try using fire-roasted tomatoes and adding 2 tablespoons of soaked and drained sun-dried tomatoes.

Nutrition Facts per serving (60 g): Calories 100, Fat Calories 55, Total Fat 6 g, Saturated Fat 1 g, Cholesterol 0 mg, Sodium 150 mg, Total Carb 10 g, Dietary Fiber 1 g, Sugars 5 g, Protein 3 g

Easy Cheezy Sauce ♥ⓖ◖

YIELD: 1 CUP SAUCE

Prep time: 5 minutes, Soak time: 20 minutes, Total time: 25 minutes, Serving size: 2 tablespoons, Number of servings: 8

On the go and need an easy cheese sauce? This is it. Six ingredients plus water makes for a sauce that is not only easy, but supplies valuable minerals, such as copper and manganese, not to mention a helping of B vitamins from old, reliable nutritional yeast. Serve on top of steamed vegetables, or toss in with pasta for a simple cream sauce. Also amazing on top of Creamy Herbed Polenta (page 170).

1 cup raw cashew pieces
¾ cup water
3 tablespoons nutritional yeast
½ teaspoon sea salt, or to taste
½ teaspoon ground turmeric (optional)
⅛ teaspoon freshly ground black pepper
Pinch of cayenne pepper or chipotle chile powder

1. Place the cashews in a bowl with ample water to cover. Allow to sit for 20 minutes, or up to a few hours. Rinse and drain well.

2. Transfer to a blender along with the remaining ingredients, including the ¾ cup of fresh water, and blend until creamy.

VARIATIONS

Add 1 tablespoon of an ethnic spice blend, such as Indian (page 106), Mexican (page 106), or Italian (page 105).

Add 1 tablespoon of minced fresh cilantro, basil, or flat-leaf parsley, or 2 teaspoons of minced fresh dill.

Blend the cheese with 1 cup of raw or roasted red bell pepper.

For Vegan Mac N Cheese, toss with elbow pasta (try rice pasta).

Nutrition Facts per serving (55 g): Calories 165, Fat Calories 110, Total Fat 12.5 g, Saturated Fat 2 g, Cholesterol 0 mg, Sodium 150 mg, Total Carb 9 g, Dietary Fiber 1 g, Sugars 1 g, Protein 6 g

Almond Dipping Sauce ⓖ◖

YIELD: ¾ CUP SAUCE

Prep time: 10 minutes, Total time: 10 minutes, Serving size: 2 tablespoons, Number of servings: 6

Versatile almonds, even when ground into butter, pack a protein punch that can't be beat in the condiment world, and adapt well as a base for other flavor accents. With lots of healthy unsaturated fatty acids, vitamin E, copper, and magnesium, adding this sauce makes any dish nutrient dense, while providing just the right amount of sweet, salty, and spicy. Be sure to adjust the water, based on the consistency of almond butter. Serve with

Grilled Plantain Kebabs (page 166) or Black Bean Tostones (page 167).

½ cup almond butter

½ cup low- or full-fat coconut milk, or soy, rice, or almond milk (for homemade, see Plant-Based Milk, page 104)

1 teaspoon wheat-free tamari or other soy sauce, or to taste

2 teaspoons pure maple syrup or Date Syrup (page 88)

1 ½ teaspoons rice vinegar

½ teaspoon tamarind paste, or 1 ½ teaspoons freshly squeezed lime juice

¼ teaspoon crushed red pepper flakes

Pinch of sea salt

1. Place all the ingredients in a bowl and whisk well. Add water, if necessary, to reach your desired consistency.

VARIATIONS

Replace the almond butter with tahini, peanut butter, or cashew butter.

Add 1 minced fresh garlic clove or peeled and minced fresh ginger.

Add 1 tablespoon of minced green onion and/or minced fresh cilantro.

♥ For a raw version, use raw almond butter; a raw sweetener, such as Date Syrup (page 88) or coconut nectar; a raw vinegar; and use your choice of a homemade Plant-Based Milk (page 104).

Nutrition Facts per serving (47 g): Calories 140, Fat Calories 105, Total Fat 12 g, Saturated Fat 1 g, Cholesterol 0 mg, Sodium 140 mg, Total Carb 6 g, Dietary Fiber 2 g, Sugars 3 g, Protein 5 g

Creamy Mexican Dipping Sauce ⊙

YIELD: 1 CUP SAUCE

Prep time: 10 minutes, Total time: 10 minutes, Serving size: 2 tablespoons, Number of servings: 8

Make your dip Mexican with the addition of classic flavors, such as antioxidant-rich cilantro, immunity-boosting garlic, and fiery chili powder. Vitamin C–rich lime juice also has unique active compounds called flavonoid glucosides, which offer antibiotic properties. Serve with Black Bean Tostones (page 167), Grilled Plantain Kebabs (page 166), or Quinoa Amaranth Cakes (page 168).

½ cup raw cashews

¼ cup plus 2 tablespoons unsweetened soy, rice, or almond milk

1 tablespoon minced fresh cilantro

2 teaspoons freshly squeezed lime juice

1 garlic clove, pressed or minced

¼ teaspoon chipotle chile powder, or ¼ teaspoon chili powder and a pinch of cayenne pepper

Pinch of chili powder

Pinch of sea salt, or to taste

Pinch of freshly ground black pepper

1. Place the cashews in a bowl with ample water to cover. Allow to sit for 20 minutes or longer. Drain, rinse, and drain well.

2. Transfer to a blender with the soy milk and blend until creamy, adding additional soy milk, if necessary, to fully blend the cashews.

3. Transfer to a small bowl. Add the remaining ingredients and mix well. Alternatively, you can process all the ingredients in a small food processor until well blended.

VARIATIONS

Add ¼ cup of mashed roasted garlic (see page 114).

For Goddess Dipping Sauce, blend with 2 tablespoons of fresh basil, 2 tablespoons of fresh flat-leaf parsley, and 1 teaspoon of fresh dill.

Go decadent and replace the cashews with vegan mayonnaise, either homemade (page 113) or Vegenaise.

Nutrition Facts per serving (30 g): Calories 85, Fat Calories6057, Total Fat 6.5 g, Saturated Fat 1 g, Cholesterol 0 mg, Sodium 25 mg, Total Carb 5 g, Dietary Fiber less than 1 g, Sugars 0 g, Protein 3 g

Roasted Red Pepper Sauce🄖

YIELD: 1 ¼ CUPS SAUCE

Prep time: 10 minutes, Cook time: 20 minutes, Cooling time: 10 minutes, Total time: 40 minutes, Serving size: 1/4 cup, Number of servings: 5

The red pepper, scientific name *Capsicum annuum*, is not only brightly colored, but super rich in antioxidant phytochemicals and loaded with vitamins A and C, as well as the essential mineral manganese. Roasting the peppers concentrates these nutrients while enhancing the flavor. The toasted coconut adds a subtle sweet and earthy tone that will rock your world. Serve on top of Creamy

Herbed Polenta (page 170), Garlicky Greens (page 191), or Broccoli Dill Quiche (page 274).

3 or 4 red bell peppers
Oil, for peppers
2 tablespoons dried shredded unsweetened coconut (optionally toasted; see page 101)
¼ teaspoon sea salt, or to taste
Pinch of freshly ground black pepper
1 teaspoon balsamic vinegar
1 teaspoon wheat-free tamari or other soy sauce (optional)

1. Preheat the oven broiler on HIGH. Slice the bell peppers in half, scoop out the seeds. Lightly oil both sides of the peppers and place, cut side down, on an oiled baking sheet.

2. Broil until char marks appear, about 8 minutes. Flip and cook for an additional 8 minutes. Transfer to a bowl and cover with a lid.

3. Allow to cool for 10 minutes. Carefully remove most of the skins, and measure out 1 ¼ cups of bell pepper for this recipe.

4. Transfer to a blender with the remaining ingredients and blend well. Serve warm.

VARIATIONS

You can grill the peppers instead of roasting them (see page 101).

Replace the red bell pepper with yellow bell pepper.

Add 1 tablespoon of coconut oil before blending.

Add six roasted garlic cloves (see page 114) or one raw garlic clove, before blending.

🌢For an oil-free version, instead of lightly oiling the peppers, add about ½ cup water or vegetable stock (see page 108) to the pan while roasting.

Nutrition Facts per serving (106 g): Calories 60, Fat Calories 35, Total Fat 4 g, Saturated Fat 3 g, Cholesterol 0 mg, Sodium 125 mg, Total Carb 5 g, Dietary Fiber 2 g, Sugars 3 g, Protein 1 g

Sweet-and-Sour Sauce🅖🌢

YIELD: 2 ½ CUPS SAUCE

Prep time: 10 minutes, Cook time: 15 minutes, Total time: 25 minutes, Serving size: 1/4 cup, Number of servings: 10

Sweet-and-sour sauce is so desirable because it hits on many of the flavor profiles, such as sweet, sour, salty, and tangy. It is believed to be native to the Chinese province of Hunan and appears often in Hunan cuisine. In most restaurants and bottled varieties, sweet-and-sour sauce is frequently oil-heavy, so give this light and clean version a try. Serve as a dipping sauce for Kentucky Baked Portobello Nuggets (page 165), Veggie Lettuce Boats (page 160), or Curried Garbanzo Cakes with Poppy Seeds (page 164).

2 cups pineapple juice

1 tablespoon Sucanat, organic sugar, or desired sweetener to taste (see page 89)

3 tablespoons rice vinegar

½ teaspoon wheat-free tamari or other soy sauce, or to taste

1 tablespoon tomato paste

1 teaspoon peeled and minced fresh ginger

¼ teaspoon crushed red pepper flakes

Pinch of sea salt, or to taste

Pinch of freshly ground black pepper

1 tablespoon plus 1 teaspoon arrowroot powder or cornstarch

2 tablespoons cold water

1. Place all the ingredients, except the arrowroot and water, in a pot over medium heat. Cook for 10 minutes, stirring occasionally. Be careful not to boil.

2. Place the arrowroot and water in a small bowl and whisk well. Add to the pot and cook until the sauce thickens, about 5 additional minutes, stirring frequently. Serve warm or cold.

Nutrition Facts per serving (62 g): Calories 45, Fat Calories 0, Total Fat 0 g, Saturated Fat 0 g, Cholesterol 0 mg, Sodium 190 mg, Total Carb 117 g, Dietary Fiber 0 g, Sugars 8 g, Protein 0 g

Simple Roasted Butternut Squash Sauce🅖

YIELD: 2 CUPS SAUCE

Prep time: 10 minutes, Cook time: 40 minutes, Total time: 50 minutes, Serving size: 1/4 cup, Number of servings: 8

Nothing says autumn quite like squash. A gourd family member, squash is actually characterized as a fruit because it has seeds. Super fibrous, and with a lovely orange color that clues us in to its heart-protecting carotenoids, butternut squash specifically also provides potassium, folate, and vitamin B_6. The roasting of the squash makes for a sauce that is totally dreamy on its own, or a nice base for herbs to add a variety of flavor possibilities. Enjoy as part of a holiday feast over steamed or roasted vegetables, and the Lentil Walnut Loaf (page 288).

1 small butternut squash (for 1 ½ cups cooked)

Oil, for baking sheet

¾ cup soy, coconut, rice, or almond milk (for homemade, see Plant-Based Milk, page 104)

½ teaspoon sea salt, or to taste

Pinch of freshly ground black pepper

Pinch of cayenne pepper

1. Preheat the oven to 425°F. Slice the squash in half lengthwise, remove the seeds with a spoon, and place on a well-oiled baking sheet or casserole dish filled with about ¼ inch of water. Place in the oven and cook until a knife can pass easily through the toughest part of the squash, about 40 minutes. Remove from the oven.

2. Carefully scoop out 1 ½ cups of the squash and place in a blender.

3. Add the remaining ingredients and blend well.

VARIATIONS

Experiment with different types of squash, such as buttercup, acorn, turban, kabocha, and delicata.

Replace the squash with sweet potatoes or pumpkin.

This sauce can serve as a base that you can take in different ethnic directions by adding 1 tablespoon of an ethnic spice blend, such as Mexican (page 106), Indian (page 106), or Italian (page 105).

Add 1 tablespoon finely chopped fresh cilantro, basil, or flat-leaf parsley.

Add 2 teaspoons of minced fresh sage or dill.

Nutrition Facts per serving (74 g): Calories 20, Fat Calories 5, Total Fat 0 g, Saturated Fat 0 g, Cholesterol 0 mg, Sodium 160 mg, Total Carb 4 g, Dietary Fiber less than 1 g, Sugars 0 g, Protein 1 g

Raw Coconut Curry Sauce ♥ⓖ♦

YIELD: 2 CUPS SAUCE

Prep time: 10 minutes, Total time: 10 minutes, Serving size: 1/4 cup, Number of servings: 8

Experience a hint of the tropics in this raw version of a coconut curry. Curry powder provides the dominant flavor with the spices turmeric, cumin, and coriander. Low on carb and high on fiber, coconut meat helps you metabolize both protein and fat due to its whopping manganese content. Serve with Raw Coconut Curry Vegetables (page 268) or as a dipping sauce for Veggie Lettuce Boats (page 160) and Raw Collard Veggie Rolls (page 260). You can even toss this sauce into a bowl of cooked rice pasta.

¾ cup medium-soft fresh coconut meat

1 ½ cups coconut water

1 tablespoon plus 1 teaspoon fresh ginger

2 tablespoons freshly squeezed lime juice

1 tablespoon raw almond butter

1 tablespoon finely chopped fresh cilantro

1 ½ teaspoons curry powder

1 teaspoon seeded and diced jalapeño pepper

1 teaspoon coconut aminos (page xv), wheat-free tamari, or other soy sauce

½ teaspoon tamarind paste

¼ teaspoon sea salt, or to taste

¼ teaspoon ground cumin

1. Place all the ingredients in a blender and blend well.

VARIATIONS

Replace the coconut meat and ½ cup of coconut water with 1 cup of coconut milk.

Replace the almond butter with peanut butter.

Nutrition Facts per serving (74 g): Calories 50, Fat Calories 35, Total Fat 4 g, Saturated Fat 2 g, Cholesterol 0 mg, Sodium 165 mg, Total Carb 4 g, Dietary Fiber 2 g, Sugars 2 g, Protein 1 g

Tahini Oat Sauce ◉ ◈

YIELD: 3 CUPS SAUCE

Prep time: 5 minutes, Cook time: 20 minutes, Total time: 25 minutes, Serving size: 1/4 cup, Number of servings: 12

This sauce proves that oats are not just for breakfast anymore. When combined with superfood tahini and its calcium, vitamin, and mineral mix, oats make a creamy, filling, and rich sauce that's both healthful and tasty. The fiber in oats helps to detoxify the digestive system as well as lower levels of cholesterol. Serve over steamed vegetables, Simple Baked Tofu (page 260), or Maple Baked Tempeh (page 262).

3 cups water

½ cup rolled oats (try gluten-free)

1 garlic clove, pressed or minced

¼ cup creamy tahini

1 ½ tablespoons freshly squeezed lemon juice

1 tablespoon wheat-free tamari or other soy sauce

¼ teaspoon crushed red pepper flakes

Pinch of sea salt

Pinch of freshly ground black pepper

1 ½ tablespoons finely chopped fresh flat-leaf parsley

1. Place the water in a small pot over medium-high heat. Add the oats, garlic, and tahini, and cook until the oats break down and the sauce thickens, about 15 minutes, stirring frequently to prevent burning.

2. Add the lemon juice, tamari, crushed red pepper flakes, salt, and black pepper, and mix well.

3. Cook for 3 minutes, stirring frequently. Add the parsley, and stir well before serving.

VARIATIONS

Replace the parsley with fresh cilantro or basil, or 2 teaspoons of minced fresh dill.

Replace the garlic with ginger.

Add 1 tablespoon of an ethnic spice blend, such as Mexican (page 106), Italian (page 105), or Moroccan (page 106).

Nutrition Facts per serving (18 g): Calories 60, Fat Calories 30, Total Fat 3 g, Saturated Fat 1 g, Cholesterol 0 mg, Sodium 100 mg, Total Carb 6 g, Dietary Fiber 1 g, Sugars 0 g, Protein 2 g

Fire-Roasted Tomato Sauce ⊙◆

YIELD: 5 CUPS SAUCE

Prep time: 10 minutes, Cook time: 35 minutes,
Total time: 45 minutes, Serving size: 1/2 cup,
Number of servings: 10

Tomatoes shine in this sublime sauce, where their lycopene and vitamin A and C content is enhanced by the addition of superherbs basil, parsley, and oregano. Many brands of canned tomatoes offer fire-roasted, which brings out the tomatoes' natural sweetness and imparts a hint of smoke. (If you can't find them in your store or prefer to make your own, you can fire roast your own tomatoes by grilling them according to the method discussed on page 101.)

Basil has antibacterial and anti-inflammatory properties, while parsley provides iron and vitamin K, and oregano gives a dollop of a strong antioxidant called rosmarinic acid, which supports the immune system. Serve over brown rice pasta, a plate of grilled vegetables (see page 101) or Three Greens with Tomato Sauce (page 197), or Simple Baked Tofu (page 260).

½ cup water
1 cup diced yellow onion
4 garlic cloves, pressed or minced
1 teaspoon dried oregano
¼ teaspoon crushed red pepper flakes
1 (28-ounce) can diced fire-roasted tomatoes, or 3 cups chopped fresh tomato with liquid
1 cup chopped tomato (½-inch pieces)
1 tablespoon tomato paste
1 tablespoon balsamic vinegar
2 tablespoons chiffonaded fresh basil
2 tablespoons finely chopped fresh flat-leaf parsley
1 tablespoon nutritional yeast
½ teaspoon sea salt, or to taste
⅛ teaspoon freshly ground black pepper

1. Place the water in a pot over medium-high heat. Add the onion and garlic and cook for 3 minutes, stirring frequently, adding small amounts of water, if necessary, to prevent sticking.

2. Lower the heat to medium. Add the oregano, crushed red pepper flakes, fire-roasted tomatoes, chopped tomato, tomato paste, and vinegar, and cook for 20 minutes, stirring frequently, lowering the temperature if the sauce begins to boil.

3. Add the basil, parsley, nutritional yeast, salt, and black pepper and cook for 15 minutes, stirring frequently.

VARIATIONS

Replace the water with 1 ½ tablespoons of melted coconut oil.

Add ½ cup of red wine along with the tomatoes.

Add additional spices or herbs, such as 2 teaspoons of fennel seeds, 2 teaspoons of fresh oregano, 2 teaspoons of chiffonaded fresh sage, 1 teaspoon of fresh thyme, and/or ½ teaspoon of minced fresh rosemary.

Add 1 cup of sliced mushrooms, ½ cup of diced olives, and/or ½ cup of chopped fennel bulb along with the tomatoes.

Add 1½ cups of cooked beans, such as fava or cannellini, or chickpeas along with the tomatoes.

Nutrition Facts per serving (114 g): Calories 40, Fat Calories 5, Total Fat 0 g, Saturated Fat 0 g, Cholesterol 0 mg, Sodium 130 mg, Total Carb 9 g, Dietary Fiber 2 g, Sugars 2 g, Protein 2 g

Oil-Free Mushroom Gravy ⊙ ◆

YIELD: 2 ½ CUPS GRAVY

Prep time: 10 minutes, Cook time: 20 minutes, Total time: 30 minutes, Serving size: 1/4 cup, Number of servings: 10

This flavorful, savory gravy highlights the unique benefits of shiitake mushrooms—namely an immune system strengthener called DEA, and beta glucan, a soluble fiber. Cashews are a seamless substitute for oil in this recipe. Besides their unmistakable creamy factor, they are a rich source of heart-friendly monounsaturated fatty acids as well as multiple minerals, including the less-often-found selenium. This immunity-supporting comfort food gravy goes well on top of Smashed Roasted Cauliflower and Parsnip (page 202), Herb-Roasted Potatoes (page 214), Simple Baked Tofu (page 260), Maple Baked Tempeh (page 262), or Lentil Walnut Loaf (page 288). Actually, this sauce goes well over almost everything!!

2 ¼ cups water or vegetable stock (see page 108)
1 ¼ cups thinly sliced yellow onion
¼ cup thinly sliced celery
4 large garlic cloves, pressed or minced
1 cup thinly sliced shiitake mushrooms
½ cup chopped raw cashews (optionally toasted; see page 101)
2 tablespoons nutritional yeast
2 teaspoons wheat-free tamari or other soy sauce, or to taste
⅛ teaspoon freshly ground black pepper
Pinch of sea salt, or to taste
Pinch of ground nutmeg
Pinch of crushed red pepper flakes
2 tablespoons finely chopped fresh flat-leaf parsley

1. Place ¼ cup of the water or stock in a pot over medium-high heat. Add the onion, celery, and garlic and cook for 2 minutes, stirring constantly, adding small amounts of water, if necessary, to prevent sticking. Add the mushrooms, and cook for 1 minute, stirring frequently. Add the remaining 2 cups of water or stock, stir well, lower the heat to medium, and cook for 2 minutes, stirring occasionally.

2. Transfer approximately half of the contents of the pot to a strong blender, add the cashews, and blend until creamy. Return to the pot.

3. Lower the heat to medium-low. Add the nutritional yeast, tamari, black pepper, salt, nutmeg, and crushed red pepper flakes, and cook for 5 minutes, stirring occasionally. Add additional water or stock if a thinner gravy is desired. Add the parsley and stir well before serving.

VARIATIONS
Experiment with different types of mushrooms.

Replace the cashews with macadamia nuts, pistachio nuts, or pecans.

Add 1 teaspoon chiffonade fresh sage along with the parsley.

You can also thicken the gravy with a roux. To do so, omit the cashews. Whisk ¼ cup of flour (try all-purpose gluten-free or the Gluten-Free Flour Mix on page 105) and ¼ cup of oil, such as safflower or sunflower, in a small bowl. Add to the gravy before adding the spices at the end of the recipe. Stir until the gravy thickens.

Nutrition Facts per serving (71 g): Calories 65, Fat Calories 40, Total Fat 4.5 g, Saturated Fat 0 g, Cholesterol 0 mg, Sodium 90 mg, Total Carb 5 g, Dietary Fiber less than 1 g, Sugars 1 g, Protein 2 g

CHAPTER 14

Soups and Stews

No book on healing would be complete without a section on soups. Many people naturally gravitate toward lighter meals of soup when they feel the need to heal, and easy-to-eat, easy-to-digest soups and broths are often the best meals to promote rest and recovery. For an added healthy benefit, all of these recipes are oil-free.

Those looking for the lightest meals can enjoy the ultralight recipes, such as Healing Broth (page 243) and Miso Vegetable Soup (page 246). Raw soups, such as Raw Cucumber Fennel Soup (page 244), Raw Carrot Brazil Nut Soup (page 245), and Watermelon Gazpacho (page 243), are perfect for warmer months. Hardier soups, such as Mexican Two-Bean Soup (page 253) and Moroccan Chickpea Stew (page 255), will be your go-to meals for the colder months. Herald the arrival of spring with Creamy Asparagus Soup with Corn (page 250), and celebrate the colors of autumn with the Ital Roasted Squash and Sweet Potato Soup (page 251). Be sure to add the Herb Croutons (page 111) for an extra crunch.

You will also find soups from ancient healing traditions. Congees are an ancient form of soup used in traditional oriental medicine. Specific herbs and vegetables are added to produce different desired results (increased digestion, decreased congestion, increased vitality, etc.). Check out the Congee with Fenugreek (page 247) for an example. Kitchari (page 257) is another ancient healing stew in the Indian Ayurvedic tradition (page 26); here, different herbs and spices are added, depending on the type of condition being addressed.

For a selection of over one hundred soups for every season, please check out my book *The 30-Minute Vegan's Soups On!* and experience for yourself a remarkable array of vegan soups for the chicken's soul!

Healing Broth☺◆

YIELD: 6 CUPS BROTH

Prep time: 10 minutes, Cook time: 30 minutes,
Total time: 40 minutes, Serving size: 1 cup,
Number of servings: 6

A plant-based equivalent to "bone broth," this easily digestible, comforting broth is full of healing, delicious medicine. Perfect for when your body needs extra nutrients and a rest from digestion, so as to move through an immune challenge. Parsnip adds folate and potassium; onions contain sulfur and the antioxidant quercetin; cabbage delivers fiber and vitamin K; carrot is an incredible source of vitamin A; and the sea vegetable arame donates trace minerals. Strain and enjoy the lightness of the broth.

7 ½ cups water or vegetable stock (see page 108)
1 ¼ cups diced yellow onion
5 garlic cloves, chopped
½ cup sliced shiitake mushrooms or dried shiitakes
1 cup chopped parsnip (½-inch pieces)
1 cup chopped potato (½-inch pieces)
1 ½ cups sliced cabbage
1 cup thinly sliced carrot
½ cup thinly sliced celery
¼ cup chopped fresh flat-leaf parsley
¼ cup arame (optional; see page 86)
Pinch of sea salt, or to taste

1. Place the water or stock in a large pot over medium-high heat. Add all the remaining ingredients, except the salt, and cook for 30 minutes.

2. Carefully pour the soup through a strainer into another pot or large bowl. Discard or enjoy the veggies on their own.

3. Add salt to taste.

VARIATIONS

Add 2 cups of chopped kale, spinach, or collards 10 minutes before straining.

Replace the parsley with fresh basil or 2 tablespoons of fresh dill.

Add 2 cups of chopped tomato along with the other vegetables.

Nutrition Facts per serving (173 g): Calories 80, Fat Calories 5, Total Fat 0 g, Saturated Fat 0 g, Cholesterol 0 mg, Sodium 60 mg, Total Carb 18 g, Dietary Fiber 5 g, Sugars 5 g, Protein 3 g

Watermelon Gazpacho♥☺◆

YIELD: 5 CUPS GAZPACHO

Prep time: 15 minutes, Total time: 15 minutes,
Serving size: 1 cup, Number of servings: 5

Watermelon soup? Why not? It may sound unusual, but watermelon is a wonderful addition to this traditional chilled soup of Mexico. A delicious and very refreshing idea for the hottest of summer days, as watermelon is so incredibly hydrating. Enter jalapeño, jicama, cilantro, and Mexican spices, offsetting watermelon's sweetness somewhat, and you have a unique twist on tomato-based gazpacho. Serve immediately, so it doesn't separate, and enjoy with other Mexican favorites, such as Tempeh Fajitas (page 279) and Maca Horchata (page 147).

6 cups chopped watermelon (1-inch cubes)

½ cup water or coconut water

¼ cup freshly squeezed lime juice

½ teaspoon seeded and diced jalapeño pepper

½ teaspoon chili powder or Mexican spice Mix (page 106)

¼ teaspoon chipotle chile powder

Pinch of sea salt

¾ cup seeded and diced cucumber

¾ cup peeled and diced jicama

1 tablespoon plus 1 teaspoon finely chopped fresh cilantro

1. Place the watermelon, water or coconut water, lime juice, jalapeño, chili powder, chipotle chile powder, and salt in a blender and blend well.

2. Add the remaining ingredients and stir well before serving.

VARIATION

Replace the cilantro with fresh mint, and replace the cucumber and jicama with blueberries and chopped strawberries.

Nutrition Facts per serving (237 g): Calories 70, Fat Calories 5, Total Fat 0.5 g, Saturated Fat 0 g, Cholesterol 0 mg, Sodium 40 mg, Total Carb 17 g, Dietary Fiber 2 g, Sugars 12 g, Protein 2 g

---

Chefs Tips and Tricks

Cooking Time

In the recipes, you will notice a prep time, cooking time, and total time. In many instances, prepping will take place while some cooking is occurring, so the total time will not necessarily equal the total of prep time and cooking time.

Raw Cucumber Fennel Soup ♥ⓖ◆

YIELD: 4 CUPS SOUP

Prep time: 20 minutes, Total time: 20 minutes, Serving size: 1 cup, Number of servings: 4

This soup is a perfect blend of flavors to satisfy a need for a light and cooling meal. Cucumbers are a beauty treatment inside and out. Used externally for healthy skin and hair, they are also an ideal pick-me-up whose replenishing qualities come from their 95 percent water content and B vitamins. Fennel delivers vitamin C, potassium, and folate. And the chromium in red onion helps steady blood sugar and has tissue-reparative benefits much like the silica in celery. Add the optional cashews if you are looking for a creamier soup. Serve as part of a raw feast with Raw Coconut Curry Veggies (page 268) and Raw Carrot Ginger Cake (page 309).

3 cups peeled, seeded, and chopped cucumber (½-inch pieces)

1 cup cold water

¼ cup raw cashew pieces (optional)

¾ cup diced fennel bulb

½ cup diced celery

¼ cup diced red onion

1 garlic clove

1 tablespoon plus 1 teaspoon freshly squeezed lime juice

¼ teaspoon sea salt, or to taste

Pinch of freshly ground black pepper

Pinch of cayenne pepper

1 cup fresh or frozen (thawed) corn

¼ cup sliced green onion

2 tablespoons chiffonaded fresh basil

1 tablespoon finely chopped fresh flat-leaf
  parsley
1 teaspoon wheat-free tamari or other soy
  sauce (optional)

1. Place the cucumber, water, cashews, if
   using, fennel, celery, red onion, garlic,
   lime juice, and salt in a blender and
   blend until smooth.

2. Transfer to a bowl along with the
   remaining ingredients and mix well
   before serving.

VARIATIONS

Replace the corn with seeded and diced
bell pepper, cabbage, or additional seeded
and diced cucumber.

Add 1 cup of diced tomato along with the
corn.

Replace the basil with fresh cilantro or
1 ½ tablespoons of minced fresh dill.

Add 1 ½ tablespoons of an ethnic spice
blend, such as Mexican (page 106), Indian
(page 106), or Ethiopian (page 106).

Go Indian by omitting the basil, and
adding 2 tablespoons of minced fresh
cilantro, 1 tablespoon of curry powder, and
2 teaspoons of ground cumin.

Go Mexican by omitting the basil, and
adding 2 tablespoons of minced cilantro,
1 tablespoon of chili powder, 1 teaspoon of
ground cumin, and ¼ teaspoon of chipotle
chile powder.

Nutrition Facts per serving (217 g): Calories 180,
Fat Calories 20, Total Fat 2 g, Saturated Fat 0 g,
Cholesterol 0 mg, Sodium 180 mg, Total Carb 37 g,
Dietary Fiber 5 g, Sugars 3 g, Protein 5 g

Raw Carrot Brazil Nut Soup ♥ⓖ♦▱

YIELD: 6 CUPS SOUP

Prep time: 15 minutes, Total time: 15 minutes,
Serving size: 1 cup, Number of servings: 6

This raw creamy and brightly colored soup,
besides being maximally tasty, is a potpourri
of ingredients and super spices that provide
maximum nutrition. Avocado and Brazil nuts
contain the healthy fats that are needed with
every meal to aid in nutrient absorption; carrot and lemon juice provide a direct shot of
vitamins A and C; and ginger and turmeric
are superfoods in a category all their own!
The soup is also delicious served warm for
a nonraw version; simply heat on the stove
over medium heat until just warm. Top with
Avocado Mousse (page 152) and/or Raw Cashew Sour Cream (page 113).

4 cups fresh carrot juice
½ cup Brazil nuts
½ cup peeled and pitted avocado
¼ cup thinly sliced green onion
1 tablespoon freshly squeezed lemon juice
1 tablespoon peeled and minced fresh ginger
2 teaspoons peeled and minced fresh
  turmeric
2 teaspoons seeded and diced jalapeño pepper
½ teaspoon sea salt, or to taste
⅛ teaspoon freshly ground black pepper
Pinch of chipotle chile powder
1 cup fresh or frozen (thawed) corn
½ cup seeded and diced red bell pepper
2 teaspoons minced fresh dill

1. Place 2 cups of the carrot juice in
   a blender. Add all the remaining

ingredients, except the corn, red bell pepper, and dill, and blend well.

2. Add the remaining 2 cups of carrot juice and blend well. Transfer to a bowl. Add the corn, red bell pepper, and dill and mix well before serving. Serve chilled.

Nutrition Facts per serving (265 g): Calories 270, Fat Calories 95, Total Fat 11 g, Saturated Fat 2 g, Cholesterol 0 mg, Sodium 255 mg, Total Carb 40 g, Dietary Fiber 6 g, Sugars 7 g, Protein 6 g

---

TEMPLATE RECIPE
Raw Vegetable Soup

- -

Base component: Replace the carrot juice with a juice of your choosing, such as tomato, or a mixed vegetable juice, such as carrot, beet, and spinach.

Creaminess component: Replace the Brazil nuts with other nuts or seeds, such as cashew, macadamia, sunflower seed, or pumpkin seed.

Vegetable component: Replace the corn and bell pepper with such vegetables as chopped celery, cucumber, purple cabbage, or zucchini.

Herb component: Replace the dill with fresh cilantro, basil, parsley, or sorrel.

Ethnic spice component: Replace the chipotle chile powder with 1 tablespoon of an ethnic spice blend, such as Mexican (page 106), Italian (page 105), or Moroccan (page 106).

Miso Vegetable Soup ☉◗

YIELD: 7 CUPS SOUP

Prep time: 20 minutes, Cook time: 30 minutes, Total time: 30 minutes, Serving size: 1 cup, Number of servings: 7

Miso paste is a salty, cultured food most commonly made from soybeans. It helps digestion by adding beneficial microorganisms to the digestive tract. Miso also has plentiful B vitamins. Many varieties are available, such as white, red, and mixed. Try them all to see how the flavor profile of the soup changes. Digestion gets a second boost in this soup with ginger, long used to remedy stomach troubles and nausea, as well as inflammation. Also perfect in this healing soup, shiitake mushrooms may be one of the most sustaining foods out there. Used medicinally in Chinese medicine for thousands of years, shiitake is now catching on as a major anticancer food, and has recently been studied as great source of bioavailable iron. Be sure to use an unpasteurized variety of miso and avoid boiling the soup, so as to preserve the maximum nutritional benefits. Serve with Nori Rolls (page 263) and Edamame Arame Salad (page 198).

5 cups water or vegetable stock (see page 108)
⅛ teaspoon dried thyme
1 tablespoon wheat-free tamari or other soy sauce, or to taste
1 tablespoon peeled and minced fresh ginger
2 garlic cloves, pressed or minced (optional)
1 cup thinly sliced shiitake or enoki mushrooms
1 cup diced carrot
½ cup peeled and thin diagonally sliced burdock root

7 ounces extra-firm tofu, cut into ¼-inch
    cubes

1 cup chopped spinach, kale, arugula, or
    watercress

¼ cup thinly sliced green onion

3 tablespoons miso paste (see page 248)

Pinch of sea salt, or to taste

1. Place the water or stock in a pot over medium-high heat. Add the thyme, tamari, ginger, garlic, if using, mushrooms, carrot, burdock root, and tofu and cook for 10 minutes, stirring occasionally.

2. Add the spinach and green onion and cook for 5 minutes.

3. Remove 1 cup of the soup liquid and place in a small bowl with the miso paste. Whisk with a fork until the miso dissolves. Return to the soup and add additional salt, if necessary.

VARIATIONS

Replace the tofu with 1 cup of edamame.

Add ¼ cup of arame or wakame sea vegetable (see page 86) along with the carrot.

Add 1 tablespoon of toasted sesame oil.

Replace the ginger with two pressed or minced garlic cloves.

Replace the carrot with parsnip, zucchini, or bell pepper.

Experiment with different types of miso, such as barley or chickpea.

Nutrition Facts per serving (100 g): Calories 50, Fat Calories 15, Total Fat 1.5 g, Saturated Fat 0 g, Cholesterol 0 mg, Sodium 190 mg, Total Carb 7 g, Dietary Fiber 2 g, Sugars 2 g, Protein 4 g

Congee with Fenugreek ⓖ ◆

YIELD: 6 CUPS CONGEE

Prep time: 10 minutes, Cook time: 40 minutes, Total time: 45 minutes, Serving size: 1 cup, Number of servings: 6

Congee, known traditionally as *hsi-fan*, is a rice water porridge commonly enjoyed in Asian countries for breakfast. It is usually cooked for hours on a very low flame or slow cooker. This is a sped-up version you can complete in less than an hour. If do you have the time, I recommend cooking it at a very low temperature for two hours or longer. The long cooking time contributes to easy digestion and, in Chinese medicine, is said to help with blood toning, regulating qi energy, which is important in treating chronically ill individuals who suffer from fatigue. Fenugreek, known as *methi* in other parts of the world, contains saponins, and cooking the seeds for a longer time brings out its particular flavor, often described as a cross between celery and maple. Spice it up by adding hot sauce (see page 109) or sriracha before serving. Have a bowl with a cup of Digestive Tea (page 133) when you are looking to give your digestive system a rest.

8 cups water

½ cup uncooked brown rice, rinsed and
    drained well

1 tablespoon fenugreek or fennel seeds

1 tablespoon peeled and minced fresh ginger

½ cup thinly sliced celery

½ cup diced carrot

½ cup sliced leek, rinsed and drained well

2 cups chopped spinach

2 teaspoons wheat-free tamari or other soy
    sauce, or to taste (optional)

Pinch of sea salt, or to taste

Chef's Tips and Tricks

Miso

Miso is a Japanese word that means "fermented beans." The beans used are almost always soybeans. Grains, such as barley, rice, or buckwheat, might be added during fermentation to achieve a certain flavor or other desired attribute.

While the thick texture of miso paste is consistent, the color and flavor can vary widely. The lightest color miso is usually white or beige, often due to inclusion of white rice during the fermentation process as well as a shorter fermentation time. A white miso may be fermented for a time period as short as several weeks, while a dark miso might be fermented for many months or even several years. White miso is usually the sweetest variety and is considered to be the most versatile for cooking since its flavor is milder. Yellow miso is produced when the soybeans are fermented with barley; it may look yellow or very light brown. Red miso is very dark brown or reddish brown in color, and it's usually saltier than white or yellow miso. The dark reddish brown color may result from steaming the soybeans prior to fermentation. Since darker-colored miso is stronger and more pungent in flavor, it is generally better suited for heavier foods, while lighter-colored miso is often more appropriate for soup, dressings, and light sauces.

Dark brown and red miso usually get their strong flavors from longer periods of fermentation. Fermentation of dark soy miso may involve three years or longer. For example, Hatcho miso, made in Okazaki, Japan, is fermented in two-hundred-year-old vats over a period of three winters.

This style of fermentation has a long and rich history, most likely having originated in China several thousand years ago, and made its way into Japan as early as the tenth century B.C.

---

1. Place the water in a pot over medium heat. Add the rice, fenugreek, and ginger, cover, and cook for 10 minutes, stirring occasionally.

2. Add the celery, carrot, and leek and cook for 30 minutes, stirring occasionally.

3. Add the spinach, tamari, if using, and salt, and stir well before serving.

VARIATIONS

Replace the rice with millet, quinoa, rye, or spelt berries.

Replace the carrot with parsnip, zucchini or gold bar squash, or burdock root.

Replace the fenugreek with poppy, sesame, or cumin seeds.

Add 1 cup of sliced mushrooms and 1 cup of corn along with the carrots.

Add ¼ cup of adzuki beans along with the rice.

Add 2 tablespoons of miso paste (see box above) before serving.

Nutrition Facts per serving (59 g): Calories 80, Fat Calories 5, Total Fat 1 g, Saturated Fat 0 g, Chole-

sterol 0 mg, Sodium 50 mg, Total Carb 16 g, Dietary
Fiber 2 g, Sugars 1 g, Protein 2 g

Asian Noodle Soup⊙◗

YIELD: 9 CUPS SOUP

Prep time: 15 minutes, Cook time: 25 minutes,
Total time: 40 minutes, Serving size: 1 1/2 cups,
Number of servings: 6

This soup goes above and beyond the timeless noodle soup by showcasing bright green
leafy vegetables, such as spicy mustard
greens, kale, and spinach: undeniably some
of the most healing foods in the world, given
their abundance of nutrients, antioxidants,
and phytochemicals in a low-calorie, high-
fiber package. Low-glycemic sweet potatoes
are also quite nutrient dense, with vitamin A,
C, B vitamins, manganese, fiber, potassium,
and iron. The soup is rounded out with shiitake mushrooms, known for their major immunity-supporting lentinan content. Serve
along with Veggie Lettuce Boats (page 160)
and Green Papaya Salad (page 175).

6 cups water or vegetable stock (see page 108)
1 tablespoon wheat-free tamari or soy sauce,
　　or to taste
¾ cup thinly sliced yellow onion
4 garlic cloves, pressed or minced
1 tablespoon peeled and minced fresh ginger
½ cup thinly diagonally cut carrot
1 ½ cups chopped sweet potato (½-inch
　　pieces)
1 cup thinly sliced shiitake mushrooms
1 teaspoon seeded and diced hot chile pepper
　　(see page 179), or ¼ teaspoon crushed red
　　pepper flakes
2 cups sliced mustard greens, kale, or spinach

4 ounces rice noodles
¼ cup thinly sliced green onion (optional)
2 tablespoons finely chopped fresh cilantro
Pinch of sea salt, or to taste

1. Place the water or stock and the tamari
   in a pot over medium-high heat. Add
   the onion, garlic, ginger, carrot, sweet
   potato, mushrooms, and chile pepper and cook for 20 minutes, stirring
   occasionally.

2. Add the mustard greens and rice
   noodles and cook for 5 minutes, or
   until the noodles are just soft, stirring
   occasionally.

3. Add the green onion, if using, cilantro,
   and salt, and stir well before serving.

VARIATIONS

Sauté the onion, garlic, and ginger in 1 tablespoon of coconut oil before adding the
water or vegetable stock (page 108).

Add 1 tablespoon of peeled fresh turmeric
along with the ginger.

Add 1 cup of cubed tofu or legumes, such
as chickpeas or adzuki beans.

Replace the sweet potato with chopped
veggies of your choice, including broccoli, asparagus, zucchini, and/or gold bar
squash.

Add 2 teaspoons of toasted sesame oil
along with the water, if you are not using
vegetable stock.

Nutrition Facts per serving (154 g): Calories 140,
Fat Calories 5, Total Fat 1 g, Saturated Fat 0 g,
Cholesterol 0 mg, Sodium 265 mg, Total Carb 31 g,
Dietary Fiber 4 g, Sugars 4 g, Protein 4 g

Creamy Asparagus Soup with Corn⊙◦▱

YIELD: 6 CUPS SOUP

Prep time: 10 minutes, Cook time: 20 minutes,
Total time: 30 minutes, Serving size: 1 cup,
Number of servings: 6

The fresh flavors of the veggies blend wonderfully in this nourishing soup with whole corn added at the end for just a bit of crunch. Our friendly cashew gives this soup its creamy richness. Asparagus features the amino acid asparagine, which detoxifies the body as a natural diuretic, especially helpful for hypertension and other heart ailments. Corn rounds out this soup by adding fiber and 10 percent of the daily requirement of folate, thiamine, phosphorus, magnesium and vitamin C. But these ingredients are just one combination possible using the same method! This is a classic template recipe with hundreds of variations possible. Enjoy with a slice of Broccoli Dill Quiche (page 274) for a lovely meal.

4 ½ cups water or vegetable stock (see page 108)
1 cup diced yellow onion
¾ cup thinly sliced celery
5 garlic cloves
3 cups chopped asparagus (½-inch pieces)
½ cup raw cashew pieces (optionally toasted; see page 101)
½ teaspoon sea salt, or to taste
⅛ teaspoon freshly ground black pepper
¼ teaspoon crushed red pepper flakes
1 ½ cups fresh or frozen (thawed) corn
1 tablespoon finely chopped fresh dill

1. Place the water or stock in a pot over medium-high heat. Add the onion, celery, garlic, and asparagus and cook until the vegetables are just tender, about 15 minutes, stirring occasionally.

2. Transfer to a blender, add the cashews, salt, black pepper, and crushed red pepper flakes, and blend until creamy. Return to the pot.

3. Add the corn and cook for 5 minutes, stirring occasionally. Add the dill and stir well before serving.

VARIATIONS

You can sauté the onion, celery, and garlic in 1 ½ tablespoons of coconut oil for 2 minutes, stirring constantly, before adding the stock.

Live on the edge and top with 1 cup of grated vegan cheese before serving.

Add 2 tablespoons of nutritional yeast before serving.

Add 1 teaspoon of wheat-free tamari or other soy sauce, along with the stock.

Try roasting the corn before adding to the soup.

Nutrition Facts per serving (203 g): Calories 285, Fat Calories 90, Total Fat 10.5 g, Saturated Fat 2 g, Cholesterol 0 mg, Sodium 225 mg, Total Carb 43 g, Dietary Fiber 6 g, Sugars 4 g, Protein 9 g

Creamy Vegan Soup

Main vegetable component: Replace the asparagus with broccoli, cauliflower, zucchini, or mixed vegetables.

Creaminess component: Replace the cashews with nuts or seeds, such as macadamia nuts, hazelnuts, or sunflower seeds; or Quinoa Milk (page 143) or soy, coconut, almond, or rice milk (for homemade, see Plant-Based Milk, page 104).

Herb and spice component: Replace the dill with fresh cilantro, basil, or parsley. Add an ethnic touch with 1 tablespoon of an ethnic spice blend, such as Ethiopian (page 106), Mexican (page 106), or Indian (page 106).

Vegetable added after blending component: Replace the corn with chopped vegetables, such as asparagus, cauliflower, bell pepper, or cabbage.

Ital Roasted Squash and Sweet Potato Soup G ◆

YIELD: 7 ½ CUPS SOUP

Prep time: 15 minutes, Cook time: 40 minutes, Total time: 55 minutes, Serving size: 1 1/4 cups, Number of servings: 6

Creamy decadence awaits in this soup brimming with the flavors of the tropics. Ital foods are those celebrated by Rastafari culture for their pure vital energy. One sip of this soup and you will see why it merits its name! Both the butternut squash and the sweet potato provide a large quantity of vitamin A, a powerful antioxidant, in this warming soup. As its name suggests, butternut squash is practically buttery, and comforting all times of year, though it appears as a side dish most often in fall and winter. Besides being delicious, coconut milk provides a particular medium-chain saturated fatty acid called lauric acid, which is converted in the body into a highly beneficial antiviral compound. Top with toasted pepitas (see page 101), and serve as part of a holiday feast with Lentil Walnut Loaf (page 288) and Oil-Free Mushroom Gravy (page 240).

1 medium-size butternut or buttercup squash (for 1¼ cups roasted)
3 ½ cups water or vegetable stock (see page 108)
1½ cups light or full-fat coconut milk
2 bay leaves
1¾ cups chopped sweet potato (½-inch pieces)
1 cup chopped yellow onion
¾ cup sliced celery
3 large garlic cloves
¼ teaspoon ground allspice
¼ teaspoon dried thyme
½ teaspoon sea salt, or to taste
⅛ teaspoon freshly ground black pepper
Pinch of crushed red pepper flakes
1 cup fresh or frozen (thawed) corn
1 tablespoon finely chopped fresh cilantro

1. Preheat the oven to 400°F. Carefully slice the squash in half lengthwise, remove the seeds, and place, cut side down, in a small casserole dish with about ½ inch of water or stock. Bake until a knife can pass easily through the

squash, about 30 minutes, depending on the size of the squash. Remove from the oven, and measure out 1 ¼ cups for this recipe.

2. Meanwhile, place the water or stock, coconut milk, bay leaves, sweet potato, onion, celery, garlic, allspice, and thyme in a pot over medium-high heat. Cook for 20 minutes, stirring occasionally. Add the salt, black pepper, and crushed red pepper and stir well. Remove the bay leaves.

3. Carefully transfer to a blender, along with the cooked squash, and blend until smooth, or use an immersion blender to puree the soup right in the pot. (Depending upon the size of your blender, you may need to blend in two or three batches. If so, have another pot or bowl on hand where you can transfer the blended soup before returning to the original pot you cooked the soup in.) Return to the pot, add the corn and cilantro, and stir well before serving.

VARIATIONS

Replace the sweet potato with potato or carrot.

Replace the coconut milk with other plant-based milk, such as soy, rice, hemp, or quinoa (see pages 104 and 143.)

Replace the corn with chopped broccoli, asparagus, or red bell pepper.

Nutrition Facts per serving (225 g): Calories 220, Fat Calories 60, Total Fat 7 g, Saturated Fat 3 g, Cholesterol 0 mg, Sodium 240 mg, Total Carb 35 g, Dietary Fiber 4 g, Sugars 3 g, Protein 4 g

Italian Spring Vegetable Stew🄖◗

YIELD: 9 CUPS SOUP

Prep time: 20 minutes, Cook time: 25 minutes, Total time: 45 minutes, Serving size: 1 1/4 cups, Number of servings: 6

Spring conjures up thoughts of green, and this soup recipe brings it on in abundance. Large portions of green beans and spinach, with touches of rosemary, basil, and parsley will ensure not only bright color, but a full spectrum of nutrient density, with the bonus of vitamin C–rich tomatoes to increase the iron absorption from the spinach, parsnip, and green beans. Serve with Smashed Roasted Cauliflower and Parsnip (page 202) and Simple Baked Tofu (page 260) with Fire-Roasted Tomato Sauce (page 239).

4 cups water or vegetable stock (see page 108)
1 (15-ounce) can diced fire-roasted tomatoes, or 1 ½ cups chopped fresh tomato with juice
½ teaspoon minced fresh rosemary (optional)
½ teaspoon dried thyme
¾ cup chopped yellow onion
½ cup sliced celery
4 garlic cloves, pressed or minced
½ cup sliced fennel bulb
1 cup chopped parsnip (½-inch pieces)
1 cup chopped green beans (½-inch pieces)
1 cup seeded and chopped red bell pepper (½-inch pieces)
1 cup chopped fresh spinach
2 tablespoons chiffonaded fresh basil
2 tablespoons finely chopped fresh flat-leaf parsley

1 teaspoon fresh summer savory (optional)

1 teaspoon fresh oregano (optional)

½ teaspoon sea salt, or to taste

¼ teaspoon crushed red pepper flakes

⅛ teaspoon freshly ground black pepper

1. Place the water or stock and fire-roasted tomatoes in a pot over medium-high heat. Add the rosemary, thyme, onion, celery, garlic, fennel, parsnip, and green beans and cook for 10 minutes, stirring frequently.

2. Add the bell pepper and cook for 10 minutes, stirring frequently.

3. Add the remaining ingredients, cook for 5 minutes, and stir well before serving.

VARIATIONS

Create a thinner soup by adding an additional cup or two of water or vegetable stock (page 108).

Replace all or some of the parsnip, green beans, and bell pepper with other veggies, such as potato, corn, mushrooms, zucchini, or cabbage.

Replace the spinach with other greens, such as thinly sliced kale, collards, or chard.

For more of a stew, add 1 cup of beans, such as chickpeas, or fava or cannellini beans. You can also add 1 cup of pasta or cubed and roasted tofu (see page 100).

Go Mexican by replacing the basil and parsley with 2 tablespoons of chopped fresh cilantro, and adding 2 teaspoons of chile powder, 1 teaspoon of ground cumin, and ¼ teaspoon of chipotle chile powder.

Go Ethiopian by adding 1½ tablespoons of Ethiopian Spice Mix (page 106).

Nutrition Facts per serving (162 g): Calories 50, Fat Calories 5, Total Fat 0 g, Saturated Fat 0 g, Cholesterol 0 mg, Sodium 220 mg, Total Carb 11 g, Dietary Fiber 3 g, Sugars 4 g, Protein 2 g

Curried Broccoli Soup with Great Northern Beans ⊙◆

YIELD: 6 CUPS SOUP

Prep time: 15 minutes, Cook time: 20 minutes, Total time: 30 minutes, Serving size: 1 cup, Number of servings: 6

Curry complements both the taste and nutrition of two plant-kingdom powerhouses in this satisfying soup. "Eat your broccoli" was good advice from Mom, after all, since eating broccoli is now well known for promoting overall health by providing an impressive amount of nutrients, including protein, all packed into its cute treelike form. The name *great northern beans* is mysterious, considering these legumes were cultivated in South America. Nonetheless, they have a delicate, nutty flavor and provide a low-fat source of iron, dietary fiber, potassium and protein. Serve with jasmine or basmati rice (page 96), Golden Rice (page 204), Unfried Rice (page 205), or Green Quinoa (page 203) for a light meal.

5 cups water or vegetable stock (see page 108)

1 cup thinly sliced onion

4 garlic cloves, pressed or minced

½ cup thinly sliced shiitake mushrooms

4 cups broccoli (small florets)

1 tablespoon curry powder

1 teaspoon cumin seeds

½ teaspoon coriander seeds

½ teaspoon garam masala (optional)

1 (15-ounce) can great northern beans, or
   1 ½ cups cooked (see page 98)

½ teaspoon sea salt, or to taste

¼ teaspoon freshly ground black pepper

Pinch of cayenne pepper

1 ½ tablespoons minced fresh cilantro

1. Place the water or stock in a pot over medium-high heat. Add the onion, garlic, mushrooms, and broccoli and cook for 10 minutes, stirring occasionally. Add the curry, cumin, coriander, and garam masala and cook for 5 minutes, stirring occasionally.

2. Add the beans and cook for 10 minutes, stirring occasionally.

3. Add the salt, black pepper, cayenne, and cilantro and stir well before serving.

VARIATIONS

Replace the broccoli with other vegetables, such as cauliflower, Romanesco, zucchini, or broccoli rabe.

Replace the beans with other beans, such as chickpeas, or kidney or pinto beans.

Replace the beans with cubed and roasted tofu or tempeh (see page 100).

Add ¾ cup of rice pasta, such as penne or elbow, along with the beans.

Nutrition Facts per serving (188 g): Calories 100, Fat Calories 10, Total Fat 1 g, Saturated Fat 0 g, Cholesterol 0 mg, Sodium 220 mg, Total Carb 19 g, Dietary Fiber 6 g, Sugars 3 g, Protein 7 g

Smoky Split Pea Soup

YIELD: 6 CUPS SOUP

Prep time: 15 minutes, Cook time: 60 minutes, Total time: 60 minutes, Serving size: 1 cup, Number of servings: 6

Talk about ancient foods! Pea remains have been found in archaeological digs in most ancient cultures, and thereby have been sustaining humans for ages with their protein and fiber prowess, not to mention their dosage of B vitamins, isoflavones, and ability to regulate blood sugar. While two kinds are included in this recipe, split peas are actually English peas or sweet peas, which, when harvested and dried, develop a natural split in the seed (hence the name). This soup also profits from a cup of celery, with its natural saltiness and issuance of major vitamin K and molybdenum, an essential trace element necessary for liver, kidney, and bone health. Healing properties are found in abundance in this pleasing pea soup. Top with Coco Bacon (page 112) and serve with Sesame Kale Salad (page 186) or Simple Chop Salad (page 174).

¾ cup dried yellow split peas

8 cups water or vegetable stock (see page 108)

1 ¼ cups diced yellow onion

1 cup thinly sliced celery

1 ½ cups chopped tomato (½-inch pieces)

4 garlic cloves, pressed or minced

¾ teaspoon dried thyme

1 cup fresh or frozen English or sweet peas

1 teaspoon liquid smoke (see page 85), or 1 tablespoon smoked paprika

1 cup thinly sliced kale

2 tablespoons finely chopped fresh flat-leaf parsley

½ teaspoon sea salt, or to taste

⅛ teaspoon freshly ground black pepper

¼ teaspoon cayenne pepper

2 teaspoons freshly squeezed lemon juice

1. Rinse and drain the split peas well. Place the water or stock in a pot over medium-high heat. Add the split peas and cook for 35 minutes, stirring occasionally.

2. Add the onion, celery, tomato, garlic, and thyme and cook for 10 minutes, stirring frequently.

3. Add the fresh or frozen peas, liquid smoke, and kale and cook for 10 minutes, stirring frequently. Add the remaining ingredients and stir well before serving.

VARIATIONS

When the soup is done cooking, carefully transfer 1 cup to a blender and blend well. Return to the pot before serving.

Add roasted and chopped tempeh (see page 100) along with the kale.

Replace the kale with spinach, arugula, dandelion greens, mustard greens, or Swiss chard.

Add 1 cup of diced carrot, parsnip, cabbage, or zucchini.

Replace the parsley with fresh cilantro, tarragon, or sorrel.

Nutrition Facts per serving (193 g): Calories 140, Fat Calories 10, Total Fat 17 g, Saturated Fat 0 g, Cholesterol 0 mg, Sodium 225 mg, Total Carb 26 g, Dietary Fiber 10 g, Sugars 7 g, Protein 9 g

Moroccan Chickpea Stew G ◆

YIELD: 8 CUPS STEW

Prep time: 10 minutes, Cook time: 25 minutes, Total time: 35 minutes, Serving size: 1 1/4 cups, Number of servings: 6

Garner the plant-strong nutrient kick of chickpeas by adding some delightful Moroccan flavorings to a hearty and sustaining soup. Chickpeas, also known as garbanzos and ceci, are full of protein, iron, fiber, manganese, and phytochemicals called saponins, which act as powerful antioxidants. The common cremini has been topping the mushroom list recently for its superior ability to calm inflammation, and it combines well with onion and carrot for added immune enhancement. Serve with Unfried Rice (page 205) and Provençal Salad (page 183) or Israeli Couscous Tabouli (page 203).

4 ½ cups water or vegetable stock (see page 108)

1 ¼ cups onion, chopped

¾ cup thinly sliced celery

3 garlic cloves, pressed or minced

1 (15-ounce) can chickpeas, or 1 ½ cups cooked (see page 98)

¾ cup diagonally sliced carrot

1 cup quartered and stemmed cremini mushrooms

¼ cup freshly squeezed orange juice

½ teaspoon sea salt, or to taste

½ teaspoon ground cumin

½ teaspoon ground coriander

¼ teaspoon ground cinnamon

¼ teaspoon ground ginger

¼ teaspoon saffron (optional)

⅛ teaspoon freshly ground black pepper

Pinch of cayenne pepper

2 tablespoons finely chopped fresh flat-leaf parsley

1. Place the water or stock, onion, celery, and garlic in a pot over medium heat. Add the chickpeas, carrot, and mushrooms and cook for 5 minutes, stirring occasionally.

2. Add all the remaining ingredients, except the parsley, and cook for 20 minutes, stirring occasionally.

3. Add the parsley, and stir well before serving.

VARIATIONS

Add 1 teaspoon of smoked paprika along with the cumin.

Replace the chickpeas with other legumes, such as navy, fava, or cannellini beans.

Add 1 cup of chopped spinach, arugula, or kale along with the parsley.

Replace the carrots and mushrooms with veggies of your choosing, such as zucchini or gold bar squash, cabbage, broccoli, or cauliflower.

Nutrition Facts per serving (161 g): Calories 100, Fat Calories 10, Total Fat 1 g, Saturated Fat 0 g, Cholesterol 0 mg, Sodium 225 mg, Total Carb 19 g, Dietary Fiber 5 g, Sugars 6 g, Protein 5 g

Mexican Two-Bean Soup ⓖ ◆

YIELD: 10 CUPS SOUP

Prep time: 15 minutes, Cook time: 20 minutes, Total time: 35 minutes, Serving size: 1 1/4 cups, Number of servings: 8

In a nutritional showdown between black beans and pinto beans, judges would be hard pressed to choose the more nutritionally dense bean. They are both packed with protein (black slightly more), potassium (pinto slightly more), good sources of healthy carbohydrates (pinto slightly more), low calorie (black slightly less), and low fat (absolutely equal). Take advantage of both in this tomato-based Mexican soup, which also adds celery and carrot to round out this commanding dish. Top with a drizzle of Raw Cashew Sour Cream (page 113) and enjoy with Mushroom Cauliflower Tacos (page 277) and a cup of Maca Horchata (page 147).

4 cups water or vegetable stock (see page 108)

1 ½ cups diced fresh tomato, or 1 (15-ounce) can fire-roasted diced tomatoes

1 ¼ cups diced onion

¾ cup thinly sliced celery

4 garlic cloves, pressed or minced

1 tablespoon chili powder or Mexican Spice Mix (page 106)

1 teaspoon ground cumin (optionally toasted; see page 101)

½ teaspoon chipotle chile powder (optional)

1 (15-ounce) can pinto beans, or 1 ½ cups cooked (see page 98)

1 (15-ounce) can black beans, or 1 ½ cups cooked (see page 98)

¾ cup sliced carrot

1 cup fresh or frozen (thawed) corn (optional)

¾ teaspoon sea salt, or to taste

¼ teaspoon freshly ground black pepper

2 tablespoons finely chopped fresh cilantro

1. Place the water or stock and the fire-roasted tomatoes in a pot over medium-high heat. Add the onion, celery, garlic, chili powder, cumin, and chipotle chile powder, if using, and cook for 10 minutes, stirring occasionally.

2. Add the beans, carrot, and corn, if using, and cook for 10 minutes, stirring occasionally.

3. Add the salt, black pepper, and cilantro and stir well before serving.

VARIATIONS

Replace the beans with other beans, such as chickpeas, or cannellini or kidney beans.

Go Indian by replacing the chili powder with curry powder, and adding 2 teaspoons of mustard seeds.

Replace the carrot and corn with other vegetables, such as mushrooms, pattypan squash, sweet potato, or bell pepper.

If you are using water instead of vegetable stock (page 108), add 1 teaspoon of wheat-free tamari or other soy sauce to taste.

For a thicker soup, add 1 cup of cooked brown rice along with the beans.

Nutrition Facts per serving (206 g): Calories 195, Fat Calories 15, Total Fat 2 g, Saturated Fat 0 g, Cholesterol 0 mg, Sodium 265 mg, Total Carb 38 g, Dietary Fiber 9 g, Sugars 3 g, Protein 9 g

Kitchari 🅖 ◆

YIELD: 8 CUPS KITCHARI

Prep time: 10 minutes, Cook time: 55 minutes, Total time: 55 minutes, Serving size: 1 cup, Number of servings: 8

The ultimate comfort food of India, *kitchari* translates as "mixture," typically including two grains. In traditional Ayurvedic cooking, different spices and herbs are added depending upon the condition being addressed. This version benefits from the nutritional properties of yellow split peas, which are loaded with protein and dietary fiber. Special in yellow split peas is tryptophan, which is connected to the brain's production of serotonin, affecting appetite, sleep, and mood. A complete protein is formed with the addition of similarly fibrous brown rice, and the greens add a nice vitamin and mineral burst. Serve with Curry Kale Salad (page 184) and Curried Garbanzo Cakes with Poppy Seeds (page 104).

2 teaspoons cumin seeds

1 teaspoon fennel seeds, or 2 teaspoons brown mustard seeds

¾ cup uncooked brown basmati rice, rinsed and drained well

¾ cup dried split peas, rinsed and drained well

10 cups water or vegetable stock (see page 108)

3 garlic cloves, pressed or minced

1 tablespoon peeled and minced fresh ginger

1 tablespoon curry powder

1 cup thinly sliced carrot

1 cup chopped spinach or arugula

2 tablespoons finely chopped fresh cilantro

¾ teaspoon sea salt, or to taste

⅛ teaspoon freshly ground black pepper
Pinch of cayenne pepper

1. Place a large pot over high heat. Add the cumin and fennel seeds and cook for 2 minutes, stirring constantly. Lower the heat to medium, add the rice and split peas, and stir well.

2. Add the water or stock, garlic, ginger, and curry powder and cook for 45 minutes, stirring occasionally.

3. Add the carrots and cook until the split peas are just soft, about 5 minutes. Add the spinach and cook for 5 minutes, stirring occasionally. For a thicker soup, cook for an additional 10 minutes. Add the cilantro, salt, black pepper, and cayenne and mix well before serving.

VARIATIONS

Add 1 cup of chopped fresh tomato along with the carrots.

Add 1 cup of chopped veggies, such as broccoli, cabbage, or Brussels sprouts, along with the carrots.

Replace the rice with quinoa or millet.

Replace the split peas with lentils or mung beans, and follow the cooking chart on pages 96–97.

Replace the spinach with kale, collards, chard, dandelion greens, or mustard greens.

Add 2 teaspoons of coriander seeds and 1 teaspoon of fenugreek seeds.

Nutrition Facts per serving (96 g): Calories 140, Fat Calories 5, Total Fat 1 g, Saturated Fat 0 g, Cholesterol 0 mg, Sodium 240 mg, Total Carb 28 g, Dietary Fiber 6 g, Sugars 2 g, Protein 6 g

CHAPTER 15

Main Dishes

Welcome to the main event. Here you will find an abundance of recipes to prepare as the centerpiece of your meal—from simple to more complex, and for nearly every occasion and palate, from more elaborate plated entrées to sandwiches, rolls, and pizza. My go-to meal is extremely simple. See my description of the Monk Bowl on pages 100 and 267. In this chapter, I provide a version of the Monk Bowl recipe for you to follow (Simple One-Pot Meal, page 266), if you are looking for a healthy and delicious meal that is easy to prepare and allows for lots of variations to keep things exciting.

Continue your world culinary tour with a range of Vegan Fusion ethnic cuisines, such as Ratatouille (page 273), Thai Curry Vegetables (page 289), Indian Creamy Lentil Saag (page 290), Middle Eastern Baked Falafel (page 262), Jamaican Patties (page 280), or Mexican Seitan-Stuffed Peppers (page 291). Those looking for raw entrées will enjoy the Raw Coconut Curry Vegetables (page 268) or Raw Collard Veggie Rolls (page 260), and the raw version of Nori Rolls (page 263).

Looking for a hardier meal? Check out the world of casseroles, including the Millet and Butternut Squash with Broccoli (page 284), Corn Casserole (page 286), and Cauliflower Casserole (page 285). For lunch, how about a veggie burger? I share two burger recipes with lots of variations. Introduce your friends to the Millet Black Bean Veggie Burgers (page 269) and Magnificent Mushroom Burgers (page 270). Sample innovative vegan twists on Sloppy Joes (pages 281), Mushroom Cauliflower Tacos (page 277), or Broccoli Dill Quiche (page 274).

Oh . . . and be sure to save room for dessert!

Raw Collard Veggie Rolls ♥Ⓖ◐

YIELD: 4 ROLLS

Prep time: 15 minutes, Total time: 15 minutes, with pâté prepared, Serving size: 1 roll, Number of servings: 4

Master your wrapping technique with a hearty, strong, colorful wrapper that holds up nicely no matter what filling you add, while keeping your heart, skin, and bones in tiptop shape as a superb source of vitamins A and K, manganese, calcium and fiber. The nut pâté and cheese provide a rich flavorful base for a fresh rainbow of veggies and a little avocado adds creamy balance. The leaves can be used raw or steamed. Serve with Curry Kale Salad (page 184), Provençal Salad (page 183) or Simple Chop Salad (page 174).

4 collard leaves
¾ cup Pecan Veggie Pâté (page 169)
¼ cup Truffled Cashew Cheese (page 159; optional)
½ cup julienned red cabbage
1 small avocado, peeled, pitted, and thinly sliced
1 medium-size tomato, thinly sliced
¼ cup shaved fennel bulb
1 cup arugula

1. Cut the bottom stem off the collard leaves and discard. Using a paring knife or vegetable peeler, carefully shave the thick part of the stem that is still part of the leaf, so that it becomes as thin as the rest of the leaf.

2. Place a small amount of pâté on the bottom portion of each collard leaf, about 1 ½ inches from the bottom of the leaf. Top with a tablespoon of the cashew cheese, if using, and one quarter of the remaining veggie fillings.

3. Fold the bottom of the leaf on top of the fillings. Fold in the sides of the leaf toward the center, and proceed to roll toward the top edge of the leaf, just like rolling a burrito, forming as tight a roll as possible.

4. Serve whole or sliced in half. If you slice in half, you may wish to hold each roll together with a toothpick.

VARIATIONS

You can steam the collard leaves until tender, about 7 minutes. Let cool and pat dry well before using in this recipe.

Experiment with different veggies, such as julienned bell pepper or jicama, sunflower or buckwheat sprouts, mixed salad greens, grated carrot, beet, or parsnip.

Replace the pâté with different spreads, such as Kalamata Rosemary Hummus (page 157), Pesto (page 215), or Sun-Dried Tomato Tapenade (page 156).

Nutrition Facts per serving (162 g): Calories 155, Fat Calories 105, Total Fat 12 g, Saturated Fat 1.5 g, Cholesterol 0 mg, Sodium 180 mg, Total Carb 12 g, Dietary Fiber 7 g, Sugars 4 g, Protein 4 g

Simple Baked TofuⒼ

YIELD: 14 OUNCES TOFU BY WEIGHT

Prep time: 10 minutes, Cook time: 20 minutes, Total time: 30 minutes, Serving size: 2.3 ounces by weight, Number of servings: 6

Tofu is the poster child for the veg protein world. A low-calorie, cholesterol-free alternative to animal proteins, it is also a source of calcium and iron. And ever-versatile tofu takes on the flavor of its marinade, making it suitable to use in so many plant-based dishes, savory or sweet. The coconut oil in this simple marinade provides a hint of the tropics. Top with Oil-Free Mushroom Gravy (page 240), Roasted Red Pepper Sauce (page 235), or Zesty Chimichurri Sauce (page 231) and serve with a selection of salads or side dishes in Chapter 12.

2 teaspoons coconut oil, melted

2 teaspoons wheat-free tamari or other soy sauce, or to taste

2 tablespoons water

2 teaspoons brown rice vinegar

1 garlic clove, pressed or minced (optional)

1 (14-ounce) package extra-firm or superfirm tofu

1. Preheat the oven or toaster oven to 375°F. Place the coconut oil, tamari, water, vinegar, and garlic, if using, on a small baking sheet and whisk well.

2. Slice the block of tofu widthwise into equal-size six cutlets and place on the baking sheet. Marinate for 6 minutes, flipping each cutlet after 3 minutes.

3. Place the baking sheet in the oven and cook for 20 minutes, flipping the cutlets after 10 minutes.

VARIATIONS

You can also slice the tofu lengthwise into three cutlets, optionally sliced again into triangles.

Try cubing the tofu before marinating and roasting (see page 100).

Replace the coconut oil with sesame oil, toasted sesame oil, olive oil, or your favorite.

Experiment with different marinades to see how the flavor of the tofu is changed.

Add 1 teaspoon of peeled and minced fresh ginger.

Replace the rice vinegar with balsamic vinegar or 2 tablespoons of red or white wine.

Replace the rice vinegar with 1 ½ tablespoons of freshly squeezed lemon or lime juice.

Add 1 tablespoon of tomato paste or ketchup to the marinade.

Add 1 tablespoon of an ethnic spice blend, such as Indian (page 106), Italian (page 105), or Mexican (page 106) to the marinade.

Add 1 tablespoon minced fresh cilantro, basil, flat-leaf parsley, or dill to the marinade.

◆ For an oil-free version, replace the coconut oil with 3 tablespoons of water or vegetable stock (see page 108).

Nutrition Facts per serving (72 g): Calories 65, Fat Calories 40, Total Fat 4 g, Saturated Fat 2 g, Cholesterol 0 mg, Sodium 180 mg, Total Carb 2 g, Dietary Fiberless than 1 g, Sugars 1 g, Protein 6 g

Maple Baked Tempeh🄖

YIELD: 8 OUNCES TEMPEH BY WEIGHT

Prep time: 10 minutes, Cook time: 20 minutes, Total time: 30 minutes, Serving size: 2 ounces by weight, Number of servings: 4

With origins in Indonesia, the powerhouse veg protein tempeh provides the base for a solid and satisfying main course. In addition to easily fulfilling protein needs, tempeh is known also to reduce cholesterol and increase bone density. As a fermented food it is easily digestible, allowing for high absorption of nutrients. Top with a sauce from Chapter 13, such as Smoky BBQ (page 231) or Ancho Chile Sauce (page 232); chop into cubes and toss with Ranch Kale Salad (page 185); or add to Smoky Split Pea Soup (page 254).

8 ounces tempeh (see page 100)

2 teaspoons wheat-free tamari or other soy sauce

2 tablespoons water

1 ½ teaspoons pure maple syrup

1 teaspoon freshly squeezed lime juice or balsamic vinegar

2 teaspoons coconut oil, melted

¼ teaspoon liquid smoke, see page 85 (optional)

1. Preheat the oven or toaster oven to 375°F. Slice the block of tempeh in half, then slice each piece in half to yield four cutlets. Place a steamer basket in a pot with about ½ inch of water over high heat. Cover and bring to a boil. Add the tempeh cutlets, lower the heat to low, cover, and cook for 3 minutes.

2. Meanwhile, place the remaining ingredients, including the 2 tablespoons of water, in a small baking dish and whisk well. Add the steamed tempeh and allow to marinate for 6 minutes, flipping each cutlet after 3 minutes.

3. Place the baking dish in the oven and cook for 20 minutes, flipping the cutlets after 10 minutes.

VARIATIONS

Add 1 teaspoon of peeled and minced fresh ginger or garlic to the marinade.

Replace the coconut oil with olive oil, toasted sesame oil, or your favorite.

Get creative with your marinade. See page 107 for alternative marinade suggestions. Also check out the variations in the Simple Baked Tofu recipe (page 260) for more ideas.

You can leave out the steaming step, if you wish.

Replace the tempeh with extra-firm or superfirm tofu.

💧For an oil-free version, replace the coconut oil with an additional 2 tablespoons of water or vegetable stock (see page 108).

Nutrition Facts per serving (66 g): Calories 140, Fat Calories 75, Total Fat 8 g, Saturated Fat 3 g, Cholesterol 0 mg, Sodium 175 mg, Total Carb 7 g, Dietary Fiber 0 g, Sugars 2 g, Protein 11 g

Baked Falafel🄖💧

YIELD: 1 ¼ CUPS FALAFEL

Prep time: 15 minutes, Cook time: 10 minutes, Total time: 25 minutes, Serving size: 2 tablespoons, Number of servings: 10

Falafel joints are omnipresent in Middle Eastern countries, offering the naturally plant-based favorite as either a substantial meal-on-the-go in a handy pita, or with side dishes as the center of a relaxed meal with friends and family. As with hummus, there is some discourse about where falafel derived, but it was likely in Egypt, where it was made with ground fava beans. Nowadays, chickpeas are usually the legume of choice in a falafel patty. By baking these yourself, you can avoid the oil puddle that can accompany some restaurant falafel patties. When you drain your canned beans, be sure to reserve some of the chickpea liquid for use in the recipe. Serve on top of Simple Chop Salad (page 174), or in pita bread with Creamy Lemon Tahini Dressing (page 228), Kalamata Rosemary Hummus (page 157), and a side of Israeli Couscous Tabouli (page 203).

1 (15-ounce) can chickpeas, or 1½ cups cooked (see page 98), 2 tablespoons chickpea liquid reserved
⅓ cup minced fresh flat-leaf parsley
2 tablespoons minced fresh cilantro (optional)
3 garlic cloves, minced or pressed
1½ tablespoons freshly squeezed lemon juice
1 tablespoon flour (try garbanzo or oat, for a gluten-free falafel)
1 teaspoon ground cumin
½ teaspoon ground coriander
½ teaspoon sea salt, or to taste
⅛ teaspoon freshly ground black pepper
¼ cup diced yellow onion
Pinch of cayenne pepper
Oil, for baking sheet (optional)

1. Preheat the oven to 400°F. Place all the ingredients in a food processor and process until just smooth. Some chunkiness is okay. Taste and add additional salt, if necessary.

2. Scoop out ten balls, using a small ice-cream scoop, and place on a parchment paper–lined or well-oiled baking sheet.

3. Bake for 5 minutes. Carefully flip and bake for an additional 5 minutes.

VARIATIONS

Replace the chickpeas with fava or cannellini beans.

Omit the parsley and add an additional 3 tablespoons of fresh cilantro.

Nutrition Facts per serving (55 g): Calories 50, Fat Calories 10, Total Fat 1 g, Saturated Fat 0 g, Cholesterol 0 mg, Sodium 120 mg, Total Carb 9 g, Dietary Fiber 2 g, Sugars 1 g, Protein 3 g

Nori Rolls☺◦

YIELD: 4 ROLLS

Prep time: 30 minutes, Cook time: 45 minutes, Cooling time: 10 minutes, Total time: 70 minutes, Serving size: 1 roll, Number of servings: 4

Nori is an edible seaweed vegetable. The sheets have prolific health benefits and function as a great wrapper, too. Nori and other sea vegetables are very low in calories and one of the best food sources of minerals: iodine, magnesium, calcium, iron, and folic acid, not to mention omega-3s. Balanced with satisfying brown rice and flavorful veggies, plant-based sushi rolls are sure to be a winner. They are easier and quicker to prepare than you might think, especially when the rice is prepared in advance. Preparing rice in advance also makes for easier rolling, as the cooler rice is easier to work with. Serve with wasabi paste and pickled ginger and a small dish of tamari for dipping. Follow the suggestions listed in the variations for a fantastic sushi party along with Miso Vegetable Soup (page 246), Edamame Arame Salad (page 198), and Mixed Fruit Kanten (page 301).

1 cup uncooked short-grain brown rice, rinsed and drained well

2 ¼ cups water

1 tablespoon rice vinegar or mirin (optional)

½ teaspoon sea salt

4 nori sheets

½ large avocado, peeled, pitted, and cut into thin strips

1 large green onion, thinly sliced lengthwise

¼ cucumber, quartered, seeded, and sliced lengthwise into ¼- to ½-inch strips

½ small red bell pepper, seeded and julienned

½ cup thinly sliced red cabbage

Grilled or roasted tofu or tempeh (see page 100), cut into ½-inch strips (optional)

Garnishes: pickled ginger, wasabi, and soy sauce

1. Place the rice, water, rice vinegar, and salt, if using, in a pot over high heat. Bring to a boil. Lower the heat to low, cover, and cook until all the liquid is absorbed, about 45 minutes. Transfer to a bowl and place in the refrigerator to cool.

2. Have ready a small bowl of cold or room-temperature water. Place a bamboo rolling mat on a clean cutting board. Place the nori sheet on the bamboo mat, shiny side down and with the long side parallel to the bottom edge

of the cutting board. If not using a mat, simply place the nori on a clean, dry surface, such as a cutting board.

3. Using a rice paddle or spatula and starting at the bottom edge of the sheet, spread about ¾ cup of the cooled rice on the nori sheet, leaving about 1 ½ inches at the top without any rice. Dip your hands in the water to prevent the rice from sticking to you.

4. Closely line up one quarter each of the avocado, strips of green onion, cucumber, red pepper, red cabbage, and tofu or tempeh, if using, on top of the rice, about 1 ½ inches from the bottom edge of the nori sheet. You can let some of the veggies stick out the ends, for a creative presentation.

5. Grab the bottom edge and roll it up, applying pressure to keep the roll as tight as possible. Dip your fingers in the water, wet the exposed 1 ½-inch strip of bare nori, and keep rolling until that edge is on the bottom. Press firmly, and leave it the seam side down while you move on to make the other three rolls.

6. When all four are rolled, start with the first roll and transfer to a cutting board. Cut a diagonal line through the middle with a serrated knife, then cut straight lines halfway through each half. Set on plates and garnish with pickled ginger, wasabi, and soy sauce.

VARIATIONS

For the tofu or tempeh, you can use the following marinade and roast according to the method described on page 100. For 14 ounces of tofu or 8 ounces of tempeh, create a marinade with 1 tablespoon of wheat-free tamari or other soy sauce, 1 tablespoon of melted coconut oil, and 2 teaspoons of rice vinegar or mirin.

Experiment with different fillings, including:

> Sautéed or grilled shiitake or portobello mushrooms, thinly sliced (see page 101).
>
> Grilled or roasted red bell pepper, thinly sliced.
>
> Carrots, thinly sliced lengthwise and steamed until just soft (see page 101).
>
> Grated veggies, such as carrot, beet, daikon, or jicama.
>
> Sliced fruit, such as mangoes or grilled pineapple (see page 101).
>
> Add a spread of umeboshi paste (see page 101), to the rice before adding the vegetables.
>
> Add a sprinkle of hemp seeds or sesame seeds, optionally toasted (see page 101), to your roll.
>
> You can add the wasabi and pickled ginger to the roll itself instead of serving on the side.

♥ For a raw version, use sun-dried nori sheets, use Pecan Veggie Pâté (page 169) or Truffled Cashew Cheese (page 159) instead of rice, and use raw fresh veggies inside the wrap.

Nutrition Facts per serving (111 g): Calories 220, Fat Calories 35, Total Fat 4 g, Saturated Fat 1 g, Cholesterol 0 mg, Sodium 300 mg, Total Carb 41 g, Dietary Fiber 3 g, Sugars 1 g, Protein 5 g

Designer Seed and Nut Crust Pizzas🌀◆

YIELD: 6 PIZZAS

Prep time: 25 minutes, Soak time: 30 minutes, Cook time: 30 minutes, Total time: 60 minutes, Serving size: about 7 tablespoons crust, Number of servings: 6

Quiz: Are the buckwheat groats in this crust a nut or a seed? They are, in fact, a seed, gluten-free, from a plant related to rhubarb and sorrel. Nuts and seeds have some of the highest nutrient density relative to their small size, and with three sets of seeds and one mega-nut, this tasty crust, enhanced by vitamin and mineral-heavy herbs and spices, will enhance any toppings. Here are some suggestions:

Choose a sauce: Fire-Roasted Tomato Sauce (page 239), Pesto (page 215), Sun-Dried Tomato Tapenade (page 156), Truffled Cashew Cheese (page 159), Smoky BBQ Sauce (page 231), Ancho Chile Sauce (page 232), Easy Cheezy Sauce (page 233), Hummus (page 159), or mashed avocado.

Choose a topping: Arugula, sliced tomatoes, sautéed mushrooms, onions, and garlic; Provençal Salad (page 183); sliced olives; sliced avocado; Simple Sauerkraut (page 176); Quick Kimchi (page 178); Garlicky Greens (page 191); or Broasted Brussels Sprouts (page 194).

3 tablespoons ground flaxseeds
¼ cup plus 2 tablespoons water
1 cup raw buckwheat groats
½ cup Brazil nuts
½ cup raw pumpkin seeds
2 tablespoons chiffonaded fresh basil
1 tablespoon finely chopped fresh flat-leaf parsley

¼ cup freshly squeezed lemon juice

2 teaspoons onion flakes

1 teaspoon garlic powder

½ teaspoon dried thyme

½ teaspoon minced fresh rosemary

½ teaspoon sea salt, or to taste

¼ teaspoon freshly ground black pepper

¼ teaspoon crushed red pepper flakes

Oil, for baking sheet

1. Preheat the oven to 400°F. Soak the flaxseeds in the water. Stir occasionally.

2. Place the buckwheat groats, Brazil nuts, and pumpkin seeds in a large bowl with ample water to cover. Allow to sit between 30 minutes and 4 hours. Drain, rinse, and drain well.

3. Place in a food processor with the remaining ingredients, including the flaxseeds and their soak water, and process until smooth.

4. Using a scoop, create six equal-size pizzas and place on a well-oiled or parchment paper–lined baking sheet. Bake for 10 minutes. Flip and bake for an additional 10–15 minutes, depending on how crispy you want the crust.

VARIATION

♥ For a raw version: Set your dehydrator to 115°F. Place the pizzas on Teflex or ParaFlexx sheets. Dehydrate for 8 hours. Flip and remove the Teflex to dehydrate directly on the dehydrator tray. Dehydrate for an additional 12 hours before serving.

Nutrition Facts per serving (107 g): Calories 210, Fat Calories 80, Total Fat 9 g, Saturated Fat 2 g, Cholesterol 0 mg, Sodium 218 mg, Total Carb 25 g, Dietary Fiber 5 g, Sugars less than 1 g, Protein 10 g

Simple One-Pot Meal ◉ ♦ ▱

YIELD: 6 CUPS QUINOA AND BEANS

Prep time: 10 minutes, Cook time: 20 minutes, Total time: 30 minutes, Serving size: 1 1/2 cups, Number of servings: 4

Ease, speed, and robust nourishment, all in one delightfully tasty package with a nutty and Asian twist. In a flash you can enjoy the combined benefits of some simple yet nutritionally potent ingredients, starting with the protein-packed goodness of quinoa and adzuki beans, and the restorative and preventative powers of onion and ginger. Succulent leafy green bok choy, or Chinese cabbage, is a perfect addition with even more protein, plus fiber, iron, magnesium, phosphorus, B vitamins, vitamin K, and even vitamin C. This meal is a joy to the senses and easy enough to make happen every day. Enjoy on its own as a complete meal, or for an extra dimension, enjoy with Smoky BBQ Sauce (page 231), Almond Dipping Sauce (page 233), Ancho Chile Sauce (page 232), or Sweet-and-Sour Sauce (page 236).

3 cups water or vegetable stock (see page 108)

½ cup uncooked quinoa, rinsed and drained (see pages 95, 144)

¼ teaspoon sea salt, or to taste

1 (15-ounce) can adzuki beans, or 1 ½ cups cooked (see page 98), drained and rinsed

½ cup diced white onion

1 tablespoon peeled and minced fresh ginger

⅛ teaspoon cayenne pepper

3 cups very thinly sliced bok choy

2 tablespoons finely chopped fresh cilantro or flat-leaf parsley

1 ½ tablespoons nutritional yeast

1 ½ tablespoons flax oil or hemp seed oil (optional)

1. Place the water or stock, quinoa, and salt in a pot over medium-high heat. Cook for 5 minutes. Add the beans, onion, ginger, and cayenne and cook for 10 minutes, stirring occasionally.

2. Add the bok choy and cook for 5 minutes, stirring frequently. Add the cilantro and gently mix well.

3. Top with nutritional yeast and flax oil, if using, before serving.

Nutrition Facts per serving (235 g): Calories 215, Fat Calories 15, Total Fat 2 g, Saturated Fat 0 g, Cholesterol 0 mg, Sodium 190 mg, Total Carb 39 g, Dietary Fiber 9 g, Sugars 2 g, Protein 11 g

TEMPLATE RECIPE
One-Pot Meal, a.k.a. Monk Bowl

Grain component: Replace the quinoa with any variety of rice, or rice pasta, millet, or buckwheat.

Veggie component: Replace the onion and bok choy with veggies of your choosing, such as broccoli, cabbage, kale, spinach, cauliflower, zucchini, chard, dandelion greens, or turnip greens.

Bean component: Replace the adzuki beans with black beans, pinto beans, chickpeas, black-eyed peas, or cannellini beans. Or replace with marinated and roasted tofu or tempeh cubes (see page 100).

Roasted Veggies and Beans⊙

YIELD: 4 CUPS VEGGIES AND BEANS

Prep time: 25 minutes, Cook time: 25 minutes, Total time: 50 minutes, Serving size: 1 cup, Number of servings: 4

This Mexican-themed one-pan meal is simple in its preparation—simply toss your vegetables and seasonings together with chickpeas and roast until done—while complex in its diverse and composite nutrient and flavor profiles. Derive five of the generally agreed-upon six components of nutrition in one pan—protein, carbohydrates, fat, vitamins, and minerals—and if you couple it with a glass of water on the side, you'll log the sixth. Serve with a fresh side salad. For a complete meal, serve with Unfried Rice (page 205), Green Quinoa (page 203), or Golden Rice (page 204).

1 (15-ounce can) chickpeas, drained well, or 1 ½ cups cooked (see page 98)
1 cup sliced parsnip (½-inch slices)
1 cup small broccoli florets
1 cup chopped portobello mushroom (½-inch pieces)
1 cup chopped zucchini (½-inch pieces)
½ cup sliced yellow onion
3 garlic cloves, pressed or minced
3 tablespoons water
2 teaspoons melted coconut or olive oil
1 teaspoon chili powder
¼ teaspoon sea salt, or to taste
⅛ teaspoon freshly ground black pepper
Pinch of crushed red pepper flakes
Oil, for baking sheet
2 tablespoons nutritional yeast (optional)

2 tablespoons finely chopped fresh cilantro

2 tablespoons freshly squeezed lime juice

1. Preheat the oven to 375°F. Place the chickpeas, parsnip, broccoli, mushroom, zucchini, onion, garlic, water, oil, chili powder, salt, black pepper, and crushed red pepper flakes in a bowl and toss well. Transfer to a lightly oiled baking sheet.

2. Bake for 25 minutes, or until the vegetables are just tender, stirring occasionally.

3. Add the remaining ingredients and mix well before serving.

VARIATIONS

◆ For an oil-free version, omit the oil, and add ¼ to ½ cup of water or vegetable stock (see page 108) to the pan when roasting.

Replace the chickpeas with other beans, such as black, pinto, fava, or kidney.

Replace the veggies with carrot, cauliflower, corn, peas, red bell pepper, or your favorites.

Replace the cilantro with fresh basil, parsley, or sorrel, or 1 tablespoon of minced fresh dill.

Add 1 tablespoon of an ethnic spice blend, such as Mexican (page 106), Italian (page 105), or Mexican (page 106).

Nutrition Facts per serving (253 g): Calories 180, Fat Calories 40, Total Fat 4 g, Saturated Fat 2 g, Cholesterol 0 mg, Sodium 180 mg, Total Carb 30 g, Dietary Fiber 8 g, Sugars 7 g, Protein 8 g

Raw Coconut Curry Vegetables ♥ⓖ◆

YIELD: 4 CUPS VEGETABLES

Prep time: 30 minutes, Total time: 30 minutes, Serving size: 1 cup, Number of servings: 4

Curries, staples of Indian cuisine, are often cooked. This raw version gives you the wonderful warm flavor of curry with the juiciness and crunch of raw vegetables and sprouts. Curry is a blend of ground spices, including cayenne or red pepper, coriander, cumin, and turmeric. Turmeric provides its signature golden color along with many of the healing benefits. Low in fat, sugar, and sodium, curry itself is a great source of vitamin B_6, folate, calcium, magnesium, phosphorus, potassium, and copper, and a very good source of dietary fiber, vitamin E (alpha tocopherol), vitamin K, iron, and manganese. A superior way to enjoy an enzyme-rich and satisfying raw veggie meal. Enjoy as part of a raw feast with raw Nori Rolls (page 263), and Raw Chocolate Pudding (page 296).

2 to 3 medium-size zucchini, spiralized (4 cups tightly packed)

1 cup tightly packed julienned red cabbage

1 medium-size red bell pepper, seeded and julienned

1 tablespoon freshly squeezed lime juice

2 teaspoons wheat-free tamari or other soy sauce, or coconut aminos (see page xv) (optional)

1 cup Raw Coconut Curry Sauce (page 237)

¼ cup thinly sliced green onion

¼ cup mung bean sprouts (optional)

1 tablespoon finely chopped fresh cilantro

¼ cup raw peanuts (optional)

1. Combine the zucchini, red cabbage, and bell pepper in a bowl. Add the lime juice, and tamari, if using. Add the Raw Coconut Curry Sauce and toss well. Portion out into four bowls, or leave in one bowl and serve family style.

2. Top with the green onion, mung bean sprouts, if using, cilantro, and peanuts, if using. Have fun!

VARIATIONS

Add other veggies, such as julienned yellow bell pepper, carrot, or beet.

Add 1 cup of raw kelp noodles (see page 87).

Add 1 cup of julienned medium-soft coconut meat.

Nutrition Facts per serving (192 g): Calories 80, Fat Calories 30, Total Fat 3.5 g, Saturated Fat 2 g, Cholesterol 0 mg, Sodium 245 mg, Total Carb 10 g, Dietary Fiber 4 g, Sugars 5 g, Protein 4 g

Millet Black Bean Veggie Burgers🄖

YIELD: 6 BURGERS

Prep time: 10 minutes, Cook time: 20 minutes, Chilling time: 10 minutes, Total time: 40 minutes, Serving size: about 1/2 cup, Number of servings: 6

Millet is an ancient grain with a lovely nutty flavor that has been cultivated for many thousands of years, and with good reason: it is full of important energizing fuel from its fiber and protein. It has emerged recently as a locally sourced, smaller-carbon-footprint, and less expensive alternative to quinoa. United with tried-and-true black beans, millet makes a premium protein to give the body all the amino acids it needs. These wholesome burgers also benefit from a colorful phytonutrient array of such additions as red bell pepper, parsley, and all the fixings. Serve with Parsnip Fries (page 199) and Broasted Brussels Sprouts (page 194).

½ cup uncooked millet

2 cups water or vegetable stock (see page 108)

½ teaspoon sea salt, or to taste

2 tablespoons chia seeds or ground flaxseeds

2 teaspoons coconut oil

¼ cup diced yellow onion

2 large garlic cloves, pressed or minced

¼ cup diced shiitake mushrooms

¼ cup seeded and diced red bell pepper

¼ teaspoon crushed red pepper flakes

¼ teaspoon freshly ground black pepper

2 tablespoons nutritional yeast (optional)

¾ teaspoon wheat-free tamari or other soy sauce, or to taste (optional)

2 tablespoons minced fresh flat-leaf parsley

1 (15-ounce) can black beans, drained and rinsed, or 1 ½ cups cooked beans (see page 98)

¼ cup oat flour

Oil, for baking sheet

Coconut oil, for sautéing (optional)

6 vegan buns

All the fixings: lettuce, thinly sliced red onion, thinly sliced tomato

1. Place the millet in a small pot over high heat. Toast for 3 minutes, stirring constantly. Add 1 ¾ cups of the water or stock, and the salt. Bring to a boil. Lower the heat to medium-low, cover, and cook until all the liquid is absorbed, about 20 minutes, stirring occasionally.

2. Meanwhile, place the chia seeds in a small bowl with the remaining ¼ cup of water or stock. Stir occasionally.

3. Place the oil in a small pan over medium-high heat. Add the onion and garlic and cook for 2 minutes, stirring frequently. Add the mushroom and bell pepper and cook for 5 minutes, stirring frequently. Add the crushed red pepper, black pepper, nutritional yeast, if using, tamari, if using, and parsley and mix well. Set aside.

4. Place the black beans in a mixing bowl and mash well with a masher, whisk, or fork. Add the oat flour and mix well. Add the millet mixture, the chia mixture, and the vegetable mixture and mix well. Taste and add additional salt, if necessary.

5. Using a slightly underfilled ½-cup measuring cup or scoop, form six ½-inch-thick patties and place on a well-oiled baking sheet. For best results, place in the freezer to cool and solidify for 10 minutes, or for up to 20 minutes in the refrigerator.

6. To cook, you can sauté the veggie burgers in a liberal amount of coconut oil in a large sauté pan. Carefully flip after 2 minutes. You can also bake the veggie burgers. To do so, preheat the oven to 400°F. Bake for 10 minutes, carefully flipping after 5 minutes.

7. To serve, carefully place your veggie burger on a bun and go to town with the fixings!

VARIATIONS

♦For an oil-free version, you can omit the coconut oil and do a water sauté with ¼ cup of water (see page 101). Add additional water, if necessary, to prevent sticking. Use parchment paper on a baking sheet, instead of oil, and bake the burgers.

For a Mexican flair, replace the parsley with fresh cilantro, and add 1 tablespoon of freshly squeezed lime juice, 2 teaspoons of chili powder, 1 teaspoon of ground cumin, and ¼ teaspoon of chipotle chile powder.

Replace the black beans with chickpeas, or cannellini or kidney beans.

Use the uncooked mixture as a filling for stuffed peppers (see page 291).

Nutrition Facts per serving (93 g): Calories 170, Fat Calories 30, Total Fat 4 g, Saturated Fat 2 g, Cholesterol 0 mg, Sodium 200 mg, Total Carb 28 g, Dietary Fiber 7 g, Sugars less than 1 g, Protein 7 g

Magnificent Mushroom Burger☺🗫

YIELD: 10 BURGERS

Prep time: 25 minutes, Cook time: 40 minutes, Total time: 60 minutes, Serving size: 1/2 cup, Number of servings: 10

This juicy, light, and nutty veggie burger is fiber loaded with its top-of-the-line ingredient list: quinoa, beans, walnuts, and mushrooms, and delivers a satisfying protein punch in a digestible and bioavailable package. Flaxseeds function as the burger binders alongside oat flour in this hold-its-shape veggie burger. Top with Caramelized Onions (page 162), and serve with Fingerling Potatoes with Pesto (page 215) and Tomato Avocado Salad (page 183).

2 tablespoons ground flaxseeds

5 tablespoons water

¾ cup uncooked quinoa, rinsed and drained (see pages 95, 144)

1 ½ cups water or vegetable stock (see page 108)

¾ teaspoon sea salt, or to taste

2 teaspoons coconut oil

½ cup diced yellow onion

2 tablespoons minced garlic

1 ½ cups diced cremini or shiitake mushrooms

⅓ cup finely chopped walnuts

1 (15-ounce) can white kidney beans, or 1 ½ cups cooked (see page 98), rinsed and drained well

½ cup peeled and grated carrot

¼ cup finely chopped fresh flat-leaf parsley

½ cup oat flour

1 tablespoon wheat-free tamari or other soy sauce (optional)

1 tablespoon dried oregano

1 teaspoon dried thyme

½ teaspoon crushed red pepper flakes

¼ teaspoon freshly ground black pepper

Oil, for baking sheet

1. Preheat the oven to 375°F. Place the flaxseeds and the 5 tablespoons of water in a small bowl. Stir occasionally.

2. Place the quinoa, the 1 ½ cups of water or stock, and ½ teaspoon of the salt in a small pot over medium-high heat. Bring to a boil. Lower the heat to simmer, cover, and cook for 15 minutes, or until the water is absorbed. Remove from the heat.

3. Meanwhile, place the coconut oil in a sauté pan over medium-high heat. Add the onion and garlic and cook for 3 minutes, stirring frequently. Add the mushrooms and remaining ¼ teaspoon of salt and cook for 7 minutes, stirring frequently. Transfer to a large bowl.

4. Mash the beans with a fork or process in a food processor until just pureed. Add to the vegetables with all the remaining ingredients, including the cooked quinoa and the flaxseed mixture, and mix well. Taste and add additional salt, if necessary.

5. Form into ten ½-cup burgers and place on a well-oiled baking sheet. Bake for 20 minutes. Carefully flip the burgers and bake for an additional 15 minutes.

6. Serve with your desired fixings!

VARIATION

🌢 For an oil-free version, use the water sauté method (see page 101). Bake on a parchment paper–lined baking sheet.

Nutrition Facts per serving (107 g): Calories 150, Fat Calories 50, Total Fat 5 g, Saturated Fat 1 g, Cholesterol 0 mg, Sodium 190 mg, Total Carb 21 g, Dietary Fiber 5 g, Sugars 1 g, Protein 7 g

Binder component: Replace the flaxseeds with chia seeds or a commercial egg replacer (see pages 84, 312).

Bean component: Replace the kidney beans with legumes, such as black beans, cannellini beans, or chickpeas.

Grain component: Replace the cooked quinoa with cooked rice or millet.

Flour component: Replace the oat flour with other flours, or bread crumbs. Add additional flour, if necessary, depending on the veggies used, to reach a moist but firm texture for the mixture.

Nut or seed component: Replace the walnuts with sunflower seeds, pecans, macadamia nuts, cashews, or your favorite.

Veggie component: Replace the mushrooms with cooked and drained chopped kale, spinach, zucchini, cabbage, chopped broccoli, or mashed potato or sweet potato. Replace the grated carrot with grated parsnip or beet. The higher the water content in the veggies, the more flour you'll need.

Spice component: Replace the oregano and thyme with an ethnic spice blend, such as Mexican (page 106), Ethiopian (page 106), or Indian (page 106).

Black Bean Grits ⓖ ◆

YIELD: 4 CUPS GRITS

Prep time: 10 minutes, Cook time: 25 minutes, Total time: 35 minutes, Serving size: 1/2 cup, Number of servings: 8

Popular in the American South and with Native American origins, creamy corn grits are not just for breakfast. Here the carb-strong grits pair up with fiber-rich black beans, both of which are enhanced with the addition of exquisite Mexican flavors: cleansing cilantro, fiery jalapeño pepper and chili powder, immunity-balancing garlic, and digestion-soothing cumin. Serve with a dollop of Vegan Sour Cream (page 112) and a side of Garlicky Greens (page 191) or Roasted Zucchini and Corn (page 192).

1 teaspoon chili powder
½ teaspoon ground cumin
3 ¼ cups water or vegetable stock (see page 108)
½ teaspoon sea salt, or to taste
¼ teaspoon freshly ground black pepper
3 garlic cloves, pressed or minced
¼ teaspoon seeded and diced jalapeño pepper
1 tablespoon coconut oil (optional)
1 cup uncooked corn grits
2 tablespoons finely chopped fresh cilantro
1 (15-ounce) can black beans, rinsed and drained well, or 1 ½ cups cooked (see page 98)
Oil, for casserole dish and pan (optional)

1. Place the chili powder and cumin in a pot over high heat and cook for 1 minute, stirring constantly. Add the water or stock, salt, black pepper, garlic,

jalapeño, coconut oil, if using, and bring to a boil.

2. Lower the heat to low, slowly add the grits, and cook for 5 minutes, stirring frequently. Cover, and cook until the grits are creamy, about 10 minutes.

3. Add the beans and cilantro and mix well.

4. You can enjoy warm as is, poured into bowls, or transfer to a well-oiled 8 by 8-inch casserole dish. Place in the refrigerator for 15 minutes, or until the grits are firm enough to slice.

5. Once sliced, you can reheat in the oven (10 minutes at 400°F) or gently sauté in oil in a skillet over high heat for a few minutes on each side.

VARIATIONS

Replace the grits with polenta (see page 96).

Replace 1 cup of the water with unsweetened soy, rice, or almond milk (for homemade, see Plant-Based Milk, page 104)

Go Italian by replacing the Mexican spices and adding 2 tablespoons of finely chopped fresh basil, 1 tablespoon of chopped fresh flat-leaf parsley, 1 teaspoon of minced fresh rosemary, and 1 tablespoon of Italian Spice Mix (page 105).

Replace the black beans with other beans of your choosing, such as pinto, kidney, or adzuki.

Indulge and add ½ cup of grated vegan cheese.

Nutrition Facts per serving (79 g): Calories 120, Fat Calories 5, Total Fat 0.5 g, Saturated Fat 0 g, Cholesterol 0 mg, Sodium 154 mg, Total Carb 24 g, Dietary Fiber 3 g, Sugars 0 g, Protein 5 g

Ratatouille Ⓖ

YIELD: 8 CUPS RATATOUILLE

Prep time: 15 minutes, Cook time: 30 minutes, Total time: 45 minutes, Serving size: 1 1/3 cups, Number of servings: 6

Prepare for a feast of Mediterranean flavors. In most ratatouille recipes, eggplant plays the starring role alongside tomato, which plays the supporting role. It seems it wasn't always this way, since in long-ago Nice, France, where it originated, zucchini were the star of the show. Nowadays, ratatouille graces the menu in many fine restaurants, but it had more humble origins as a peasant's stew using a potpourri of summer vegetables. Eggplant provides ample copper, fiber, and thiamine. The rich tomato base provides an abundance of lycopene, shown to benefit heart health. Serve over rice or Green Quinoa (page 203) and a Caesar Salad (page 181) with chopped Maple Baked Tempeh (page 262).

2 teaspoons olive oil

1 ½ cups chopped onion

2 tablespoons minced garlic

2 teaspoons dried oregano

1 ½ teaspoons dried thyme

1 cup seeded and diced green or red bell pepper

¾ cup quartered cremini mushrooms

½ cup diced fennel bulb

5 ½ cups chopped eggplant (1-inch pieces)

¾ teaspoon sea salt, or to taste

3 cups chopped fresh tomato or chopped fire-roasted tomatoes (1 [28-ounce] can)

½ cup red wine (optional)

3 tablespoons chiffonaded fresh basil

2 tablespoons finely chopped fresh flat-leaf parsley

2 tablespoons balsamic vinegar

¼ teaspoon freshly ground black pepper

¼ teaspoon crushed red pepper flakes

1. Place the oil in a large sauté pan over medium-high heat. Add the onion, garlic, oregano, and thyme and cook for 2 minutes, stirring frequently. Add the bell pepper, mushrooms, and fennel and cook for 3 minutes, stirring frequently. Add the eggplant and salt and cook for 7 minutes, stirring frequently and adding small amounts of water, if necessary, to prevent sticking.

2. Add the fire-roasted tomatoes and red wine, if using, and cook until the eggplant is just tender, about 10 minutes, stirring frequently.

3. Add the remaining ingredients and stir well before serving.

VARIATIONS

Add ½ teaspoon of fresh rosemary and ½ teaspoon of minced fresh sage.

Add 1 cup of chopped zucchini along with the tomatoes.

◆ For an oil-free version, use the water sauté method (see page 101).

Nutrition Facts per serving (361 g): Calories 105, Fat Calories 20, Total Fat 2 g, Saturated Fat 0 g, Cholesterol 0 mg, Sodium 325 mg, Total Carb 20 g, Dietary Fiber 7 g, Sugars 9 g, Protein 3 g

---

TEMPLATE RECIPE
Quiche

Thickener component: Replace the cashews with macadamia or Brazil nuts.

Binder component: Replace the flaxseeds with chia seeds or commercial egg replacer (see page 84, 312).

Veggie component: Replace the broccoli and shiitake mushrooms with vegetables of your choosing, such as cauliflower, Romanesco, carrot, parsnip, zucchini, or corn.

Herb component: Replace the dill with fresh basil, parsley, cilantro, or sorrel.

Spice component: Add 1 tablespoon of an ethnic spice blend, such as Herbes de Provence (page 106), Moroccan (page 106), Mexican (page 106), or Indian (page 106).

Broccoli Dill Quiche Ⓖ ◁

YIELD: 1 QUICHE

Prep time: 15 minutes, Soak time: 25 minutes, Cook time: 30 minutes, Total time: 60 minutes, Serving size: 1 slice, Number of servings: 8

Quiche's creamy cheesiness and flowery broccoli seem to go hand in hand. Everyone's favorite cancer-fighting crucifer, broccoli, is not only fun to eat but also doles out loads of vitamins A, C, and K, folate, and potassium. Perky dill teams up with sweet fennel to promote carminative, antihistamine, and relaxing properties. And along with flavorful marjoram, dill is also helpful to the respiratory system and provides calcium, B complex, vitamin

C, and oils that help balance neurological hormones. Shiitake mushrooms further expand this delectable dish into a treat for your body on all levels. Enjoy with a simple salad and cup of Moroccan Chickpea Stew (page 255) or Raw Carrot Brazil Nut Soup (page 145).

½ cup raw cashew pieces

1 tablespoon ground flaxseeds 3 tablespoons water

1 premade vegan piecrust, or Breakfast Tart crust (page 129)

2 teaspoons coconut oil

½ cup diced shallot

4 garlic cloves, minced or pressed

½ cup diced shiitake mushroom

¼ cup finely chopped fennel bulb

4 cups finely chopped broccoli florets

3 tablespoons nutritional yeast

2 tablespoons freshly squeezed lemon juice

½ cup thinly sliced green onion

1 tablespoon minced fresh dill

1 teaspoon chopped fresh marjoram, or ½ teaspoon dried

½ teaspoon sea salt, or to taste

1 teaspoon wheat-free tamari or other soy sauce (optional)

½ teaspoon truffle oil (optional; see page 88)

½ teaspoon crushed red pepper flakes

¼ teaspoon freshly ground black pepper

1. Place the cashews in a bowl with ample water to cover. Allow to sit for 25 minutes or longer. Place the flaxseeds in a small bowl with the 3 tablespoons of water.

2. Meanwhile, if using premade piecrust, defrost the pie shell according to the package instructions. Preheat the oven to 375°F. Poke a few holes in the pie

shell, using a fork. Bake for 15 minutes. Remove from the oven and set aside. If using the Breakfast Tart crust, prepare it according to directions on page 129.

3. Meanwhile, place the coconut oil in a sauté pan over medium-high heat. Add the shallot and garlic and cook for 3 minutes, stirring frequently. Add the mushrooms and fennel and cook for 3 minutes, stirring frequently. Add the broccoli and cook for 7 minutes, stirring frequently, adding small amounts of water, if necessary, to prevent sticking. Transfer one cup of vegetable mixture to a strong blender.

4. Rinse and drain the cashews. Add to the blender and blend until the cashews are completely pureed. Add small amounts of water, if necessary, to reach the consistency where there is little to no grittiness. Return to the pan with the remaining ingredients, including the flaxseed mixture, and mix well. Taste the mixture and add additional salt or tamari to taste, if necessary.

5. Transfer to the pie crust and bake for 30 minutes, or until golden brown on top. Allow to cool slightly before slicing.

VARIATION

◆ For an oil-free version, use the water sauté method (see page 101) and omit the truffle oil.

Ⓖ For a gluten-free version, use the crust from the Sun-Dried Tomato Fennel Breakfast Tart (see page 129).

Nutrition Facts per serving (148 g) for filling: Calories 140, Fat Calories 75, Total Fat 8.5 g, Saturated Fat 3 g, Cholesterol 0 mg, Sodium 315 mg, Total Carb 12 g, Dietary Fiber 3 g, Sugars 3 g, Protein 6 g

Nutrition Facts per serving (178 g) with crust from Breakfast Tart: Calories 290, Fat Calories 165, Total Fat 19 g, Saturated Fat 6 g, Cholesterol 0 mg, Sodium 326 mg, Total Carb 23 g, Dietary Fiber 6 g, Sugars 5 g, Protein 11 g

Lemon Tempeh with Kale and Rice Noodles ◆

YIELD: 4 ½ CUPS TEMPEH, KALE, AND NOODLES

Prep time: 15 minutes, Cook time: 20 minutes, Total time: 35 minutes, Serving size: 1 cup plus 2 tablespoons, Number of servings: 4

With roots in Indonesia, soy-based tempeh, in a light lemon marinade, is the protein source in this filling pasta and veggie dish. Tempeh offers the same abundance of nutritionals of tofu but with a hardier texture and nuttier taste, and possibly more—the culturing process may extract more B vitamins and even vitamin K. A perfect addition to this dish is some thinly sliced greenery in the form of kale or spinach, veritable superstars in the plant kingdom, and gluten-free carbs in rice pasta, which help complete a well-rounded, light, yet satisfying meal. Serve with a drizzle of Almond Dipping Sauce (page 233) or Zesty Chimichurri Sauce (page 231) and Super Sprout Salad (page 173).

8 ounces rice pasta

3 cups very thinly sliced kale or spinach

¼ cup plus 1 ½ tablespoons freshly squeezed lemon juice

3 tablespoons water

1 teaspoon stone-ground mustard

1 ½ tablespoons fresh dill

1 teaspoon pure maple syrup

1 ½ teaspoons wheat-free tamari or other soy sauce, or to taste

¼ teaspoon freshly ground black pepper

Pinch of crushed red pepper flakes

8 ounces chopped tempeh, cut into ½-inch cubes

1 cup chopped tomato (½-inch pieces)

1 ½ tablespoons hemp or flax oil (optional)

2 tablespoons nutritional yeast

1. Preheat the oven or toaster oven to 375°F. Place a pot of water over high heat and bring to a boil. Add the pasta and cook according to the package instructions. Rinse and drain well. Return to the pot. Add the kale and gently toss to combine.

2. Meanwhile, place ¼ cup of the lemon juice and the water, mustard, 1 ½ teaspoons of the dill, maple syrup, 1 teaspoon of the tamari, black pepper, and crushed red pepper flakes in a small baking dish and mix well. Add the tempeh and allow to sit for 5 minutes, or up to 1 hour, stirring occasionally. Place in the oven and bake for 10 minutes. Carefully stir well, and bake for an additional 10 minutes.

3. Portion out the pasta and kale or place in a bowl to serve family style. Top with the tempeh and tomatoes and drizzle with the remaining tamari, the remaining 1 ½ tablespoons of lemon juice, and oil, if using. Top with the nutritional yeast and the remaining 1 tablespoon of dill before serving.

VARIATIONS

Top with chopped avocado.

Replace the tempeh with tofu, seitan, or portobello mushrooms.

Replace the rice noodles with quinoa or rice.

Replace the kale with collards, spinach, chard, or arugula.

Experiment with different marinades for the tempeh (see page 107).

Nutrition Facts per serving (234 g): Calories 205, Fat Calories 60, Total Fat 7 g, Saturated Fat 1 g, Cholesterol 0 mg, Sodium 175 mg, Total Carb 24 g, Dietary Fiber 4 g, Sugars 4 g, Protein 15 g

Mushroom Cauliflower Tacos ⓖ

YIELD: 6 TACOS; 3 CUPS FILLING

Prep time: 15 minutes, Cook time: 10 minutes, Total time: 25 minutes, Serving size: 1 taco with 1/2 cup filling, Number of servings: 6

If mushroom and cauliflower are not the first ingredients that come to mind for a taco filling, you will quickly see that this delightful combination of flavors held together in a lightly sweet corn tortilla works in so many ways. Cauliflower, the "new broccoli," is chock-full of vitamins and minerals, including iron, potassium, and vitamin C. Equally health preserving, vitamin D–containing mushrooms add to the mega-nutrient mix in this supersatisfying dish. What a yummy way to keep your body healthy and vibrant. Serve with Smoky Salsa (page 151), Glorious Guacamole (page 151), and Raw Cashew Sour Cream (page 113). To serve family style, place the tortillas on a small plate, covered with a clean cloth napkin. For a grain-free version, serve the filling in lettuce or cabbage wraps.

2 teaspoons coconut oil
½ cup diced yellow onion
3 garlic cloves, pressed or minced
½ cup diced red bell pepper
1 cup diced mushrooms (try shiitake, cremini, or button)
½ teaspoon sea salt, or to taste
⅛ teaspoon freshly ground black pepper
2 cups diced cauliflower
1 teaspoon chili powder
½ teaspoon ground cumin
Pinch of chipotle chile powder or cayenne pepper
2 tablespoons freshly squeezed lime juice
1 ½ tablespoons minced fresh cilantro
6 vegan corn tortillas

1. Place the coconut oil in a pan over medium heat. Add the onion and cook for 1 minute, stirring frequently. Add the garlic, bell pepper, mushrooms, salt, and pepper and cook for 3 minutes, stirring frequently.

2. Add the cauliflower, chili powder, cumin, and chipotle chile powder and cook until the cauliflower is just tender, about 10 minutes, stirring frequently. Add the lime juice and cilantro and mix well. Lower the heat to low to keep filling warm.

3. Warm the tortillas briefly by placing them one at a time in a dry sauté pan over high heat, flipping with tongs until just warmed through.

4. Place the mushroom cauliflower filling inside the tortillas, top with your condiments of choice, and enjoy!

VARIATIONS

Add ½ teaspoon of seeded and diced jalapeño pepper and ½ teaspoon of paprika.

Add ½ cup of chopped walnuts.

Replace 1 cup of the cauliflower with diced tempeh or tofu.

Replace the tortillas with hard taco shells.

◆ For an oil-free version, use the water sauté method (see page 101).

Nutrition Facts per serving (139 g): Calories 90, Fat Calories 20, Total Fat 2.5 g, Saturated Fat 1.5 g, Cholesterol 0 mg, Sodium 230 mg, Total Carb 16 g, Dietary Fiber 3 g, Sugars 2 g, Protein 3 g

BBQ Roasted Tofu with Collards⊙

YIELD: 4 CUPS TOFU AND COLLARDS

Prep time: 20 minutes, Cook time: 30 minutes, Total time: 40 minutes, Serving size: 1 cup, Number of servings: 4

Take mildly flavored tofu to a new level with the pizzazz of a rich smoky barbecue sauce. Tofu's amino acid, calcium, iron, and protein is complemented well by a helping of greens—and collards are among the most nutrient-dense foods out there: rich in supply of fiber; vitamins A, C, and K; as well as folate, manganese, and calcium. Serve over rice or quinoa and top with Vegan Sour Cream (page 112).

2 teaspoons coconut oil, melted

1 teaspoon wheat-free tamari or other soy sauce, or to taste

1 (14-ounce) package extra-firm or superfirm tofu

¼ cup water

1 cup thinly sliced yellow onion

4 cups stemmed and chopped collards (½-inch pieces)

1 cup Smoky BBQ Sauce (page 231)

1. Preheat the oven or toaster oven to 375°F. Place the coconut oil and tamari on a small baking sheet and whisk well.

2. Slice the block of tofu lengthwise into three cutlets. Stack the cutlets on top of each other. Make three cuts lengthwise and three cuts widthwise to yield a total of sixteen cubes per cutlet.

3. Place the baking dish in the oven and cook for 20 minutes, stirring occasionally. For a crisper cube, you can heat the oven broiler on HIGH and cook for an additional 5 minutes. Set aside.

4. Place the water in a pot over medium-high heat. Add the onion and cook for 3 minutes, stirring frequently and adding additional water, if necessary, to prevent sticking.

5. Add the collards and cook for 3 minutes, stirring frequently and adding additional water, if necessary, to prevent sticking.

6. Lower the heat to low, add the BBQ sauce, and cook for 5 minutes, stirring frequently. Add the tofu cubes and gently stir well before serving.

Replace the tofu with tempeh, seitan, or chopped Beyond Meat or Gardein (see page 84).

Replace the collards with kale, chard, arugula, or spinach and cook for less time.

◆ For an oil-free version, marinate and cook the tofu cubes in 3 tablespoons of water or vegetable stock (see page 108).

See page 107 for suggestions on altering the marinade.

Replace the collards with kale.

Nutrition Facts per serving (225 g): Calories 175, Fat Calories 60, Total Fat 7 g, Saturated Fat 3 g, Cholesterol 0 mg, Sodium 220 mg, Total Carb 21 g, Dietary Fiber 4 g, Sugars 13 g, Protein 11 g

Tempeh Fajitas◉

YIELD: 6 FAJITAS; 18 OUNCES FIXINGS BY WEIGHT

Prep time: 25 minutes, Cook time: 15 minutes, Total time: 30 minutes, Serving size: 4 ounces by weight, Number of servings: 6

Tempeh- and veggie-stuffed fajitas are a perfect go-to for plant-based eaters because of the abundance of vegetables tossed alongside protein powerhouse tempeh. In these Mexican-spiced fajitas, glean the benefits of potent onions, vitamins A and C–rich red and green peppers, and the selenium and copper contained in portobello mushrooms. If you have the time for a full-blown fiesta, serve with Glorious Guacamole (page 151), Smoky Salsa (page 151), and Vegan Sour Cream (page 112).

BROILED TEMPEH

8 ounces tempeh, cut into ¼-inch slices

¼ cup plus 1 tablespoon water

2 teaspoons wheat-free tamari or other soy sauce, or to taste

2 teaspoons melted coconut oil

¼ teaspoon chili powder

⅛ teaspoon chipotle chile powder

VEGETABLES

2 teaspoons coconut oil

1 cup sliced onion (¼-inch slices)

1 cup seeded and sliced red bell pepper (¼-inch slices)

1 cup seeded and sliced green bell pepper (¼-inch slices)

2 cups sliced portobello mushroom (½-inch slices)

1 teaspoon wheat-free tamari or other soy sauce, or to taste

1 teaspoon chili powder

½ teaspoon ground cumin

⅛ teaspoon chipotle chile powder or cayenne pepper

1 ½ tablespoons finely chopped fresh cilantro

1 ½ tablespoons freshly squeezed lime juice

Pinch of sea salt, or to taste

¼ teaspoon liquid smoke, see page 85 (optional)

FIXINGS

1 ½ cups thinly sliced lettuce, spinach, or arugula

1 thinly sliced tomato, cut into ½-inch strips

6 corn tortillas

1. Prepare the broiled tempeh: Preheat the oven broiler on HIGH. Place all the broiled tempeh ingredients, except for the tempeh itself, on a small baking sheet and stir well. Add the tempeh and

toss until evenly coated. Place in the oven and broil for 3 minutes. Remove from the oven, carefully flip the tempeh, and return to the oven. Broil for 3 minutes, remove from the oven, and set aside.

2. Prepare the vegetables: Place the onion in a large sauté pan or cast-iron pan over medium-high heat and cook until translucent, about 3 minutes, stirring frequently. Add the red and green bell pepper and cook for 3 minutes, stirring frequently. Add the portobello mushroom and cook for 5 minutes, stirring frequently and adding small amounts of water, if necessary, to prevent sticking.

3. Lower the heat to low, add the chili powder, cumin, chipotle chile powder, cilantro, lime juice, salt, and liquid smoke, if using, and stir well.

4. Prepare the fixings, including warming the tortillas. To warm tortillas, wrap in foil or a slightly damp towel and heat in a 350°F oven for 7 minutes. Alternatively, place a sauté pan over high heat. Add the tortillas one by one and heat each side for 1 minute, or until the tortillas are soft.

5. Assemble your fajitas by adding a few strips of tempeh, a serving of vegetables, and a serving of fixings to each tortilla. Or serve family style and let your guests create their own fajita.

VARIATIONS

Replace the tempeh with tofu, or Gardein or Beyond Meat (see page 84).

Replace the tempeh with seitan (see page 100).

Replace the vegetables with your favorites, including roasted or grilled eggplant, carrots, baby bok choy.

Add 1 cup of grated vegan mozzarella-style cheese along with the vegetables.

⬥For an oil-free version, replace the coconut oil in the marinades with water, and use the water sauté method (see page 101) for the vegetables.

Nutrition Facts per serving (205 g): Calories 190, Fat Calories 70, Total Fat 8 g, Saturated Fat 4 g, Cholesterol 0 mg, Sodium 335 mg, Total Carb 22 g, Dietary Fiber 4 g, Sugars 4 g, Protein 11 g

Jamaican Patties

YIELD: 6 PATTIES

Prep time: 30 minutes, Cook time: 40 minutes, Total time: 70 minutes, Serving size: 1 patty, Number of servings: 6

Jamaican patties are traditionally a filled crust thought to be a cross between Jamaican cuisine and the British pasty, created when the British arrived in Jamaica. With a nutritionally balanced trio of bean, grain, and carb in the form of lentil or pigeon peas, potato, and spinach, experience the taste of Jamaica straight from your own oven. Serve warm out of the oven with Raw Tamarind Sauce (page 230), Smoky BBQ Sauce (page 231), Cilantro Mint Chutney (page 229), or your sauce of choice.

FILLING

2 small Yukon gold or red bliss potatoes, chopped small

½ cup finely chopped spinach or arugula

1 ½ tablespoons freshly squeezed lemon juice

½ cup cooked lentils or pigeon peas (see page 98) or garden peas

¾ teaspoon cumin seeds

2 garlic cloves, pressed or minced

½ teaspoon sea salt, or to taste

⅛ teaspoon freshly ground black pepper

½ teaspoon dried thyme

1 teaspoon curry powder

1 tablespoon minced fresh cilantro

DOUGH

2 cups white spelt flour or Gluten-Free Flour Mix (page 105)

Pinch of sea salt, or to taste

½ teaspoon ground turmeric

2 tablespoons coconut oil

6 tablespoons to ½ cup water

1. Prepare the filling: Preheat the oven to 350°F. Prepare the filling. Place a pot with a steamer basket and 1 inch of water over medium-high heat. Add the potatoes, cover, and cook until just tender, about 10 minutes. Transfer to a bowl and mash well. Measure out 1 ¼ cups for this recipe. Add the remaining filling ingredients, and mix well.

2. Prepare the dough: Place the flour, salt, and turmeric in a bowl and whisk well. Add the coconut oil and water and knead into a ball. The dough should hold together and be slightly moist.

3. Roll out the dough into a log and divide into six equal-size pieces. Roll out each piece into a 5-inch-diameter circle. Place about 3 ounces (just under ¼ cup) of filling on the center of each circle.

Fold the circle in half, and pinch the edges together to form your patties.

4. Place on a parchment paper–lined baking sheet. You can optionally baste each patty with additional coconut oil. Bake for 30 minutes, or until golden brown. Serve warm.

VARIATIONS

Replace the potatoes with sweet potatoes.

Add 1 tablespoon of Indian Spice Mix (page 106) or Mexican Spice Mix (page 106).

Replace the peas with cooked black-eyed peas, black beans, or pinto beans.

Replace the potatoes with Smashed Roasted Cauliflower and Parsnip (page 202).

🝆 Replace the oil with additional water or mashed banana.

Ⓖ For a gluten-free version, use Gluten-Free Flour Mix (see page 105).

Nutrition Facts per serving (183 g): Calories 245, Fat Calories 70, Total Fat 8 g, Saturated Fat 4.5 g, Cholesterol 0 mg, Sodium 540 mg, Total Carb 41 g, Dietary Fiber 6 g, Sugars 2 g, Protein 7 g

Sloppy Joes Ⓖ

YIELD: 4 CUPS FILLING

Prep time: 15 minutes, Cook time: 30 minutes, Total time: 45 minutes, Serving size: 2/3 cup, Number of servings: 6

In this version of old-school sloppy joes, which are said to have originated in Iowa or

Key West in the 1950s, tempeh and mushrooms do a stellar job of giving this comfort dish a fresh new vibrancy. Their earthy flavors combine with onions, garlic, and tomatoes for a truly superfood meal, providing ample protein, fiber, essential vitamins and minerals as well as protective antioxidants and bioflavonoids that stay active even when cooked. Serve with Cream of Kale (page 201) and Herb-Roasted Potatoes (page 214).

2 teaspoons coconut oil

1 ½ cups diced yellow onion

2 tablespoons minced garlic

1 cup diced tempeh

2 ½ cups chopped cremini mushrooms (½-inch pieces)

3 ½ cups crushed fire-roasted tomatoes (1 [28-ounce] can) or fresh tomatoes

1 tablespoon freshly squeezed lime juice

2 teaspoons raw apple cider vinegar

1 ½ teaspoons wheat-free tamari or other soy sauce

Pinch of sea salt, or to taste

¼ teaspoon chipotle chile powder

¼ teaspoon ground cumin

¼ teaspoon ground coriander (optional)

¼ teaspoon freshly ground black pepper

⅛ teaspoon crushed red pepper flakes

6 vegan buns

Fixings of choice (sliced tomato, sliced onion, sliced pickles, lettuce)

1. Place the oil in a sauté pan over medium-high heat. Add the onion and garlic and cook for 3 minutes, stirring frequently. Add the tempeh and cook for 3 minutes, stirring frequently and adding small amounts of water, if necessary, to prevent sticking.

2. Add the mushrooms and cook for 3 minutes, stirring frequently. Add the remaining ingredients, except the buns and fixings, and cook for 10 minutes, stirring frequently. Lower the heat to low, and cook until most of the liquid is absorbed, about 10 minutes.

3. Place the buns on individual plates. Top with about ⅔ cup of sloppy joe filling and the fixings. Serve warm.

VARIATIONS

Add 1 tablespoon of molasses and 2 teaspoons of vegan Worcestershire sauce.

Add 1 cup of seeded and diced bell pepper along with the onion.

Replace the tempeh with chopped walnuts, cashews, or Brazil nuts.

Replace the tempeh with tofu, seitan, or Beyond Meat (see page 84).

♦ For an oil-free version, use the water sauté method (page 101).

Nutrition Facts per serving (242 g) for filling: Calories 135, Fat Calories 45, Total Fat 5 g, Saturated Fat 2 g, Cholesterol 0 mg, Sodium 290 mg, Total Carb 18 g, Dietary Fiber 4 g, Sugars 8 g, Protein 9 g

Grilled Eggplant Towers with Cashew Ricotta ⊖ ♦

YIELD: 4 TOWERS

Prep time: 20 minutes, Soak time: 20 minutes, Cook time: 15 minutes, Total time: 45 minutes, Serving size: 1 tower, Number of servings: 4

In the 18th century, Europeans named this round fruit an eggplant because it resembled large goose eggs—in fact, more so because it was a white or yellow variety, rather than the purple, tear-shaped aubergine we see most commonly today. Eggplant is a very good source of dietary fiber; vitamins B_1, B_6, and K; copper, manganese, niacin, potassium, and folate. It contains phytonutrient nasunin, which specifically protects lipids in the brain, and also helps balance blood sugar to promote healthy weight loss. Here, slices of eggplant are grilled and stacked with vegan cheese for an impressive (and delicious!) presentation that would make Michelangelo proud. For the cheese, cashews are transformed with the help of miso, lemon, and a perfect blend of aromatic herbs into a rich and tangy, true Italian ricotta. Top with Fire-Roasted Tomato Sauce (page 239) or a dollop of Pesto (page 215) and serve with Waldorf Salad (page 180) and Green Quinoa (page 203) or Pearled Barley with Mushrooms and Corn (page 210).

CASHEW RICOTTA CHEESE

¾ cup raw cashew pieces

¼ cup water

2 tablespoons nutritional yeast

1 tablespoon white miso paste (optional) (see page 248)

1 tablespoon freshly squeezed lemon juice

1 tablespoon minced fresh flat-leaf parsley

1 tablespoon minced fresh basil

1 clove garlic

½ teaspoon sea salt

½ teaspoon dried oregano (optional)

½ teaspoon dried thyme (optional)

½ teaspoon dehydrated onion flakes (optional)

⅛ teaspoon freshly ground black pepper

⅛ teaspoon crushed red pepper flakes

GRILLED EGGPLANT

¼ cup water

1 tablespoon balsamic vinegar

1 tablespoon olive oil (optional)

1 tablespoon Italian spice mix (page 105), or 1 teaspoon dried oregano and ½ teaspoon dried thyme

Pinch of sea salt

Pinch of freshly ground black pepper

1 medium-size eggplant, cut into eight ½-inch slices

1 medium-size tomato, cut into 4 slices

4 fresh parsley leaves

Black sesame seeds

1. Prepare the cheese: Place the cashews in a bowl of water with ample room to cover. Allow to sit for 20 minutes, or up to a few hours. Rinse and drain well. Place in a blender with the remaining Cashew Ricotta ingredients, including the ¼ cup of fresh water, and blend until just creamy. Some chunkiness is okay.

2. Meanwhile, prepare the eggplant: Preheat a grill. Place the water, vinegar, olive oil, if using, Italian Spice Mix, salt, and black pepper on a baking sheet with raised edges and whisk well. Add the eggplant and allow to sit for 10 minutes, or up to 30 minutes, flipping periodically.

3. Grill until char marks appear and the eggplant is just tender, about 5 minutes on each side, depending upon the heat of the grill.

4. To assemble your towers, select the largest four slices of eggplant as the bottom layer. Top each with ⅛ cup of the cheese, then another slice of eggplant,

followed by ⅛ cup of cheese. Top each tower with a slice of tomato, a sprinkle of black sesame seeds, and a parsley leaf before serving. You can optionally reheat in the oven before serving.

VARIATIONS

You can broil the eggplant instead of grilling. Place the marinade ingredients in a baking dish and mix well. Add the eggplant and broil until just tender, about 7 minutes per each side, depending upon the heat of the broiler.

Replace the cashews in the Cashew Ricotta Cheese with macadamia nuts or Brazil nuts.

Nutrition Facts per serving (276 g): Calories 300, Fat Calories 175, Total Fat 20 g, Saturated Fat 3.5 g, Cholesterol 0 mg, Sodium 305 mg, Total Carb 24 g, Dietary Fiber 7 g, Sugars 7 g, Protein 11 g

Millet and Butternut Squash with Broccoli🟢◆

YIELD: 6 ½ CUPS SQUASH AND BROCCOLI

Prep time: 10 minutes, Cook time: 40 minutes, Total time: 50 minutes, Serving size: 1 heaping cup, Number of servings: 6

Of North African origin, millet is an easily digestible and gluten-free grain that is full of fiber and protein, along with niacin, copper, and manganese. It also has a prolific amount of lignans, phytonutrients known to ward off heart disease, and phosphorus, important for tissue growth and repair. Toasting the millet brings out more of a nutty flavor. This comforting casserole also includes beta-carotene-rich, energy-sustaining butternut squash and adds broccoli, carrots, and both dried and fresh herbs to provide an abundant balance of healthful nutrients. After you combine the roasted squash, millet, and steamed vegetables, the dish can be served as it is, or optionally chilled, sliced, and baked to serve in individual squares. Top with Roasted Red Pepper Sauce (page 235) or Oil-Free Mushroom Gravy (page 240) and serve along with a simple salad or Black Bean and Corn Salad (page 189).

1 small butternut squash
Oil, for baking sheet (optional)
1 ½ cups uncooked millet
4 cups water or vegetable stock (see page 108)
4 garlic cloves, pressed or minced
1 teaspoon sea salt, or to taste
2 teaspoons dried oregano
1 teaspoon dried thyme
¼ teaspoon freshly ground black pepper
¼ teaspoon crushed red pepper flakes
1 ½ cups small broccoli floret
1 cup thinly sliced carrot
2 tablespoons chiffonaded fresh basil
1 tablespoon finely chopped fresh flat-leaf parsley

1. Preheat the oven to 425°F. Slice the squash in half lengthwise, remove the seeds, and place on a well-oiled baking sheet or a casserole dish filled with about ¼ inch of water. Place in the oven and cook until a knife can pass easily through the thickest part of the squash, about 40 minutes. Remove from the oven. Carefully scoop out 1 ½ cups of the squash and place in a large bowl.

2. Meanwhile, place the millet in a pot over high heat and cook for 2 minutes,

stirring frequently to prevent burning. Add the water or stock. Lower the heat to medium-low. Add the garlic, salt, oregano, thyme, black pepper, and crushed red pepper flakes and cook covered until the millet is soft and the liquid is absorbed, about 25 minutes, stirring occasionally. Add to the squash.

3. Meanwhile, place a steamer basket in a pot filled with about ½ inch of water over high heat. Bring to a boil. Lower the heat to low. Add the broccoli and carrots and cook until the vegetables are just tender, about 5 minutes. Add to the squash along with the basil and parsley, and mix well. Taste and add additional salt to taste, if necessary.

4. Transfer to an 8 by 8-inch casserole dish. You can enjoy warm as is, and serve with a spoon. You can also place in the refrigerator for 30 minutes, or until the casserole is firm enough to slice. Once sliced, you can reheat in the oven (10 minutes at 400°F) before serving.

VARIATIONS

Turn this into a casserole by baking for 20 minutes at 350°F. Allow to cool before slicing.

Add 1 teaspoon of minced fresh rosemary and 1 tablespoon chopped fresh marjoram.

Replace all or some of the broccoli and carrot with your favorite veggies, including parsnip, bell pepper, corn, or cauliflower. Enjoy the vegetables steamed, sautéed, roasted, or grilled (see page 101).

Add 2 tablespoons of an ethnic spice blend, such as Moroccan (page 106), Indian (page 106), or Mexican (page 106).

Replace the basil with fresh cilantro or 1 ½ tablespoons of minced fresh dill.

Nutrition Facts per serving (195 g): Calories 230, Fat Calories 20, Total Fat 2.5 g, Saturated Fat 0 g, Cholesterol 0 mg, Sodium 320 mg, Total Carb 46 g, Dietary Fiber 7 g, Sugars 2 g, Protein 7 g

Cauliflower Casserole Ⓖ ◆

YIELD: 6 CUPS CASSEROLE

Prep time: 30 minutes, Cook time: 30 minutes, Total time: 60 minutes, Serving size: 1 1/2 cups, Number of servings: 4

Cauliflower power stars in this luscious, home-style casserole, but "the other white vegetable" or "the white carrot"—parsnip—plays an important role as an excellent source of fiber, trace minerals, vitamin C, and B vitamins, including folate. Accenting the creamy comforting shades of white are flashes of red and vitamins A, B_6, and C from the red pepper; vibrant spring green and flavonoids from the fresh dill; and striking yellow carotenoid and anti-inflammatory effects from the turmeric. Serve with Chili Lime Grilled Asparagus with Red Bell Pepper (page 193) or Ginger Rainbow Chard (page 189), and Grilled Mediterranean Vegetables and Quinoa (page 212).

¾ cup raw cashew pieces
3 cups small cauliflower florets
1 cup chopped parsnip (½-inch pieces)
½ cup seeded and diced red bell pepper
¼ cup diced yellow onion

¼ cup nutritional yeast

2 garlic cloves, pressed or minced

2 tablespoons tahini

1 ½ tablespoons freshly squeezed lemon juice

1 tablespoon minced fresh dill

½ teaspoon sea salt, or to taste

½ teaspoon ground turmeric

⅛ teaspoon smoked paprika

⅛ teaspoon freshly ground black pepper

Pinch of crushed red pepper flakes

1 cup unsweetened almond, soy, or rice milk (for homemade, see Plant-Based Milk, page 104)

Oil, for casserole (optional)

1. Preheat the oven to 400°F. Place the cashews in a bowl with ample water to cover. Allow to sit for 20 minutes, or up to a few hours.

2. Meanwhile, place all the remaining ingredients, except the almond milk and the oil, if using, in a bowl and mix well.

3. Rinse and drain the cashews well. Transfer to a blender along with the almond milk and blend until creamy. Pour into the cauliflower mixture and mix well. Taste and add additional salt to taste, if necessary.

4. Transfer to a well-oiled or nonstick 8 by 8-inch casserole dish and bake until golden brown, about 30 minutes. The dish will solidify as it cools. Serve warm.

VARIATIONS

Add 1 teaspoon Dijon mustard along with the tahini.

Replace the cashews with macadamia nuts or Brazil nuts.

Replace the cauliflower with broccoli or Romanesco, or mixed vegetables, such as zucchini, corn, and asparagus.

Replace the dill with 2 tablespoons of minced fresh cilantro, basil, sorrel, or parsley.

Add 1 tablespoon of an ethnic spice blend, such as Ethiopian (page 106), Herbes de Provence (page 106), or Mexican (page 106).

Nutrition Facts per serving (318 g): Calories 370, Fat Calories 210, Total Fat 24 g, Saturated Fat 4 g, Cholesterol 0 mg, Sodium 385 mg, Total Carb 29 g, Dietary Fiber 7 g, Sugars 7 g, Protein 14 g

Corn Casserole◆

YIELD: 4 ½ CUPS CASSEROLE

Prep time: 15 minutes, Cook time: 45 minutes, Total time: 55 minutes, Serving size: 1 1/8 cups, Number of servings: 4

Corn (also known as maize) is the featured ingredient in this buttery casserole, and is one of the most popular cereals in the world and forms the staple food in many countries, including the United States and many African countries. Since corn is one of the most highly GMO crops around (see page 60), you'll want to be sure to purchase only organic corn. Phosphorous, along with magnesium, manganese, zinc, iron, and copper, are found in all varieties of corn, and unlike many other foods, cooking actually increases its amount of usable antioxidants. Corn provides significant levels of iron, folate, and beta-carotene. Health benefits of corn include controlling diabetes, prevention of heart ailments, lowering hypertension, and maintenance of good vision and skin. Serve with Quinoa Chickpea Pilaf (page 211) and Sesame Kale Salad (page 186), or a bowl of Ital Roasted Squash and Sweet Potato Soup (page 251).

3 cups fresh or frozen (thawed) corn

1 ½ cups unsweetened almond, soy, or coconut milk (for homemade, see Plant-Based Milk, page 104)

2 tablespoons nutritional yeast

¼ cup plus 2 tablespoons garbanzo or tapioca flour

2 tablespoons arrowroot powder or cornstarch

2 tablespoons tahini (optional)

¼ teaspoon sea salt, or to taste

½ teaspoon ground turmeric (optional)

¼ teaspoon chipotle chile powder

¼ teaspoon freshly ground black pepper

Oil, for casserole dish (optional)

1 cup diced yellow onion

1 large garlic clove, pressed or minced

½ teaspoon seeded and diced jalapeño pepper

2 tablespoons finely chopped fresh cilantro

1. Preheat the oven to 350°F. Place 1 ½ cups of the corn and the almond milk, nutritional yeast, flour, arrowroot, tahini, if using, salt, turmeric, if using, chipotle chile powder, and black pepper in a blender and blend until creamy.

2. Transfer to a well-oiled or nonstick 8 by 8-inch casserole dish along with the remaining corn, onion, garlic, jalapeño, and cilantro, and mix well. Taste and add additional salt if necessary.

3. Bake for 45 minutes, or until golden brown. Allow to cool slightly before slicing.

VARIATIONS

Add 1 teaspoon of smoked paprika.

Replace the corn with cauliflower, broccoli, chopped zucchini, or parsnip.

🔸 For an oil-free version, use the water sauté method (see page 101) and use a nonstick pan for baking.

Nutrition Facts per serving (293 g): Calories 530, Fat Calories 70, Total Fat 7.5 g, Saturated Fat 1 g, Cholesterol 0 mg, Sodium 270 mg, Total Carb 104 g, Dietary Fiber 11 g, Sugars 3 g, Protein 15 g

---

TEMPLATE RECIPE
Vegan Loaf

Legume component: Replace the lentils with chickpeas, or black or pinto beans.

Grain component: Replace the rice with millet, buckwheat, quinoa, polenta, or amaranth. (See page 96 for grain-cooking instructions.)

Nut component: Replace the walnuts with pecans, pistachios, macadamia nuts, or sunflower seeds.

Ethnic spice component: For Italian, add 1 tablespoon of Italian Spice Mix (page 105), and add additional fresh herbs, such as 2 tablespoons of chiffonaded basil, 1 teaspoon of oregano and 1 teaspoon of thyme. For Mexican, replace the parsley with fresh cilantro and add 2 tablespoons of Mexican Spice Mix (page 106). For Indian, replace the parsley with fresh cilantro and add 2 tablespoons of Indian Spice Mix (page 106).

Lentil Walnut Loaf ⓖ ▱

YIELD: 1 (8 BY 4-INCH) LOAF; 4 ½ CUPS

Prep time: 15 minutes, Cook time: 45 minutes,
Total time: 50 minutes, Serving size: 3/4-cup
portion, Number of servings: 6

Lentils are a favorite for their nutty and earthy flavor, ease and speed of cooking, and stellar nutritional profile: loaded with fiber, folate, iron, protein, and then some. They nicely blend with rich walnuts, which have the highest quantity of alpha-linolenic acid of any nut, not to mention protein, trace minerals, and lecithin, making them a potent brain food. The result is a delightful loaf that, completed by onion, celery, garlic, oats, parsley, sage, and mushrooms, is both filling and flavorful. Serve as part of a holiday feast with Oil-Free Mushroom Gravy (page 240), Green Beans with White Bean Fennel Sauce (page 217), and Pumpkin Pudding (page 307).

¾ cup uncooked short-grain brown rice
1 ½ cups water or vegetable stock (see page 108)
¾ teaspoon sea salt, or to taste
2 teaspoons coconut oil
¾ cup diced yellow onion
4 garlic cloves, pressed or minced
½ cup thinly sliced celery
¾ cup diced shiitake mushrooms
2 (15-ounce) cans lentils, or 3 cups cooked (see page 98)
¾ cup rolled oats (try gluten-free)
½ cup chopped walnuts (optionally toasted; see page 101)
¼ cup water or vegetable stock (see page 108)
2 tablespoons finely chopped fresh flat-leaf parsley
1 tablespoon chiffonaded fresh sage

1 teaspoon wheat-free tamari or other soy sauce (optional)
¼ teaspoon freshly ground black pepper
¼ teaspoon cayenne pepper
Oil, for loaf pan (optional)

1. Preheat the oven to 375°F.

2. Place the rice, water, and ¼ teaspoon of the salt in a pot over medium-high heat. Bring to a boil. Cover, lower the heat to a simmer, and cook until all liquid is absorbed, about 40 minutes.

3. Meanwhile, place the coconut oil in a sauté pan over medium-high heat. Add the onion and cook for 1 minute, stirring frequently. Add the garlic and celery and cook for 2 minutes, stirring frequently. Add the mushrooms and cook for 5 minutes, stirring frequently and adding a small amount of water, if necessary, to prevent sticking.

4. Place the lentils, rolled oats, walnuts, and water or stock in a food processor and process until smooth. Transfer to the pan along with the remaining ingredients, including the cooked rice and remaining ½ teaspoon of salt, and mix well. Taste and add additional salt or tamari to taste, if necessary.

5. Transfer to a lightly oiled or parchment paper–lined 8 by 4-inch loaf pan and bake for 30 minutes. Allow to cool slightly before slicing.

VARIATION

◆ For an oil-free version, use the water sauté method (see page 101).

Nutrition Facts per serving (215 g): Calories 370, Fat Calories 85, Total Fat 9.5 g, Saturated Fat 1.5 g, Cholesterol 0 mg, Sodium 458 mg, Total Carb 57 g, Dietary Fiber 13 g, Sugars 4 g, Protein 17 g

Thai Curry Vegetables

YIELD: 4 ¼ CUPS VEGETABLES

Prep time: 15 minutes, Cook time: 25 minutes, Total time: 40 minutes, Serving size: 1 cup plus 1 tablespoon, Number of servings: 4

This recipe is an exceptionally pleasurable way to enjoy your favorite veggies, gently bathed in the delectable combination of curry spices and coconut. Curry is a staple food and is often considered a "medicine" because it is so comforting and nourishing. Its main flavoring is turmeric, known as queen of the medicinal plant kingdom, complemented further by the healing qualities of cayenne, cumin, and coriander, all combined into a low-sodium blend of incredible flavor. Lemongrass and kaffir lime both add to the dish's flavor as well as its ability to calm and clear the body. The kaffir lime leaves will maintain their rejuvenating potency even after long storage. Serve over Golden Rice (page 204) with Green Papaya Salad (page 175) or Asian Cucumber Salad (page 175).

1 (14-ounce) can light or full-fat coconut milk
3 garlic cloves
1 tablespoon peeled and minced fresh ginger
1 stalk lemongrass, very bottom removed, white and light green part only, cut into ½-inch pieces
2 teaspoons seeded and diced hot chile pepper (see Scoville scale, page 179)
5 kaffir lime leaves
1 ½ teaspoons cumin seeds

1 ½ teaspoons curry powder
¼ teaspoon sea salt, or to taste
1 teaspoon ground coriander
¼ teaspoon freshly ground black pepper
1 ½ cups chopped zucchini (½-inch pieces)
1 cup cubed eggplant (½-inch pieces)
1 cup quartered cremini mushrooms
1 cup chopped potato or parsnip (½-inch pieces)
¾ cup thinly sliced carrot, cut diagonally
½ cup chopped tomato
2 cups stemmed and sliced Swiss chard or bok choy (1-inch pieces)
2 tablespoons finely chopped fresh cilantro
1 teaspoon wheat-free tamari or other soy sauce, or to taste (optional)

1. Place the coconut milk, garlic, ginger, lemongrass, chile pepper, and kaffir lime leaves in a strong blender and blend until creamy. Transfer to a pot over medium-high heat.

2. Add the cumin, curry, salt, coriander, and black pepper and mix well. Add the zucchini, eggplant, mushrooms, potato, carrot, and tomato and cook for 15 minutes, stirring occasionally.

3. Add the chard and cook for 5 minutes, stirring occasionally. Add the cilantro and tamari, if using, and stir well to incorporate before serving.

VARIATIONS

Spice it up: add an extra teaspoon (or two) of diced chile pepper.

Add 1 cup of cubed and roasted tofu or tempeh (see page 100).

Add ½ cup of thinly sliced onion along with the zucchini.

Replace the zucchini, eggplant, potato, mushrooms, and carrot with veggies of your choosing, such as cabbage, bell pepper, gold bar squash, broccoli, and/or cauliflower.

Replace the chard with collards, kale, spinach, or dandelion greens.

Nutrition Facts per serving (397 g): Calories 150, Fat Calories 70, Total Fat 8 g, Saturated Fat 5 g, Cholesterol 0 mg, Sodium 210 mg, Total Carb 17 g, Dietary Fiber 5 g, Sugars 5 g, Protein 3 g

Creamy Lentil Saag ⊙ ◊

YIELD: 4 CUPS LENTIL SAAG

Prep time: 5 minutes, Cook time: 20 minutes, Total time: 25 minutes, Serving size: 1 cup, Number of servings: 4

Saag means "spinach" in several South Asian languages. No matter the name, spinach doesn't disappoint: it is loaded with more than twenty nutrients and more than twelve flavonoid compounds, rendering it beneficial to almost every part of the body. Chief among its nutrient list are vitamins A and K, manganese, folate, and magnesium. Paired with the fiber, lean protein, iron, and folate of brown lentils, this heavenly South Asian specialty will satisfy your stomach and your palate. Top with toasted coconut (see page 101) and serve with rice, quinoa, or brown rice pasta (see page 96). Enjoy with Curry Kale Salad (page 184).

1 ½ teaspoons curry powder
1 teaspoon ground cumin

⅛ teaspoon cayenne pepper
2 cups unsweetened soy, rice, or coconut milk (for homemade, see Plant-Based Milk, page 104) or coconut milk beverage
½ cup diced yellow onion
3 garlic cloves, pressed or minced (optional)
1 (15-ounce can) brown lentils, or 1 ½ cups cooked (see page 98)
2 ½ cups tightly packed chopped spinach (7.5 ounces)
¼ teaspoon sea salt, or to taste
⅛ teaspoon freshly ground black pepper
2 teaspoons freshly squeezed lemon juice
1 tablespoon finely chopped fresh cilantro

1. Place the curry powder, cumin, and cayenne in a pot over medium-high heat and cook for 1 minute, stirring constantly.

2. Lower the heat to medium. Add the soy milk, onion, and garlic, if using, and cook for 5 minutes, stirring frequently. Add the lentils and cook for 10 minutes, stirring occasionally. Add the spinach, salt, and pepper and cook until just wilted, about 5 minutes, stirring occasionally.

3. Add the lemon juice and cilantro and mix well before serving.

VARIATIONS

Add 1 cup of diced grilled tempeh or tofu (see page 191).

Add 1 cup of diced tomato or fire-roasted tomatoes.

Add 2 teaspoons of brown mustard seeds and/or coriander seeds along with the curry powder.

Replace the lentils with yellow split peas, red lentils, black lentils, or chickpeas (see cooking chart on page 98).

Replace the spinach with arugula, kale, collards, or chard; you may need to increase or decrease the cook time, depending on how fast your greens wilt.

You can add 1 ½ tablespoons of coconut oil or sesame oil before adding the spices.

Nutrition Facts per serving (241 g): Calories 145, Fat Calories 25, Total Fat 3 g, Saturated Fat 1 g, Cholesterol 0 mg, Sodium 210 mg, Total Carb 20 g, Dietary Fiber 8 g, Sugars 3 g, Protein 11 g

Mexican Seitan-Stuffed Peppers

YIELD: 3 ¼ CUPS FILLING

Prep time: 10 minutes, Cook time: 30 minutes, Total time: 40 minutes, Serving size: appropriately 1/2 cup filling in 1/2 bell pepper, Number of servings: 6

If you tolerate gluten, savory seitan can be a superior way to get your essential amino acids. Made with whole wheat flour and usually cooked in a broth with the sea vegetable kombu and soy sauce, it provides a whopping 16 grams of protein per serving, while also supplying ample amounts of vitamin C, thiamine, riboflavin, niacin, and iron. It also absorbs flavors nicely. Here, spicy seitan and fire-roasted tomatoes stuffed into phytochemical-rich red bell peppers, plus the immunity-boosting qualities of onion and garlic, make an artful and satisfying addition to any Mexican meal. Top with a dollop of Vegan Sour Cream (page 112), Glorious Guacamole (page 151), and toasted pepitas (see page 101).

3 large bell peppers, seeded and sliced in half

MEXICAN SEITAN

2 teaspoons coconut oil

1 cup diced yellow onion

4 garlic cloves, pressed or minced

16 ounces chopped seitan (¼-inch pieces)

1 ½ cups chopped fresh tomatoes (½-inch pieces) or 1 (15-ounce can fire-roasted tomatoes)

1 teaspoon wheat-free tamari or other soy sauce (optional, depending on saltiness of the seitan)

1 tablespoon rice vinegar, raw cider vinegar, or coconut vinegar

1 teaspoon chili powder

¼ teaspoon chipotle chile powder

2 tablespoons nutritional yeast (optional)

Pinch of sea salt (optional, depending on saltiness of the seitan)

¼ teaspoon freshly ground black pepper

2 tablespoons finely chopped fresh cilantro

¾ cup grated vegan mozzarella-style cheese (optional)

1. Preheat the oven to 400°F. Place the bell peppers, cut side down, in a casserole dish with about ¼ inch water. Place in the oven and cook for 10 minutes. Remove from the oven.

2. Meanwhile, prepare the seitan: Place the oil in a large sauté pan over medium-high heat. Add the onion and cook for 2 minutes, stirring frequently. Add the garlic and cook for 1 minute, stirring frequently. Add the seitan and cook for 5 minutes, stirring frequently and adding a small amount of water, if necessary, to prevent sticking.

3. Add the tomatoes, tamari if using, rice vinegar, chili powder, chipotle chile powder, nutritional yeast, if using, salt, and black pepper and cook for 5 minutes, stirring frequently and adding a small amount of water, if necessary, to prevent sticking. Add the cilantro and mix well.

4. Scoop a little over ½ cup of the seitan mixture into each bell pepper half. Top with vegan cheese, if using, and bake for 5 minutes, or until the cheese melts, if using. Serve warm.

VARIATIONS

Ⓖ Replace the seitan with tempeh, tofu, or chopped Beyond Meat (see page 84).

◆ For an oil-free version, use the water sauté method (see page 101).

Take your dish in an Indian direction by replacing the chili powder with 1 tablespoon of curry powder and 2 teaspoons of ground cumin powder.

Nutrition Facts per serving (204 g): Calories 155, Fat Calories 35, Total Fat 4 g, Saturated Fat 1 g, Cholesterol 0 mg, Sodium 380 mg, Total Carb 12 g, Dietary Fiber 3 g, Sugars 7 g, Protein 19 g

Broccoli Rabe Penne Pasta with Oil-Free Cream Sauce ◆▯

YIELD: 6 CUPS PASTA AND SAUCE

Prep time: 15 minutes, Cook time: 15 minutes, Total time: 30 minutes, Serving size: 1 1/2 cups, Number of servings: 4

Broccoli rabe has smaller flowering heads (and a more pungent flavor) than broccoli, bright green tender leaves (which are eaten along with the heads), and the same cancer-fighting elements as the other cruciferous veggies. Popular in Italian cuisine, this vegetable gives a wholesome portion of our daily dose of vitamins A and C, and folate to this creamy pasta dish, which is even further accentuated by superpowered shiitakes. The sauce makes enough for 16 ounces of pasta, should you have a 16- instead of 12-ounce package. Enjoy as a part of hardy meal with Italian Spring Vegetable Soup (page 252) and Provençal Salad (page 183).

12 ounces dried penne pasta (try brown rice; see page 96)

¼ cup water

4 garlic cloves, pressed or minced

1 cup thinly sliced shiitake mushrooms

2 cups chopped broccoli rabe (½-inch pieces)

2 tablespoons chiffonaded fresh basil

SIMPLE VEGAN CREAM SAUCE

2 cups unsweetened soy, rice, coconut, or almond milk (for homemade, see Plant-Based Milk, page 104).

½ cup raw cashew pieces, optionally soaked in hot water to cover for 20 minutes, drained, and rinsed well

3 tablespoons nutritional yeast

¼ teaspoon sea salt, or to taste

¼ teaspoon freshly ground black pepper

¼ teaspoon crushed red pepper flakes

1. Bring a large pot of water to a boil over high heat. Add the pasta and cook according to the package instructions. Place in a large bowl.

2. Meanwhile, place the ¼ cup of water in a large sauté pan over medium-high

heat. Add the garlic and cook for 1 minute, stirring frequently. Add the shiitake mushrooms and cook for 2 minutes, stirring frequently and adding small amounts of water, if necessary, to prevent sticking. Add the broccoli rabe, lower the heat to low, and cook for 3 minutes, stirring occasionally and adding small amounts of water, if necessary, to prevent sticking.

3. Prepare the sauce: Place all the sauce ingredients in a strong blender and blend until creamy. Pour into the vegetable mixture.

4. Cook until the broccoli rabe is just tender, about 5 minutes, stirring occasionally. Transfer to the pasta, add the basil, and mix well before serving.

VARIATIONS

You can sauté the garlic and mushrooms in 1½ tablespoons of coconut oil for 2 minutes over medium-high heat, stirring constantly, before adding the remaining ingredients.

Top with 1 cup of grated vegan cheese before serving.

Add additional herbs, such as 2 tablespoons of chopped fresh flat-leaf parsley, ½ teaspoon of minced fresh rosemary, and ½ teaspoon of fresh thyme.

Replace the broccoli rabe with broccoli, cauliflower, bok choy, or your favorites.

Nutrition Facts per serving (345 g): Calories: 540, Fat Calories: 145, Total Fat 16 g, Saturated Fat 2 g, Cholesterol 0 mg, Sodium 210 mg, Total Carb 79 g, Dietary Fiber 7 g, Sugars 5 g, Protein 20 g

TEMPLATE RECIPE
Simple Vegan Cream Sauce

Plant-based milk component: Use different plant-based milks, such as soy, rice, hemp, almond, coconut, or quinoa (see page 104).

Nut component: Replace the cashews with macadamia nuts, hemp seeds, or pine nuts.

Optional herb component: Add 2 tablespoons of minced fresh basil, parsley, cilantro, or sorrel; or 1 tablespoon fresh dill.

Optional ethnic spice component: Add 1 tablespoon of Mexican Spice Mix (page 106), Indian Spice Mix (page 106), Italian Spice Mix (page 105), or Moroccan Spice Mix (page 106).

CHAPTER 16

Desserts and Sweet Snacks

Here is where we get our sweet on—and it is in fact possible to indulge in delectable goodness without all of the sugar we are accustomed to. Remember, not all sugars are created equal. The overconsumption of refined white sugar and high-fructose corn syrup is implicated in many behavior disorders, obesity, and other diseases, but there are many nonrefined, more natural options to provide sweetness, including syrups and coconut or date sugar, among others. Please see the chart on page 89 as a guide to some of the more whole food–based alternatives.

While the following desserts are a healthier choice compared to those loaded with animal fats, moderation is the key when dealing with treats made from concentrated sweeteners. The most healthful choice for a sweet treat is, of course, whole fresh fruit (including dates, which are nature's candy). Everyone loves a bowl of colorful, fresh, organic fruit. Those with blood sugar issues (see section on diabetes on page 6) will need to minimize and regulate all sugar intake, including that from fresh fruit, although berries can be a good choice as they are lower on the glycemic index and can actually help rebuild blood vessels.

This chapter will show you how to prepare delicious fruit-based desserts, such as Banana Mango Ice Cream (page 298) and Fruit-Sweetened Baked Pears (page 303), or other fruit-sweetened desserts, such as Fruit-Sweetened Black Bean Brownies (page 312) and Mixed Fruit Kanten (page 301). For raw foodies, a full contingent of raw food desserts includes Raw Carrot Ginger Cake (page 309), Choco-Chia Pudding (page 295), and Raw Hemp Energy Balls (page 298). For a healthy end to your holiday feasts, enjoy the Pumpkin Pudding (page 307) or Raw Apple Crumble (page 300).

As with the other sections, these recipes are either naturally oil-free or easily adaptable to become oil-free.

As you prepare the recipes, remember to enjoy a beverage from Chapter 10 while partaking of your dessert.

Superfood Trail Mix ♥ⓖ◊▱

YIELD: 2 CUPS TRAIL MIX

Prep time: 5 minutes, Total time: 5 minutes, Serving size: 2 tablespoons, Number of servings: 16

This combo creates a satisfying handful of nutrients that you can easily take on the go! In this superfood, low-sugar snack, you get the mood-lifting benefit of magnesium rich cacao, plus the ample protein, vitamins, minerals, and the hormone-supporting oil of pumpkin seeds. Sweet coconut adds extra brain power and stamina, and the exciting yet lesser-known goji berries and mulberries provide major fiber, antioxidants, flavonoids, and an array of extra phytonutrients. A perfect travel snack as well as a topping for Açai Power Bowl (page 120), Multigrain Grits (page 126), or Iron-Rich Morning Glory Steel-Cut Oats (page 127).

1 cup dried mulberries
1 cup raw pumpkin seeds
½ cup goji berries
¼ cup raw cacao nibs
¼ cup dried or shredded unsweetened coconut

1. Place all the ingredients in a bowl and mix well.

Nutrition Facts per serving (25 g): Calories 90, Fat Calories 70, Total Fat 8 g, Saturated Fat 3.5 g, Cholesterol 0 mg, Sodium 8 mg, Total Carb 5 g, Dietary Fiber 3 g, Sugars 1 g, Protein 4 g

---

TEMPLATE RECIPE
Superfood Trail Mix

- -

Dried fruit component: Replace the mulberries with golden berries, raisins, currants, or dried apricots.

Seed and nut component: Replace the pumpkin seeds with the seeds or nuts of your choosing, including pecans, almonds, cashews, or sunflower seeds.

Indulge and add vegan dark chocolate chips to your mix.

Choco-Chia Pudding ♥ⓖ◊

YIELD: 3 CUPS PUDDING

Prep time: 10 minutes, Soak time: 30 minutes, Total time: 30 minutes, Serving size: 1/2 cup, Number of servings: 6

Who knew that the chia pets of old featured what is now considered a superfood of the future. Chia pudding is a fun and delicious way to partake of the nutrient powers concentrated in this tiny seed of a desert plant. The seeds are supercharged with omega-3 fatty acids, carbs, protein, fiber, antioxidants, and calcium. The freshly made, creamy Brazil nut milk provides the trace minerals selenium, copper, and phosphorous, and the dates and cacao add a helping of fiber and magnesium for a low-glycemic and high-protein chocolate treat. Serve with fresh berries and Cashew Cream (page 297).

½ cup Brazil nuts
2 ½ cups water

3 pitted dates

3 tablespoons raw cacao powder

¼ cup raw coconut nectar (see page 89),
   raw agave nectar, or desired sweetener
   to taste

1 teaspoon pure vanilla extract

¼ teaspoon ground cinnamon

⅛ teaspoon ground nutmeg

Pinch of sea salt

½ cup chia seeds

Fresh fruit

1. Rinse and drain the Brazil nuts. Place in a strong blender with 1¼ cups of the water and blend until creamy. Add the remaining 1¼ cups of water and blend well. Pour through a fine strainer or sprout bag (see page 82). Save the pulp for use in homemade crackers (see page 139). Return the liquid to the blender.

2. Add the dates, cacao powder, coconut nectar, vanilla, cinnamon, nutmeg, and salt and blend well. Pour into a large bowl.

3. Add the chia seeds and stir well. Allow to sit on the counter or in the refrigerator for 30 minutes, stirring occasionally.

4. Transfer to parfait cups and top with fresh fruit before serving.

VARIATIONS

See the Chia Pudding Template Recipe on page 117.

Nutrition Facts per serving (55 g): Calories 215, Fat Calories 120, Total Fat 14 g, Saturated Fat 3 g, Cholesterol 0 mg, Sodium 30 mg, Total Carb 22 g, Dietary Fiber 10 g, Sugars 9 g, Protein 5 g

Raw Chocolate Pudding ♥ Ⓖ ◆

YIELD: 1 ½ CUPS PUDDING

Prep time: 25 minutes, Total time: 25 minutes, Serving size: 2 tablespoons, Number of servings: 6

Prepare to have your world rocked with three basic ingredients and a couple of pinches of spice, which create a rich and raw chocolate pudding. Cacao, the bean responsible for our beloved chocolate, comes from a small evergreen tree native to Mexico and South America and is known for its mood-enhancement properties and high antioxidant content. Almond butter and dates provide a perfect balance of nutrient impact and decadence that make this a great, easy, anytime dessert or snack. Top with fresh fruit and a dollop of Cashew Cream (page 297). Serve at the end of a raw feast, including Veggie Lettuce Boats (page 160) and Raw Coconut Curry Vegetables (page 268).

½ cup pitted dates (try Medjool)

1 cup water

¼ cup raw cacao powder

¼ cup raw almond butter

Pinch of ground cinnamon

Pinch of ground nutmeg

1. Place the dates and water in a bowl. Allow to sit for 20 minutes, and up to overnight.

2. Place all the ingredients, including the soak water, in a food processor and process until smooth.

For a frozen treat version, and an added crunch, soak ½ cup of raw buckwheat groats in water with ample room to cover for 30 minutes or longer, drain, and rinse well. Add to the above ingredients after processing and mix well. Place in the freezer to solidify.

Replace the dates with dried figs or apricots, and add additional sweetener to taste (see page 89).

Nutrition Facts per serving (26 g): Calories 110, Fat Calories 60, Total Fat 6.5 g, Saturated Fat 1 g, Cholesterol 0 mg, Sodium 2 mg, Total Carb 13 g, Dietary Fiber 3 g, Sugars 8 g, Protein 3 g

Strawberry Cashew Cream ♥☺◌

YIELD: 1 ½ CUPS CREAM

Prep time: 10 minutes, Soak time: 20 minutes, Total time: 30 minutes, Serving size: 2 tablespoons, Number of servings: 10

Cashews transform again, this time into a sweet cream in a delicacy that can be eaten alone or as a topping for other lovely dessert items. The health benefits of cashews are many. They supply iron, phosphorus, selenium, phytochemicals, antioxidants, and protein. This cream is sweetened with the addition of bonbon-sweet, nutrient-rich, energy-supplying dates. For a lighter color, replace the dates with raw coconut nectar or raw agave nectar. Use as a topping on fresh fruit or such desserts as Raw Carrot Ginger Cake (page 309), Fruit-Sweetened Baked Pears (page 303), or Mixed Fruit Kanten (page 301).

CASHEW CREAM
¾ cup raw cashew pieces
5 large pitted Medjool dates (see page 125)
½ teaspoon pure vanilla extract (optional)
Pinch of sea salt, or to taste
½ to ¾ cup water

1 cup chopped fresh strawberries
⅛ teaspoon ground cardamom

1. Prepare the Cashew Cream: Place the cashews in a bowl with ample water to cover. Allow to sit for at least 20 minutes, and up to a few hours. Rinse and drain well.

2. Place in a strong blender along with the dates, vanilla, if using, salt, and ½ cup of the water. Blend until very creamy, adding additional water, if necessary, to reach your desired consistency.

3. Add the strawberries and cardamom, and blend well.

VARIATIONS

Replace the dates with sweetener to taste, such as coconut nectar, raw agave nectar, xylitol, or pure maple syrup (see page 89).

Replace the strawberries with mango, blueberries, peach, or papaya.

Nutrition Facts per serving (47 g): Calories 130, Fat Calories 70, Total Fat 7.5 g, Saturated Fat 1.5 g, Cholesterol 0 mg, Sodium 17 mg, Total Carb 15 g, Dietary Fiber 2 g, Sugars 10 g, Protein 3 g

Banana Mango Ice Cream ♥🅖♦

YIELD: 3 CUPS ICE CREAM

Prep time: 10 minutes, Total time: 10 minutes + freeze time, Serving size: 1/2 cup, Number of servings: 6

Utilizing frozen bananas as a base for a vegan ice cream has made many a plant-based eater's life sweeter and creamier. Made with only natural fruit sugars, this ice cream is healthful enough to have for breakfast, supplying the day ahead with mega potassium, magnesium, and folate. In this recipe, mango is the flavor du jour, but experimenting with whatever fruits are handy or local is encouraged. This will only work in a strong blender or a gear juicer, such as a Champion. You may need to slightly thaw the bananas to get them to process. You can also use small amounts of a plant-based milk, such as almond or coconut (for homemade, see page 104) to reach the desired consistency. Serve on its own or on top of warmed Fruit-Sweetened Black Bean Brownies (page 312).

3 large peeled and chopped bananas (3 cups), frozen
1 cup chopped mango
1 teaspoon pure vanilla extract
Pinch of ground cinnamon
Pinch of ground nutmeg or cardamom

1. Place all the ingredients in a strong blender.

2. Starting on low speed, begin to blend. Increase the speed, and blend until pureed, using the tamper constantly to reach desired consistency.

VARIATIONS

Add ½ cup of strawberries, blueberries, raspberries, or blackberries.

Replace the mango with strawberry, papaya, blueberries, strawberries, jackfruit, or peaches.

Replace the mango with cherries, and add ½ cup of vegan chocolate chips or cacao nibs after pureeing.

Nutrition Facts per serving (96 g): Calories 80, Fat Calories 5, Total Fat 0 g, Saturated Fat 0 g, Cholesterol 0 mg, Sodium 1 mg, Total Carb 20 g, Dietary Fiber 2 g, Sugars 12 g, Protein 1 g

Raw Hemp Energy Balls ♥🅖♦▱

YIELD: 16 ENERGY BALLS

Prep time: 20 minutes, Total time: 20 minutes, Serving size: 1 tablespoon, Number of servings: 16

These versatile, wholesome, and travel-friendly fruit-sweetened bites get their punch from a plethora of stamina-supplying ingredients: almond, date, coconut, and hemp. Hemp seeds are rare in the plant kingdom for containing all essential amino acids, which makes for stellar fuel. Coconut's fat is a generous energy supplier that also has added immune supporting benefits.

1 cup raw almonds
⅔ cup pitted Medjool dates (see box, page 125)
¼ cup dried shredded unsweetened coconut
2 tablespoons raw almond butter (optional)
½ teaspoon ground cinnamon
½ teaspoon ground cardamom

Pinch of sea salt

¾ teaspoon culinary-grade rose water (optional)

⅓ cup raw cacao nibs

¼ cup hemp seeds

1. Place the almonds in a food processor and process until finely ground.

2. Add the dates, coconut, almond butter, if using, cinnamon, cardamom, salt, and rose water, if using, and process until smooth. Transfer to a bowl.

3. Add the cacao nibs and mix with your hands until evenly distributed. Form into sixteen small balls.

4. Place the hemp seeds in a small dish. Roll each ball in the hemp seeds until coated. Store in a glass jar in the refrigerator for up to a week.

Nutrition Facts per serving (24 g): Calories 115, Fat Calories 75, Total Fat 9 g, Saturated Fat 2 g, Cholesterol 0 mg, Sodium 13 mg, Total Carb 8 g, Dietary Fiber 3 g, Sugars 4 g, Protein 4 g

TEMPLATE RECIPE
Raw Energy Balls

Nut or seed component: Replace the almonds with pecans, pumpkin seeds, or sunflower seeds.

Superfood add-on component: Replace the cacao nibs with goji berries. Add ½ cup of sunflower seeds, pumpkin seeds, or raisins along with the cacao nibs.

Add 1 tablespoon of maca powder and/or spirulina.

Sweetener component: Replace the dates with dried figs, raisins, dried apricots, or your desired sweetener to taste (see page 89).

Nut butter component: Replace the almond butter with macadamia butter, cashew butter, or coconut butter.

Topping component: Replace the hemp seeds with sesame seeds or raw cacao powder.

Crunchy Chocolate Buckwheat Clusters ⑥ ◆

YIELD: 10 CLUSTERS

Prep time: 25 minutes, Cook time: 5 minutes, Chill time: 20 minutes, Total time: 50 minutes, Serving size: 2 tablespoons, Number of servings: 10

These chocolatey, almondy, chewy bites have a nice surprise crunch, courtesy of raw buckwheat groats. Buckwheat is a fully versatile seed that can be used sprouted, cooked, raw, or soaked, and is often found in the bulk bin. But the buck(wheat) doesn't stop there—in all forms, buckwheat groats are high in fiber, magnesium, copper, zinc, and manganese, and contain eight essential amino acids. Enjoy with a cup of Warming Herbal Chai (page 133).

½ cup raw buckwheat groats

½ cup vegan dark chocolate chips

3 tablespoons almond butter

¼ cup raisins

½ teaspoon pure vanilla extract

Pinch of ground cardamom

1. Place the buckwheat groats in a bowl with ample water to cover. Allow to sit for 20 minutes. Drain, rinse, and drain well. Return to the bowl.

2. Meanwhile, melt the chocolate chips in a double boiler (see Chef's Tips and Tricks). When melted, add to the buckwheat groats along with the remaining ingredients and mix well.

3. Form into ten small clusters, and place on a parchment paper–lined dish. Place in the refrigerator until cooled, about 20 minutes.

VARIATIONS

Replace the buckwheat groats with chopped nuts, such as almonds, walnuts, or pecans; or seeds, such as sunflower, pumpkin, sesame, or hemp.

Add additional sweetener to taste, depending on sweetness of the chocolate chips.

Nutrition Facts per serving (28 g): Calories 130, Fat Calories 55, Total Fat 6 g, Saturated Fat 2.5 g, Cholesterol 0 mg, Sodium 0 mg, Total Carb 17 g, Dietary Fiber 2 g, Sugars 9 g, Protein 3 g

Raw Apple Crumble ♥ ⓖ ♦

YIELD: 5 CUPS CRUMBLE

Prep time: 30 minutes, Total time: 30 minutes, Serving size: 1/2 cup, Number of servings: 10

There's some truth to the saying that an apple a day keeps the doctor away, mostly

because of the antioxidant flavonoids contained in the peel. Another important health component in apples is a special fiber called pectin, making for a unique fiber-plus-phytonutrient combination. This is a raw version of the commonly baked dessert, so you get all the health-boosting properties of the ingredients without having to turn on your oven (and a toothsome, crispy texture, to boot!). Raisins are energy boosters with all their natural sugar, not to mention iron and potassium. Walnuts are a favorite for their cancer-fighting, heart-healing, brain-boosting nutrients, and combining forces with dates, coconut, and spices, they create a perfect crumble topping for a healthy spin on this classic dessert. Enjoy this with a dollop of Strawberry Cashew Cream (page 297).

APPLE LAYER

4 cups unpeeled, cored and thinly sliced apple (about 3 apples)

1 cup raisins

½ cup pitted Medjool dates (see page 125)

½ cup water

¾ cup freshly squeezed apple or orange juice

¼ teaspoon orange zest

¼ teaspoon ground cinnamon

Pinch of ground nutmeg

Pinch of ground allspice

Pinch of sea salt

CRUMBLE

1 ¼ cups chopped walnuts

¼ cup pitted Medjool dates

2 tablespoons dried shredded unsweetened coconut

Pinch of ground cinnamon

Pinch of ground cardamom

1. Prepare the apple layer: Place the apples and raisins in a bowl.

2. Place the dates, water, apple juice, orange zest, cinnamon, nutmeg, allspice, and sea salt in a blender and blend until creamy. Add to the apple mixture and mix well. Transfer to an 8 by 8-inch casserole dish.

3. Prepare the crumble: Place all the ingredients in a food processor and pulse chop until the walnuts are finely ground. Do not overprocess. Sprinkle on top of apple layer.

VARIATIONS

Replace the apples with pears, peaches, or pineapple.

Replace the walnuts with hazelnuts, pistachio nuts, or sunflower seeds.

Replace the dates with dried figs or apricots.

Nutrition Facts per serving (122 g): Calories 250, Fat Calories 105, Total Fat 12 g, Saturated Fat 3 g, Cholesterol 0 mg, Sodium 19 mg, Total Carb 38 g, Dietary Fiber 5 g, Sugars 29 g, Protein 4 g

Mixed Fruit Kanten ⊙ ◆

YIELD: 5 CUPS KANTEN

Prep time: 5 minutes, Cook time: 15 minutes, Chill time: 40 minutes, Total time: 55 minutes, Serving size: 1/2 cup, Number of servings: 10

Bananas and blueberries strut their stuff in this kanten—"the Jell-O of Japan"—jelled with a type of seaweed called agar (or agar agar) in the United States. Bananas are well known to elevate energy and contribute to heart health, and they also provide a source of tryptophan, which regulates mood. Blueberries score a sky high antioxidant content, working to keep blood vessels strong and healthy. Adding the flavonoid antioxidant content of apple juice, this kanten contains a plethora of health-giving nutrients. Top with Cashew Cream (page 297) and additional fresh fruit.

4 cups apple juice

¼ cup plus 1 tablespoon agar flakes

1 cup sliced banana

1 cup fresh blueberries or pitted and chopped plums (½-inch pieces)

1 teaspoon pure vanilla extract

½ teaspoon orange zest (optional)

½ teaspoon ground cinnamon

⅛ teaspoon ground cardamom

Pinch of sea salt

1. Place a pot over high heat. Pour in the apple juice. Add the agar, whisk well, and bring to a boil.

Chef's Tips and Tricks

An Apple a Day

Did you know that there are more than 7,500 varieties of apples in the world? Some of the more popular and commonly available varieties are listed below. Be sure to purchase organically grown whenever possible, as apples have high pesticide residues if not grown organically (see page 61).

Gala—Crisp and mildly sweet with a thin skin. Eating or salad apple. Popular with kids. Originated in New Zealand.

Fuji—Firm, crisp, sweet. Eating, baking, or salad apple. Applesauce from a Fuji needs little or no sugar. Originated in Japan.

Pink Lady—Tart and tending toward more expensive, very pink/light green exterior. Likes to stay on the tree longer than any other apple!

Braeburn—Superfirm, tart, and sweet all in one, with yellow flesh. Eating, baking, sauce, or salads. Came from New Zealand.

Stayman Winesap—Sweet apple, good for everything.

Granny Smith—Very tart and crispy. Good for eating, baking, or salads. Originated in Australia.

Rome—Tart with a green/white inside. Best for sauce, baking, or freezing.

Jonagold—Sweet/tart combo. Great for baking, freezing, eating, salads, or applesauce. Originated in the USA.

McIntosh—Sweet and tart with a lot of juice. Good for eating, baking, apple sauce, or salads. Originated in the USA.

Red Delicious—Crunchy and mildly sweet with a yellow inside. Good eating apple and salad apple.

Golden Delicious—Crunchy and sweet. Related only in name to Red. Freezes well. Eating, baking, or salad apple, also used in applesauce.

Honeycrisp—Sweet, supercrisp, and tart. Great for eating, cooking, baking, salads, or applesauce. Originated in the USA.

At an apple a day, it would take over twenty years to sample all the different varieties. Better get started!

2. Lower the heat to medium and cook until the agar dissolves, about 5 minutes. Add the remaining ingredients and mix well.

3. Carefully transfer to an 8 by 8-inch casserole dish.

4. Place in the refrigerator and chill until just cool. Transfer to the freezer and allow to cool until firm enough to cut, about 40 minutes. If placing in the refrigerator, allow about 2 hours or more to set.

VARIATIONS

Experiment with different types of fruit juices and fresh and dried fruits.

Nutrition Facts per serving (143 g): Calories 100, Fat Calories 0, Total Fat 0 g, Saturated Fat 0 g, Cholesterol 0 mg, Sodium 26 mg, Total Carb 25 g, Dietary Fiber 2 g, Sugars 15 g, Protein less than 1 g

Fruit-Sweetened Baked Pears ⊖♦

YIELD: 3 STUFFED PEARS

Prep time: 10 minutes, Cook time: 30 minutes,
Total time: 40 minutes, Serving size: 1/2 pear,
Number of servings: 6

Exquisite pears are fiber-plentiful and also have the benefits of potassium and vitamins A, C, and K. This fruity baked treat additionally derives the nutritional benefits of three of nature's other varieties of candy: iron-rich and energy-lifting dates and raisins as well as vitamin C-famous oranges. If your pears are superfirm before baking, allow an extra 5 to 20 minutes to cook. Serve warm topped with vegan ice cream or coconut yogurt, and enjoy with a cup of warmed Brazil Nut Milk (page 104).

¼ cup pitted and chopped dates (try Medjool)
½ cup water
3 ripe pears
½ teaspoon orange zest
1 cup apple juice or freshly squeezed orange juice
1 teaspoon pure vanilla extract
½ teaspoon ground cinnamon
¼ teaspoon ground nutmeg
Pinch of sea salt
¼ cup chopped pecans or walnuts
¼ cup raisins
1 tablespoon dried shredded unsweetened coconut (optional)
Chiffonaded fresh mint

1. Preheat the oven to 400°F. Place the dates and water in a small bowl and allow to sit for 5 minutes.

2. Slice the pears in half lengthwise and scoop out the seeds with a tablespoon, leaving at least a tablespoon-size hole in each pear half. Place, scooped-out side up, in an 8 by 8-inch casserole dish.

3. Place the dates, their soak water, and the orange zest, apple juice, vanilla, cinnamon, nutmeg, and salt in a blender and blend until smooth. Pour over the pears.

4. Place in the oven and bake for 20 minutes, occasionally basting the pears with the sauce. Meanwhile, place the pecans, raisins, and coconut, if using, in a small bowl and mix well.

5. Remove the pears from the oven and place about 1 ½ tablespoons of the pecan mixture in the scooped-out hole in each pear.

6. Return to the oven and bake for an additional 10 minutes, or until the pears are just tender.

7. To serve, place the pears on individual plates and top with any remaining liquid from the casserole dish. Garnish with mint.

VARIATIONS

Replace the pears with apples.

Replace the raisins with dried currants. Replace the pecans with chopped walnuts, hazelnuts, macadamia nuts, or cashews.

For a lower-fat version, omit the nuts.

For a decadent version, top the pears with a teaspoon of vegan butter before baking.

Nutrition Facts per serving (158 g): Calories 150,
Fat Calories 30, Total Fat 3.5 g, Saturated Fat 0 g,
Cholesterol 0 mg, Sodium 27 mg, Total Carb 32 g,
Dietary Fiber 4 g, Sugars 23 g, Protein 3 g

QUICKER AND EASIER

Grilled Fruit

For a simple, sweet treat, try grilling fruit, such
as pineapple, peaches, or pears, to bring out
a deep and caramelized flavor. Grill until char
marks appear. Chop up and top with a dollop
of Cashew Cream (page 297) and a pinch each
of ground cinnamon and ground cardamom.

Chocolate Pecan Dipped Fruit ⊙ ◆

YIELD: 24 PIECES FRUIT

Prep time: 20 minutes, Cook time: 15 minutes,
Total time: 30 minutes, Serving size: 2 pieces fruit,
Number of servings: 12

For your next romantic evening, or when
you just have to have chocolate, look no further for a decadent dessert that satisfies the
sweet tooth while providing antioxidants as
well as all the nutrients found in fresh fruit.
These confections share the health benefits
of strawberries, a natural anti-inflammatory,
and bananas, yummy mineral suppliers. Adding to the richness are buttery pecans, with
their wealth of vitamin E and manganese.
The optional flavoring of chili powder makes
these an unusual, fun dessert to serve at the
end of a dinner party, where guests can create their own, following the variations below.

CHOCOLATE DIPPING SAUCE
¾ cup vegan dark chocolate chips
¼ teaspoon ground cinnamon

¼ teaspoon chili powder (optional)

PECAN COCONUT TOPPING
3 tablespoons finely chopped pecans
   (optionally toasted; see page 101)
3 tablespoons dried shredded unsweetened
   coconut (optionally toasted; see page 101)
⅛ teaspoon ground cardamom

FRUIT
2 bananas, cut into 1-inch slices (16 pieces)
8 strawberries

1. Begin the chocolate dipping sauce: Melt
   the chocolate in a double boiler. If no
   double boiler is available, place an inch
   of water in a small pot and bring to a
   boil. Lower the heat to medium. Place a
   dry metal or glass bowl on top of the pot
   and add the chips. Allow to heat until
   the chips are melted, about 10 minutes,
   depending upon the type of chips.

2. Meanwhile, prepare the topping: Combine all the topping ingredients in a
   small bowl and mix well.

3. When the chips are melted, remove the
   top pan of the double boiler or the bowl
   from the pot. Add the cinnamon and
   chile powder, if using, and stir well.

4. Dip the fruit: Using a fork, dip the bananas and strawberries in the chocolate, coating them well.

5. Liberally coat with the topping and
   place on a clean plate. Refrigerate until
   the chocolate is solid, about 15 minutes.

VARIATIONS

Feel free to dip other fruit. such as cherries, pineapple, and even candied ginger.

Expand your dippables into the decadent realm and dip pretzels, Almond Butter Chocolate Chip Cookie pieces (page 310), and Fruit-Sweetened Black Bean Brownie pieces (page 312).

Replace the pecans with cashews, macadamia nuts, hazelnuts, or sesame seeds.

Replace the vanilla extract with other flavored extracts, such as raspberry, hazelnut, almond, orange, or coffee.

Replace the chocolate chips with vegan carob chips.

Replace the chocolate chips with an equivalent amount of chopped-up vegan chocolate bar. Go crazy with the multitude of varieties of bars, each one creating a different dip.

Nutrition Facts per serving (45 g): Calories 110, Fat Calories 70, Total Fat 8 g, Saturated Fat 4 g, Cholesterol 0 mg, Sodium 0 mg, Total Carb 12 g, Dietary Fiber 3 g, Sugars 7 g, Protein 2 g

Cranberry Walnut Power Krispy Bars ⊙◦

YIELD: 10 KRISPY BARS

Prep time: 10 minutes, Chill time: 40 minutes, Total time: 50 minutes, Serving size: 1/4 cup, Number of servings: 10

Make your own energy bar and skip over the packaged ones at the supermarket—especially if you are spending time label-reading to determine if there are added sugars, salt, or oil. This bar is also another reason to bring out the cranberries outside of holiday seasons, and with good reason: they are an incredibly low-calorie superfood with a whopping content of vitamins C and E and phytonutrients. Their counterpart, walnuts, are a top-notch source of anti-inflammatory omega-3 fatty acids. Enjoy this sweet and tart bar as an afternoon snack while sipping some warm Gold Milk (page 144) or Sunrise Carrot Juice (page 137).

½ cup Date Syrup (page 88), coconut nectar, or agave nectar
½ cup creamy almond butter
2 ½ cups puffed brown rice cereal (not powdered or ground rice)
½ cup dried cranberries
¼ cup chopped walnuts
2 tablespoons hemp seeds (optional)
1 teaspoon pure vanilla extract
½ teaspoon ground cinnamon
¼ teaspoon ground nutmeg
Pinch of sea salt
Oil, for casserole dish (optional)

1. Place the date syrup and almond butter in a pan over medium heat. Cook for 3 minutes, stirring frequently. Add the remaining ingredients and stir well until evenly incorporated.

2. Transfer to a well-oiled or parchment paper–lined 8 by 8-inch casserole dish. Place in the refrigerator until solidified, about 30 minutes.

3. Cut into ten equal-size pieces and enjoy!

VARIATIONS

Replace the almond butter with peanut, cashew, or macadamia butter.

Replace the cranberries with vegan chocolate chips or other dried fruit, such as raisins, currants, chopped figs, or apricots.

Power it up with 1 tablespoon of maca powder and 1 tablespoon of spirulina powder.

Add an extra ¼ cup of chopped walnuts.

Replace the walnuts with other chopped nuts, such as hazelnuts or pistachios, or seeds, such as pumpkin or sunflower.

Nutrition Facts per serving (80 g): Calories 340, Fat Calories 95, Total Fat 11 g, Saturated Fat 1 g, Cholesterol 0 mg, Sodium 22 mg, Total Carb 54 g, Dietary Fiber 6 g, Sugars 3 g, Protein 8 g

Sweet and Spicy Baked Plantain◉

YIELD: 2 ½ CUPS PLANTAIN

Prep time: 5 minutes, Cook time: 30 minutes, Total time: 35 minutes, Serving size: 1/2 cup, Number of servings: 5

Starchy plantains are classified as vegetables, but when ripe with some black spots can be enticingly sweet. They pack in similar nutritional value to that of bananas and then some—containing more vitamins A, B$_6$, and C, and potassium. Spice up the sweetness with the capsicum-supplying heat of cayenne pepper, known for increasing circulation and metabolism. This and a cup of Maca Horchata (page 147) is a perfect way to finish off your Mexican meals.

Oil, for baking sheet
3 cups diagonally sliced ripe plantains
    (½-inch pieces; for more about plantains,
    see box on page 167)
1 tablespoon melted coconut oil
½ teaspoon ground cinnamon

¼ teaspoon ground nutmeg
⅛ teaspoon cayenne pepper, or to taste
Pinch of sea salt
Pinch of ground allspice
Pinch of ground mace (optional)

1. Preheat the oven to 400°F. Place all the ingredients on a well-oiled baking sheet and toss well.

2. Bake for 15 minutes and gently flip the plantains.

3. Return to the oven and bake for 15 minutes, or until golden brown.

VARIATIONS

Replace the plantains with just-ripe bananas.

Add ½ cup of coconut milk and/or 2 tablespoons of pure maple syrup, and toss well before baking.

◗ For an oil-free version, replace the coconut oil with coconut milk or soy milk and add a small amount of water to the baking dish before baking.

Nutrition Facts per serving (92 g): Calories 135, Fat Calories 30, Total Fat 3 g, Saturated Fat 2.5 g, Cholesterol 0 mg, Sodium 33 mg, Total Carb 29 g, Dietary Fiber 2 g, Sugars 13 g, Protein 1 g

QUICKER AND EASIER

Crazy Good Banana Chocolate Treat◗

Preheat the oven to 350°F. Slice a banana lengthwise, leave in its skin, place on a baking sheet or small casserole dish, and fill with vegan chocolate chips. Bake for 15 minutes and enjoy warm with vegan ice cream.

Pumpkin Pudding ⓖ ◗

YIELD: 4 ½ CUPS PUDDING

Prep time: 20 minutes, Cook time: 30 minutes,
Total time: 50 minutes, Serving size: 1/2 cup,
Number of servings: 9

Much more than a Halloween symbol, pumpkins are well worth bringing into the kitchen for this pudding or pie. Pumpkins provide generous quantities of vitamins, minerals, and fiber, as well as carotenoids, such as beta-carotene, which give the vibrant orange color and contribute a twinkle to our eyesight. The allspice that gives pumpkin pie its traditional flavor has benefits as well: used over time as an aid for various digestive ailments. Enjoy warm topped with Cashew Cream (page 297) and a cup of warm Choco-Maca Elixir (page 145).

2 (15-ounce) cans pure pumpkin puree, or
   3 cups cooked pumpkin
½ cup arrowroot powder or cornstarch
¼ cup almond butter
¼ cup soy or coconut milk
¼ cup pure maple syrup, coconut nectar, or
   Date Syrup (page 88), or to taste
1 teaspoon pure vanilla extract
¾ to 1 teaspoon ground cinnamon
¼ teaspoon ground nutmeg or cardamom
¼ teaspoon ground allspice
⅛ teaspoon sea salt (optional)
Pinch of ground cloves
Pinch of ground mace (optional)
Oil, for casserole dish (optional)

1. Preheat the oven to 375°F. Place all the ingredients, except the oil, in a food processor or strong blender and process until smooth.

2. Transfer to an 8 by 8-inch lightly oiled or nonstick casserole dish and bake for 30 minutes.

3. Remove from the oven and serve warm.

VARIATIONS

Add ½ cup of soaked and drained cashews. Place in the blender with the soy milk and maple syrup and blend until creamy.

For pumpkin pie, place in a 9-inch vegan piecrust (store-bought or see Breakfast Tart crust recipe on page 129) and bake for 50 minutes at 375°F. Allow to cool before slicing.

Replace the soy milk with rice milk, hemp milk, or almond milk (for homemade, see Plant-Based Milk, page 104).

Replace the pumpkin with cooked sweet potato or acorn squash.

Nutrition Facts per serving (125 g): Calories 130, Fat Calories 40, Total Fat 4 g, Saturated Fat 4 g, Cholesterol 0 mg, Sodium 9 mg, Total Carb 22 g, Dietary Fiber 4 g, Sugars 9 g, Protein 3 g

QUICKER AND EASIER

For a superquick and easy, sweet snack, place 1/4 cup of tahini, a pinch each of ground cinnamon and ground cardamom, and your desired sweetener to taste (see page 89) in a small bowl and stir well. You can add a couple of tablespoons of raisins or dried currants, if you wish. Tahini is one of my favorite foods, providing iron and unique lignans called sesamin and sesamol, which may assist in lowering cholesterol and promoting heart health. Its high levels of calcium and magnesium also contribute to bone health. Enjoy with a spoon!

Apricot Oat Bars◉♦

YIELD: 8 BARS

Prep time: 30 minutes, Cook time: 15 minutes,
Chill time: 60 minutes, Total time: 105 minutes,
Serving size: 1/2 cup, Number of servings: 8

Nuts and dried fruits are the name of the game for these bars, which profit from a hearty crust full of magnesium-rich almonds and soothing oats, famed for their cholesterol-lowering properties. Furthermore, "reconstituting" dried fruit results in a gooey topping chock-full of apricots' health-promoting phytochemicals and dates' famous digestion and mood-balancing qualities. Also doubles as a breakfast bar; enjoy with a cup of Digestive Tea (page 133).

TOPPING

1 cup chopped dried apricots (¼-inch pieces)
1 cup pitted and chopped dates (try Medjool)
1 ½ cups water
1 tablespoon freshly squeezed lemon juice
½ teaspoon lemon zest
½ teaspoon ground cinnamon
⅛ teaspoon ground cardamom
1 teaspoon pure vanilla extract
3 tablespoons dried shredded unsweetened coconut

CRUST

¾ cup raw almonds
¾ cup rolled oats (try gluten-free)
1 cup dried currants or raisins
¼ cup tightly packed pitted and chopped dates (try Medjool)
Pinch of ground cinnamon
Pinch of ground allspice
Pinch of ground mace (optional)
Oil, for casserole dish (optional)

1. Prepare the topping: Place all the topping ingredients, except the coconut, in a pan over medium heat. Cook for 15 minutes, or until the dates thoroughly break apart.

2. Meanwhile, prepare the crust: Place the almonds in a food processor and process until finely ground. Add the oats, currants, dates, cinnamon, allspice, and mace, if using, and process until ground.

3. Press the crust ingredients into a parchment paper–lined or lightly oiled 8 by 8-inch casserole dish, forming a ¼- to ½-inch-thick crust.

4. Pour the topping ingredients on top of the crust, creating an even layer. Top with the coconut. Place in the refrigerator until the topping solidifies enough to cut into bars, about 30 minutes.

5. Enjoy chilled or slightly warmed in the oven.

VARIATIONS

♥ For a raw version, soak the dates and apricots in water until soft, then blend in a strong blender along with other topping ingredients.

Replace the apricots with other fruit, such as blueberries, bananas, figs, or mango.

Nutrition Facts per serving (78 g): Calories 280, Fat Calories 90, Total Fat 10 g, Saturated Fat 4 g, Cholesterol 0 mg, Sodium 25 mg, Total Carb 47 g, Dietary Fiber 6 g, Sugars 35 g, Protein 5 g

Raw Carrot Ginger Cake ♥ ◆

YIELD: 8 SERVINGS

Prep time: 35 minutes, Setting in freezer: 4 hours,
Total time: 4 hours 35 minutes, Serving size: about
2 by 4 inches, Number of servings: 8

For a twist on traditional carrot cake, try this
no-bake version where the "flour" consists of
ground buckwheat and hazelnuts, and the
cake is placed in the freezer instead of the
oven to set. Hazelnuts, a lesser-used nut also
known as filberts, provide an earthy flavor with
a hefty protein, fiber, and healthy fat content.
They are also the tree nut with the highest
folate and proanthocyanidin (condensed tannins and sturdy antioxidants) content. Not to
mention, you also get the beta-carotene that
can't be beat in carrots. Break out this recipe
for your next raw birthday party and top it off
with a glass of Brazil Nut Milk (page 104).

CASHEW CREAM FROSTING

⅔ cup raw cashew pieces

¼ cup water

1 tablespoon raw agave nectar, coconut
   nectar, or Date Syrup (page 88)

Pinch of ground cardamom

RAW CARROT GINGER CAKE

1 cup raw buckwheat groats

½ cup pitted and chopped dates (try
   Medjool)

½ cup plus 2 tablespoons water

½ cup hazelnuts

1 cup peeled and diced carrot

1 teaspoon peeled and minced fresh ginger

1 teaspoon orange zest (optional)

¼ teaspoon ground cinnamon

¼ teaspoon ground allspice

Pinch of sea salt

1. Prepare the frosting: Place the cashews
   in a bowl with ample water to cover.
   Allow to sit for 20 minutes, or up to
   3 hours. Rinse and drain well. Transfer
   to a blender with the 2 tablespoons of
   fresh water, agave nectar, and cardamom, and blend until creamy. Depending upon the strength of your blender,
   you may need to add slightly more water to reach your desired consistency.
   Set aside.

2. Meanwhile, prepare the cake: Place the
   buckwheat groats in a bowl with ample
   water to cover. Allow to sit for 30 minutes, up to 2 hours.

3. Place the dates in a bowl with ½ cup
   plus 2 tablespoons of water. Allow to sit
   for 15 minutes.

4. Drain the buckwheat groats, rinse, and
   drain well. Transfer to a food processor
   with the remaining cake ingredients,
   including the dates and the date soak
   water, and process until well pureed.
   Transfer to a small loaf pan (8 ½ by
   4 ½ by 2 ⅝ inches) or a similarly sized
   baking dish, and spread out evenly.

5. Top with the frosting and spread out
   evenly.

6. Place in the freezer until the frosting
   solidifies, about 4 hours. If you over-
   freeze, allow to defrost before slicing.
   Can be stored in the refrigerator.

VARIATIONS

Replace the hazelnuts with almonds, pecans, or walnuts.

Replace the dates with raisins, dried apricots, or dried figs.

Nutrition Facts per serving (74 g): Calories 290, Fat Calories 180, Total Fat 20 g, Saturated Fat 2.5 g, Cholesterol 0 mg, Sodium 33 mg, Total Carb 25 g, Dietary Fiber 4 g, Sugars 16 g, Protein 7 g

TEMPLATE RECIPE
Simple Cookie Recipe

Flour component: Replace the spelt flour with whole wheat pastry flour.

Oil component: Replace the banana with applesauce, coconut, or safflower or sunflower oil.

Nut butter component: Replace the almond butter with another nut butter, such as cashew butter, or peanut butter or tahini.

Chip or add-on component: replace the chocolate chips with vegan carob chips, raisins, dried currants, nuts, or seeds.

Almond Butter Chocolate Chip Cookies ⊙ ◆

YIELD: 16 COOKIES

Prep time: 10 minutes, Cook time: 15 minutes, Total time: 25 minutes, Serving size: 1 cookie, Number of servings: 16

Indulge your sweet tooth with these rich and nutty cookies that surprise with a burst of chocolate goodness. These treats benefit from the richness of almond butter: heart-healthy, wholesome, and filling, with vast quantities of vitamin E, protein, and omega-3 fatty acids. Almond butter can help lower bad cholesterol and maintain blood sugar as well. Spelt flour, containing gluten, is often more easily digestible than wheat. Another bonus is that spelt flour is richer in protein and minerals than wheat flour, making for a healthier cookie. Enjoy with a cup of Sesame Hemp Revitalizer (page 146) or Gold Milk (page 144).

DRY

½ cup vegan dark chocolate chips
¼ cup spelt flour
¼ cup rolled oats (try gluten-free)
3 tablespoons dried shredded unsweetened coconut
1 teaspoon baking powder
⅛ teaspoon sea salt (optional)
⅛ teaspoon ground cardamom

WET

1 cup almond butter
¼ cup mashed banana
¼ cup finely chopped dates
1 tablespoon chia seeds mixed with 3 tablespoons water
1 teaspoon pure vanilla extract

1. Preheat the oven to 350°F. Combine the dry ingredients in a bowl and whisk well.

2. Combine the wet ingredients in another bowl and mix well. Add the wet to dry and mix well.

3. Use a heaping tablespoon to form eighteen cookies and place them on a parchment paper–lined baking sheet. Bake for 12 to 15 minutes.

4. Allow to cool slightly before transferring to a plate or cooling rack.

G For gluten free, use the Gluten-Free Flour Mix (page 105) and certified gluten-free rolled oats.

Nutrition Facts per serving (50 g): Calories 150, Fat Calories 85, Total Fat 9.5 g, Saturated Fat 1 g, Cholesterol 0 mg, Sodium 117 mg, Total Carb 13 g, Dietary Fiber 3 g, Sugars 2 g, Protein 5 g

Fruit-Sweetened Pistachio Peach Cobbler **G** ◆ ▱

YIELD: 3 ½ CUPS COBBLER

Prep time: 10 minutes, Cook time: 45 minute, Total time: 55 minutes, Serving size: 1/2 cup, Number of servings: 6

If you are on an "only fruit sugar" plan, here is the dessert that satisfies in the sweet department, thanks to its behind-the-scenes date content blended in. Front and center are peaches: the fuzzy fruit that is native to parts of China. Besides sweetness, peaches offer portions of your daily vitamin A and C intake. Pistachios, originally from the Middle East, are a rich gourmet treat on their own, but here they form a unique crust that also adds protein, potassium, and vitamins A and B$_6$ to this cobbler. Enjoy with a tall glass of Basil Rosemary Lemonade (page 141) on a hot summer's day.

FILLING

1 tablespoon freshly squeezed lemon juice
⅓ cup pitted and chopped dates (try Medjool)
1 tablespoon arrowroot
1 cup water or fruit juice, such as apple, peach, or pineapple

1 teaspoon pure vanilla extract
¼ teaspoon ground cinnamon
⅛ teaspoon ground nutmeg
Pinch of ground mace (optional)
Pinch of sea salt
4 cups sliced fresh peaches, or 2 (10-ounce) bags frozen
Oil for casserole dish (optional)

TOPPING

¾ cup roasted unsalted pistachio nuts
¾ cup rolled oats (try gluten-free)
⅛ teaspoon ground cinnamon
Pinch of ground nutmeg
Pinch of sea salt
¼ cup applesauce or coconut oil

1. Prepare the filling: Preheat the oven to 350°F. Place all the filling ingredients, except the peaches and oil, in a blender and blend until creamy. Transfer to a lightly oiled or nonstick 8 by 8-inch casserole dish, add the peaches, and mix well.

2. Prepare the topping: Place the pistachio nuts in a food processor and process until finely chopped. Add the oats, cinnamon, nutmeg, and salt and process until the oats are slightly chopped, about 30 seconds, being careful not to overprocess. Transfer to a bowl with the applesauce and mix well. Distribute the topping evenly over the filling.

3. Bake for 45 minutes, or until the top is golden brown. Serve warm.

VARIATIONS

Go decadent by replacing the applesauce with vegan butter.

G For a gluten-free version, use certified gluten-free rolled oats.

Nutrition Facts per serving (133 g): Calories 195, Fat Calories 60, Total Fat 7 g, Saturated Fat 1 g, Cholesterol 0 mg, Sodium 40 mg, Total Carb 31 g, Dietary Fiber 5 g, Sugars 16 g, Protein 6 g

TEMPLATE RECIPE
Fruit Cobbler

Topping component: Replace the pistachios with nuts or seeds of your choosing, such as pecans, macadamia nuts, walnuts, sunflower seeds, pumpkin seeds, or hemp seeds.

Filling component: Replace the peaches with any fruit of your choosing, such as apples, pineapple, mangoes, pears, nectarines, or plums.

Sweetener component: Replace the dates with your desired sweetener of choice (see page 89).

Fruit-Sweetened Black Bean Brownies **G** ◆

YIELD: MAKES 12 BROWNIES

Prep time: 15 minutes, Cook time: 45 minutes, Total time: 60 minutes, Serving size: about 2 1/2 by 2 inches, Number of servings: 12

The secret ingredient in this recipe is low-calorie, fiber- and protein-rich black beans, making these brownies into a fudgy healthy temptation. They are naturally sweetened with dates, which add additional fiber as well as significant potassium. The chocolate fix comes from cocoa powder, which contains endorphin and serotonin boosters for mood as well as heart-healthy flavonoids. Our egg replacer is in the form of ground flaxseeds or chia seeds, rich in the omegas, which form a gel when soaked in water. Serve warm topped with a scoop of vegan ice cream or Cashew Cream (page 297).

¼ cup water
2 tablespoons ground flaxseeds or chia seeds
1 (15-ounce) can black beans, drained and rinsed well, or 1 ½ cups cooked (see page 98)
1 cup soy, rice, or almond milk (for homemade, see Plant-Based Milk, page 104)
½ cup mashed banana
¾ cup tightly packed pitted and chopped Medjool dates (see page 125)
½ cup unsweetened cocoa powder
1 cup rolled oats
½ cup almond flour or flour of choice
2 teaspoons pure vanilla extract
¼ teaspoon ground cinnamon
⅛ teaspoon ground nutmeg
Pinch of sea salt

1. Preheat the oven to 375°F. Place the water in a small bowl. Add the ground flaxseeds and mix well. Allow to sit until a gel forms, about 15 minutes, stirring occasionally.

2. Meanwhile, place the black beans in a food processor with the soy milk, banana, dates, and cocoa powder and process until pureed. Transfer to a bowl.

3. Place ½ cup of the oats in a strong blender and blend until well ground. Transfer to the black bean mixture.

4. Add the remaining ½ cup of oats, almond flour, vanilla, cinnamon, nutmeg, and salt and mix well. Add the soaked flaxseeds and mix well.

5. Pour the mixture into a parchment paper–lined 8 by 8-inch casserole dish and bake for 45 minutes. Allow to cool before slicing.

VARIATIONS

Go for it and add 1 cup of vegan dark chocolate chips to the batter. Mix well before transferring to the baking dish.

Really boost the chocolate flavor by adding 2 tablespoons of brewed espresso and 1 teaspoon of coffee extract along with the soy milk.

For a sweeter brownie, replace all or some of the dates with Sucanat, or your sweetener of choice (see page 89).

Replace the banana with coconut oil or vegan butter.

For a nuttier brownie, remove from the oven after 25 minutes. Top with ½ cup of chopped walnuts or pecans, return to the oven, and bake for an additional 20 minutes.

Ⓖ For gluten-free, use the Gluten-Free Flour Mix (page 105) and certified gluten-free rolled oats.

Nutrition Facts per serving (90 g): Calories 175, Fat Calories 40, Total Fat 5 g, Saturated Fat 1 g, Cholesterol 0 mg, Sodium 21 mg, Total Carb 30 g, Dietary Fiber 7 g, Sugars 11 g, Protein 7 g

Vegan Fusion

Vegan Fusion is a style of cuisine that celebrates the culinary contributions from around the world. This means that I often combine ingredients from different ethnic foods in the same dish or menu. Vegan Fusion cuisine also represents a return to the natural methods of growing food and utilizes organic ingredients whenever possible. Organic food is grown without the use of chemical fertilizers and pesticides, most of which have not been fully tested for their long-term effects on humans. For maximum food safety, go organic. Please see page 60 for more information on organics.

I also recommend using a minimum of processed and packaged ingredients. This is much better for your health and is the environmentally sustainable way to go. Also, eating locally grown foods whenever possible ensures optimal flavor and freshness and conserves resources. Growing foods in your own garden or participating in community-supported agriculture programs (CSAs) are the best way to go if you have the opportunity. It's quite fulfilling to see something grow from seed to plant. Farmers' markets, where you can meet the people growing your food, are the next best choice. Stock up on what is fresh and in season. Using a Template Recipe format (see page 93), many of the recipes in *Healing the Vegan Way* can be adapted to include whatever ingredients are available.

Peace Begins in the Kitchen

I believe that the time we spend preparing food can be a calming and healing experience for us. Do what you can to create a clean and peaceful environment. Play your favorite music, decorate the table with flowers, and let your creative juices flow. Use your time in the kitchen as an opportunity to cultivate mindfulness and gratitude. Leave your cares at the door, and focus on the present moment experience of preparing the food. Notice the colors, textures, and aromas of the ingredients. Think lovingly of the people for whom you will be preparing the food. They will notice it!

Remember that food is art. The plate is your canvas and nature provides all of the colors, textures, and flavors for you to create your culinary masterpiece. Have fun with it!

Want to Know More?

Our company, Vegan Fusion, promotes the benefits of plant-based cuisine for our health, the preservation of our planet, and a more peaceful world. In addition to our award-winning cookbooks, we offer workshops, chef trainings and immersions (see page 356), vegan chef certifications, the Doctor and the Chef wellness programs (www.doctorandchef.com), and vegan culinary retreats around the world. We also offer consulting services, and can assist in menu and recipe development with this innovative global cuisine. For inspiration surrounding the vegan lifestyle, to check out our online culinary course, and to sign up for our free online newsletter, please visit our website, www.veganfusion.com.

The Three Doors and the Why Factor

Typically when you ask people why they went vegan, they give answers that can fit into one or more of three general categories: (1) health or medical, (2) environmental or political, or (3) ethical or spiritual. These three categories are all like doors leading into the same room. You may have entered the room through one door, but once you are in the room, you meet people who have entered through other doors, and you can each embrace one another's motivations for living a plant-based lifestyle.

Most people enter through the first door, and the vast majority of the information in this book addresses this topic and the multitude of the health benefits of a plant-based lifestyle. In this section, I would like to explain briefly the other two doors. I personally entered through the third door, due to my connection to and love for animals. At the time I became vegetarian, I was not aware of the health benefits or the environmental benefits of a plant-based diet. Over time I became educated on those topics and that has fortified my convictions.

Door #2 Why Vegan for the Earth?

I feel that a vegan diet is the future of food, and is the key to a sustainable future for humanity. *Vegan* describes a diet and lifestyle that does not include the use or consumption of any animal-based products, including dairy or eggs. Vegans also avoid wearing fur, leather, and silk, and products tested on animals. The phrase *plant-based* is often used instead of the word *vegan*.

Eating vegan foods happens to be one of the most effective steps we can take to protect the environment. The environmental footprint of a vegan diet is a fraction of that of a meat-based diet. It takes 16 pounds of grain and 2,500 gallons of water to produce 1 pound of beef. It's astonishing to realize this, when we see so much in the news about food and water shortages and people going to bed hungry. Vegan foods represent the best use of the earth's limited resources.

We must use the resources of our planet wisely if we are to survive. World scientists agree that climate change poses a serious risk to humanity, and to life as we know it. The key to reducing global warming is to reduce activities that produce the greenhouse gases that cause the Earth's temperature to rise. According to a 2006 report by the UN's Food and Agriculture Organization titled "Livestock's Long Shadow," raising livestock for food consumption is responsible for 18 percent of all greenhouse gases emitted—more than the entire world's transportation industry combined.

Not convinced? Consider these figures:

- The livestock population of the United States consumes enough grain and soybeans each year to feed over five times the human population of the country. Animals are fed over 80 percent of the corn and 95 percent of the oats that are grown on our soil.

- According to the USDA, 1 acre of land can produce 20,000 pounds of vegetables. This same amount of land can only produce 165 pounds of meat.
- It takes 16 pounds of grain to produce 1 pound of meat.
- It requires 3 ½ acres of land per person to support a meat-centered diet, 1 ½ acres of land to support a lacto-ovo vegetarian diet, and ⅙ of an acre of land to support a plant-based diet.
- If Americans were to reduce meat consumption by just 10 percent, it would free up 12 million tons of grain annually.
- Half of the water used in the United States goes to irrigate land growing feed and fodder for livestock. It takes about 2,500 gallons of water to produce a single pound of meat. Similarly, it takes about 4,000 gallons of water to provide a day's worth of food per person for a meat-centered diet, 1,200 gallons for a lacto-ovo vegetarian diet, and 300 gallons for a plant-based diet.
- Developing nations use land to raise beef for wealthier nations instead of utilizing that land locally for sustainable agriculture practices.
- Topsoil is the dark, rich soil that supplies the nutrients to the food we grow. It takes five hundred years to produce an inch of topsoil. This topsoil is rapidly vanishing, due to clear cutting of forests and cattle-grazing practices.
- For each acre of forestland cleared for human purposes, 7 acres of forest is cleared for grazing livestock or growing livestock feed. This includes federal land that is leased for cattle-grazing purposes. This policy greatly accelerates the destruction of our precious forests.
- To support cattle grazing, South and Central America are destroying their rainforests. These rainforests contain close to half of all the species on Earth and numerous medicinal plants. Over a thousand species a year are becoming extinct and most of these are from rainforest and tropical settings. This practice also causes the displacement of indigenous peoples who have been living in these environments for countless generations.
- The factory farm industry is one of the largest polluters of our ground water, due to the chemicals, pesticides, and run-off waste that is inherent in its practices.
- Over 60 million people die of starvation every year. This means that we are feeding grain to animals while our fellow humans are dying of starvation in mind-staggering numbers.

When you look at the disproportionate amount of land, water, and resources it takes to support a meat-based diet, it makes a lot of sense for us to introduce more plant-based foods into our way of life. Whether by going completely vegan or simply including more vegan meals each week, every little bit helps.

Much of this environmental information is provided from the landmark book *Diet for a New America*, written by John

Robbins, a pioneer in the promotion of the health and environmental benefits of a plant-based lifestyle. Robbins founded EarthSave International to educate, inspire, and empower people around the world. He is also the author of *The Food Revolution* and his latest book, *No Happy Cows*.

Door #3: Choosing to Be Kind

Many people adopt a vegan diet out of a commitment toward nonviolence. For them, we are meant to be stewards and caretakers of the Earth and its inhabitants and do not wish to support practices that inflict suffering on any creature that has the capacity to feel pain.

The small family farm where husbandry practices engendered a certain respect for the animals that were used for food is becoming a thing of the past. Today, most of the world's meat, dairy, and egg production occur on massive factory farms that are owned by agribusiness conglomerates. This has brought about practices that view the raising and transportation of farm animals solely in terms of their ability to generate profits.

Animals are routinely given chemicals and antibiotics to keep them alive in these conditions. To increase the weight of cows, many are fed sawdust, plastic, tallow, grease, and cement dust seasoned with artificial flavors and aromas. Mother pigs on factory farms are kept in crates that are so small they are unable to turn around. Dairy cows are forced to remain pregnant most of their lives and are injected with hormones to increase milk production for human consumption.

To sum it up, choosing to eat plant-based foods is a triple win: it's good for the environment, good for the animals, and good for you.

Metric Conversions Chart

The recipes in this book have not been tested with metric measurements, so some variations might occur.

Remember that the weight of dry ingredients varies according to the volume or density factor: 1 cup of flour weighs far less than 1 cup of sugar, and 1 tablespoon doesn't necessarily hold 3 teaspoons.

Oven Temperature Equivalents,
Fahrenheit (F) and Celsius (C)

100°F = 38°C
200°F = 95°C
250°F = 120°C
300°F = 150°C
350°F = 180°C
400°F = 205°C
450°F = 230°C

General Formulas for Metric Conversion

Ounces to grams → ounces × 28.35 = grams
Grams to ounces → grams × 0.035 = ounces
Pounds to grams → pounds × 453.5 = grams
Pounds to kilograms → pounds × 0.45 = kilograms
Cups to liters → cups × 0.24 = liters
Fahrenheit to Celsius → (°F − 32) × 5 ÷ 9 = °C
Celsius to Fahrenheit → (°C × 9) ÷ 5 + 32 = °F

Weight (Mass) Measurements

1 ounce = 30 grams
2 ounces = 55 grams
3 ounces = 85 grams
4 ounces = ¼ pound = 125 grams
8 ounces = ½ pound = 240 grams
12 ounces = ¾ pound = 375 grams
16 ounces = 1 pound = 454 grams

Volume (Liquid) Measurements

1 teaspoon = ⅙ fluid ounce = 5 milliliters
1 tablespoon = ½ fluid ounce = 15 milliliters
2 tablespoons = 1 fluid ounce = 30 milliliters
¼ cup = 2 fluid ounces = 60 milliliters
⅓ cup = 2 ⅔ fluid ounces = 79 milliliters
½ cup = 4 fluid ounces = 118 milliliters
1 cup or ½ pint = 8 fluid ounces = 250 milliliters
2 cups or 1 pint = 16 fluid ounces = 500 milliliters
4 cups or 1 quart = 32 fluid ounces = 1,000 milliliters
1 gallon = 4 liters

Volume (Dry) Measurements

¼ teaspoon = 1 milliliter
½ teaspoon = 2 milliliters
¾ teaspoon = 4 milliliters
1 teaspoon = 5 milliliters
1 tablespoon = 15 milliliters
¼ cup = 59 milliliters
⅓ cup = 79 milliliters
½ cup = 118 milliliters
⅔ cup = 158 milliliters
¾ cup = 177 milliliters
1 cup = 225 milliliters
4 cups or 1 quart = 1 liter
½ gallon = 2 liters
1 gallon = 4 liters

Linear Measurements

½ inch = 1½ cm
1 inch = 2½ cm
6 inches = 15 cm
8 inches = 20 cm
10 inches = 25 cm
12 inches = 30 cm
20 inches = 50 cm

Comprehensive Nutrient Reference Guide

The following chart illustrates the macro and micronutrients needed for optimal health, as well as their plant sources. Please refer to this frequently on your journey of healing the vegan way!

Chapter 1 showed how plant foods have the power to combat common diseases and chronic conditions. The nutrients in plants directly affect your overall wellness by fulfilling their important biochemical roles to ensure that your body systems function optimally. The body has an amazing capacity to adapt and compensate for a lack of nutrients for a period of time, and many people are living in this compensatory state simply because they are not eating enough pure whole foods. Whether you have a diagnosis or are looking for ways to support your body's regular functioning, this chart is meant to help highlight specific foods that can provide direct support to certain body systems, either during a healing phase or as a preventative practice in keeping the body in optimal shape from the inside out!

Nutrition Chart

Nutrients	How Does It Work?	Plant Sources
BLOOD AND CIRCULATORY SYSTEM		
Vitamin K (phylloquinone and menaquinones)	Vitamin K is found in the blood and along vessel walls and is crucial for blood coagulation as a cofactor to several vitamin K–dependent clotting factors.	Spinach, kale, collards, lettuce, parsley, cabbage, broccoli, Brussels sprouts, soybeans, grapes, berries
Magnesium	Magnesium is involved in the regulation of blood clotting by balancing the effect of calcium, which promotes the formation of clots. The ratio of magnesium to calcium is very important for this reason. Magnesium also relaxes arterial smooth muscle, helping to regulate blood pressure and decrease strain on the heart.	Dark leafy greens, pumpkin seeds, almonds, sunflower seeds, sesame seeds, black beans, quinoa, Brazil nuts, cashews, soybeans, avocado, bananas, chocolate
Vitamin B_9 (folate)	Folate creates and maintains red blood cells, preventing anemia.	Lentils, pinto beans, collard greens, chickpeas, asparagus, spinach, black beans, broccoli, cauliflower, parsley, beets
Vitamin C (ascorbic acid)	Vitamin C increases the absorption of iron, which is important in manufacturing hemoglobin, the molecule in red blood cells that carries oxygen.	Citrus fruits, papaya, Brussels sprouts, pineapple, peppers, tomatoes, broccoli, spinach, greens, cauliflower, strawberries

Nutrients	How Does It Work?	Plant Sources
Vitamin E (tocopherol)	Tocopherol helps form red blood cells and also acts as a blood thinner.	Sunflower seeds, almonds, vegetable oils, greens, olives, avocado, peanuts, asparagus
Copper	Copper is a mineral that helps prevent anemia as a cofactor to the enzyme involved in the body's storage and absorption of iron.	Sesame seeds, cashews, soybeans, shiitake mushrooms, sunflower seeds, tempeh, chickpeas, lentils, walnuts
Iron	Iron manufactures hemoglobin, which helps red blood cells carry oxygen throughout the body.	Dark leafy greens, prunes, raisins, dates, beans, lentils, chickpeas, soybeans, artichokes, pumpkin seeds, chocolate, thyme, blackstrap molasses, apricots, potatoes, quinoa, tempeh, tofu, tahini, broccoli
Calcium	Calcium helps keep the smooth muscles that line your blood vessels toned so as to move blood through the body.	Kale, broccoli, spinach, fortified cereals and plant-based milks, seaweeds, pistachios, sesame seeds, almonds, beans, and tofu
Allicin	Allicin in garlic can reduce atherosclerosis, or fatty deposits in the arteries, as an antioxidant as well as by modifying lipoproteins. It is also known to decrease blood pressure.	Garlic
Isoflavones (genistein and daidzein)	Isoflavones reduce blood pressure and increase vessel dilation.	Soybeans
Lutein	Lutein supports blood vessels by inhibiting lipid peroxidation, a likely factor in the etiology of cardiovascular disease.	Kale, spinach, other greens, peas, corn
Zeaxanthin	Zeaxanthin, like lutein, may prevent athero-sclerosis of carotid arteries by inhibiting LDL-induced migration of monocytes to artery cell walls.	Green vegetables, citrus
Rutin	Rutin helps strengthen capillary walls if they become weakened, potentially useful for varicose veins, hemorrhoids, and preventing heart attacks and strokes.	Kasha, black tea, apple peels, onion, citrus
Selenium	Selenium is known to increase blood flow, which in turn can help to improve blood pressure, hasten wound healing, and enhance natural defense against disease.	Brazil nuts, sunflower seeds, mushrooms, asparagus, tofu

Nutrients	How Does It Work?	Plant Sources
Chlorophyll	Chlorophyll is very similar in structure to human blood cells. It provides a source of magnesium, and supports healthy circulation, helping to bring oxygen to tissues.	Parsley, green leafy vegetables, sea vegetables, spirulina, basil, broccoli
Sodium	Sodium in the blood helps the body regulate blood pressure, volume, and fluid balance. This is important in electrolyte balance for preventing dehydration and hypotension. Sodium is also important for proper muscle and nerve function, including heart and blood vessel muscles.	Beets, celery, carrots, spinach, chard, most fruits
Phytosterols	Phytosterols are plant compounds similar in structure to cholesterol, well documented to lower LDL cholesterol and triglycerides.	Vegetable oils, beans, nuts, some fruits and veggies
Protein	Albumins and globulins, protein molecules in the blood, are critical factors in maintaining the proper fluid balance between cells and extracellular space. This balances fluid in the body to prevent edema.	Nuts, flaxseeds, beans, brown rice, tofu, tempeh, miso, soy milk, brewer's yeast, quinoa, amaranth, chlorella, spirulina, sprouted seeds
Potassium	Potassium is an electrolyte needed to help keep water balanced between cells and body fluids. It is needed in proper proportion to sodium levels to regulate blood pressure.	White beans, leafy greens, baked potato, apricots, squash, avocado, mushrooms, bananas, sweet potato, soybeans, lentils
Omega-3 fatty acids	Omega-3s reduce inflammation throughout the body, also reducing damage to your blood vessels to potentially prevent heart disease. In addition, they have been shown to decrease triglycerides, lower blood pressure, reduce blood clotting, decrease stroke and heart failure risk, and reduce irregular heartbeats.	Walnuts, flaxseeds, olive oil, chia seeds
Omega-6 fatty acids	Omega-6s help relax smooth muscles, improving blood flow and lowering blood pressure.	Sunflower oil, corn oil, soybean oil, avocado oil, walnuts, Brazil nuts, sesame seeds, pumpkin seeds
Vitamin D (calciferol)	Recent studies show that vitamin D may lower blood pressure by causing blood vessels to relax, allowing for more and easier blood flow.	Vitamin D is manufactured by exposure to sunlight, but is also found in store-bought fortified plant-based milks and orange juice.

Nutrients	How Does It Work?	Plant Sources
BONES AND TEETH		
Omega-3 fatty acids	Linoleic acid and alpha-linolenic acid can help increase bone formation and reduce bone resorption by lowering inflammatory prostaglandins.	Walnuts, flaxseeds, olive oil, chia seeds, hemp seeds
Vitamin C (ascorbic acid)	Vitamin C is needed for the formation and activation of collagen, which holds cells together. It is necessary for the health of connective tissues, such as cartilage, dentin for tooth enamel, gum tissue, skin, and bones.	Citrus fruits, papaya, Brussels sprouts, pineapple, peppers, tomatoes, broccoli, spinach, greens, cauliflower, strawberries
Vitamin K (phylloquinone and menaquinones)	Vitamin K builds strong bones and supports bone density by making a protein called osteocalcin, which binds calcium.	Spinach, kale, collards, lettuce, parsley, cabbage, broccoli, Brussels sprouts, soybeans, grapes, berries
Calcium	Calcium is stored in the structures of bones and teeth, essential to their strength by adding hardness to the bone matrix.	Kale, broccoli, spinach, fortified cereals and plant-based milks, seaweeds, pistachios, sesame seeds, almonds, beans, tofu
Iodine	Iodine is essential to thyroid health; indirectly implicated in bone health caused by hyperthyroidism.	Sea vegetables such as kelp, arame, dulse, and nori; iodized salt, strawberries, cranberries, navy beans, potatoes
Manganese	Manganese is an important cofactor to the enzymes required for the formation of healthy cartilage and bones.	Hazelnuts, pumpkin seeds, whole wheat, tofu, spinach, kale, black tea, cloves, oats, chickpeas, brown rice, pineapple
Phosphorus	Phosphorus is concentrated in bones and teeth, working closely with calcium to form and maintain healthy teeth and bones as well as adding rigidity.	Pumpkin seeds, sunflower seeds, Brazil nuts, tofu, lentils, peanuts, whole wheat, corn, broccoli, garlic
Isoflavones (genistein and daidzein)	Isoflavones may offer protection against osteoporosis by improving bone mineral density.	Soybeans
Vitamin D (calciferol)	Adequate vitamin D is essential for directing calcium to bones and teeth, rather than being absorbed into the blood.	Vitamin D is manufactured by exposure to sunlight, but is also found in store-bought fortified plant-based milks and orange juice.

Nutrients	How Does It Work?	Plant Sources

BRAIN—MENTAL AND COGNITIVE

Nutrients	How Does It Work?	Plant Sources
Omega-3 fatty acids	Omega-3s may slow mental decline and stabilize mood. DHA is found in nerve tissue, and is therefore potentially linked to prevention of both dementia and depression.	Walnuts, flaxseeds, olive oil, chia seeds, hemp seeds
Omega-6 fatty acids	Omega-6s are important for brain growth and development. They also support brain function by helping with transmission of nerve impulses.	Sunflower oil, corn oil, soybean oil, avocado oil, walnuts, Brazil nuts, sesame seeds, pumpkin seeds
Essential amino acids	Certain amino acids—namely trytophan, phenylalamine, and threonine—boost memory and learning, enhance mood, and counter depression as precursors to serotonin.	Nuts, flaxseeds, beans, brown rice, tofu, tempeh, miso, soy milk, brewer's yeast, quinoa, amaranth, chlorella, spirulina, sprouted seeds
Vitamin B_1 (thiamine)	Thiamine's key role in brain health is in central nervous system energy production, helping the body's cells to convert carbs into energy for the brain. Alcohol can interfere with its intestinal absorption, which can lead to a type of encephalopathy and psychosis seen in alcoholics. Along with other B vitamins, Vitamin B_1 is important to replace after indulging in alcohol.	Very small amounts are in virtually all foods. Good sources are sunflower seeds, flaxseeds, asparagus, black beans, green peas, split peas, barley, lentils, oats, lima beans, brown rice, soybeans, pistachio, peanuts, Brazil nuts, pecans, raisins, blackstrap molasses.
Vitamin B_5 (pantothenic acid)	B_5 helps the central nervous system communicate with the brain. It is known as an antistress vitamin because it provides energy and has positive effects on mood and brain function.	Avocado, whole grains, legumes, broccoli, molasses, mushrooms, corn
Phenylethylamine	Phenylethylamine is a brain chemical known to increase alertness and concentration. It stimulates the actions of dopamine (well-being and feeling pleasure), norepinephrine (wakefulness and higher performance), acetylcholine (for memory and mental activity), and serotonin (for better mood emotion and impulse control).	Cacao, soy, lentils, peanuts, almonds, chickpeas, flaxseeds, sesame seeds, walnuts
Selenium	Selenium has been associated with improved mood and lowered risk of depression, perhaps because of its essential role in regulating thyroid hormone.	Brazil nuts, sunflower seeds, mushrooms, asparagus, tofu

Nutrients	How Does It Work?	Plant Sources
DETOXIFICATION—LIVER AND KIDNEYS		
Molybdenum	Molybdenum, a trace mineral, produces enzymes that facilitate phase 2 detoxification in the liver.	Kidney and navy beans, lentils, split peas, cereals, leafy vegetables, oats
Sulfur	Sulfur compounds provide protection from environmental threats and help rid the body of toxins and heavy metals. They are important in forming glutathione, a major detoxifying agent and powerful antioxidant.	Nuts, flaxseeds, sunflower seeds, durian fruit, garlic, onions, asparagus, cabbage, Brussels sprouts, broccoli, kale, turnips
Isothiocyanates	A group of highly bioavailable sulfur-containing compounds that contain phytochemicals that neutralize toxins and may prevent cancers by promoting the elimination of certain carcinogens.	Broccoli, cauliflower, kale, Brussels sprouts, cabbage, watercress
Chlorophyll	Binding of chlorophyll may interfere with the gastrointestinal absorption of potential carcinogens, reducing the amount that reaches susceptible tissues. Chlorophyll also stimulates one of the liver's important detoxification pathways.	Parsley, green leafy vegetables, sea vegetables, spirulina, basil, broccoli
Eugenol	Eugenol is the chemical component responsible for cloves' powerful effects and potent scent. It is known traditionally as a blood purifier for its antimicrobial action. Research has repeatedly shown that eugenol-containing plants are effective at establishing an environment that is unfriendly to harmful organisms.	Cloves, basil, cinnamon, oregano, nutmeg, turmeric
DIGESTIVE		
Fiber	Fiber is a polysaccharide, made of sugar units bonded together in such a way that they pass through to the large intestine intact, rather than being broken down and digested. This structure is important in helping to speed digestive transit times, promoting the removal of toxins and wastes from the body.	Beans, lentils, whole grains, brown rice, artichokes, corn, nuts, potato, berries, oatmeal, avocado, chia seeds, flaxseeds, broccoli, cabbage, apples, Brussels sprouts
Essential amino acids	Amino acids produce gastric enzymes in the body, promoting proper digestion and optimizing absorption of nutrients.	Nuts, flaxseeds, beans, brown rice, tofu, tempeh, miso, soy milk, brewer's yeast, quinoa, amaranth, chlorella, spirulina, sprouted seeds
Vitamin B$_3$ (niacin)	Niacin has shown to help with digestive disturbances, such as IBS, potentially by helping to increase stomach acid in cases of hypochlorhydria, which causes bloating and pain.	Cremini mushrooms, lentils, tomatoes, bell peppers, sweet potatoes, peas, peanuts, beans, fortified cereals, beets, sunflower seeds, asparagus

Nutrients	How Does It Work?	Plant Sources
Chromium	Chromium regulates the metabolism of glucose, lowering blood sugar, helping with proper carbohydrate digestion and energy usage. It is said to also help curb sugar cravings.	Broccoli, oats, grapes, whole grains, mushrooms, tomatoes, asparagus, green beans, potatoes, bananas, molasses
Chlorophyll	Chlorophyll is detoxifying and also provides a source of magnesium, which helps prevent constipation.	Parsley, green leafy vegetables, sea vegetables, spirulina, basil, broccoli
"Vitamin U"	Vitamin U is another name for the compound S-methylmethionine. It is not a true vitamin, but was given the name "U" for its role in speeding the healing of peptic ulcers. It seems to have overall protective effects in the gastrointestinal mucosa and in the liver.	Cabbage, especially as juice

ENDOCRINE/HORMONAL

Nutrients	How Does It Work?	Plant Sources
Fiber	Fiber helps maintain steady glucose levels, providing more sustained energy, slowing blood sugar spikes, and reducing diabetes risk.	Beans, lentils, whole grains, brown rice, artichokes, corn, nuts, potato, berries, oatmeal, avocado, chia seeds, flaxseeds, broccoli, cabbage, apples, Brussels sprouts
Vitamin D (calciferol)	Calciferol has been shown to reduce the risk of diabetes and slow its progression, potentially by keeping pancreatic beta cells that produce insulin around longer and also helping tissues to be more sensitive to insulin.	Vitamin D is manufactured by exposure to sunlight, but is also found in store-bought fortified plant-based milks and orange juice
Manganese	Manganese is needed for insulin response and helps the body regulate blood sugar.	Hazelnuts, pumpkin seeds, whole wheat, tofu, spinach, kale, black tea, cloves, oats, chickpeas, brown rice, pineapple
Essential amino acids	Amino acids are the building blocks of all hormones in the body.	Nuts, flaxseeds, beans, brown rice, tofu, tempeh, miso, soy milk, brewer's yeast, quinoa, amaranth, chlorella, spirulina, sprouted seeds
Vitamin B_2 (riboflavin)	Riboflavin supports the function of the adrenal glands, small glands that produce hormones you can't live without (including sex hormones and cortisol, involved in stress management).	Cremini mushrooms, asparagus, broccoli, spinach, greens, buckwheat, fortified cereals, soybeans, almonds

Nutrients	How Does It Work?	Plant Sources
EYE HEALTH		
Vitamin A	Vitamin A prevents eye problems and enhances vision through its action with rods and cones in the retina.	Dark orange vegetables, such as carrot, pumpkin, squash, and sweet potato; green leafy vegetables, such as kale, collards, bok choy, and spinach; orange fruits, such as melon, peach, papaya, and mango; red pepper; fortified cereals
Vitamin B$_3$ (niacin)	Niacin contributes to maintenance of healthy eyes by helping to maintain the health of small blood vessels, such as those in the eye.	Cremini mushrooms, lentils, tomatoes, bell peppers, sweet potatoes, peas, peanuts, beans, fortified cereals, beets, sunflower seeds, asparagus
Vitamin E (tocopherol)	Vitamin E contributes to eyes by protecting the retina from oxygen generated damage.	Sunflower seeds, almonds, vegetable oils, greens, olives, avocado, peanuts, asparagus
Zinc	Zinc is required for healthy vison. It regulates the release of vitamin A from the liver to facilitate the protective action of retinol.	Sesame seeds, pumpkin seeds, lentils, chickpeas, cashews, quinoa, almonds, peanuts, fortified cereals
Beta-carotene	Beta-carotene is the carotenoid precursor to vitamin A that protects eyes from cataract formation and other eye problems.	Broccoli, sweet potato, pumpkin, carrots, apricots, asparagus, grapefruit
Lutein	Lutein supports the health of the retinas. It is thought to function as a light filter, protecting the eye tissues from sunlight damage.	Kale, spinach, other greens, peas, corn
Zeaxanthin	Zeaxanthin protects and improves vision as a strong antioxidant along with lutein.	Green vegetables, citrus
HEART HEALTH		
Omega-3 fatty acids	Omega-3 fats are the precursors for anti-inflammatory molecules, important in balancing the heightened inflammatory state responsible for many diseased states, particularly atherosclerosis.	Walnuts, flaxseeds, olive oil, chia seeds, hemp seeds
Fiber	Fiber binds with cholesterol from the diet to help the body process and excrete it. Many studies have shown swift reductions in cholesterol with increased dietary soluble fibers.	Beans, lentils, whole grains, brown rice, artichokes, corn, nuts, potato, berries, oatmeal, avocado, chia seeds, flaxseeds, broccoli, cabbage, apples, Brussels sprouts

Nutrients	How Does It Work?	Plant Sources
Vitamin B$_3$ (niacin)	Niacin helps the body to process cholesterol and lowers lipoprotein (a), a significant risk factor in cardiovascular disease.	Cremini mushrooms, lentils, tomatoes, bell peppers, sweet potatoes, peas, peanuts, beans, fortified cereals, beets, sunflower seeds, asparagus
Vitamin B$_5$ (pantothenic acid)	Pantothenic acid helps the body balance its lipid profile by helping to increase HDL and to inhibit platelet aggregation, which can lead to clots.	Avocado, whole grains, legumes, broccoli, molasses, mushrooms, corn
Selenium	Selenium is a strong antioxidant that protects endothelial cells of the arteries against oxidative damage. It has been used in the treatment of cardiomyopathy.	Brazil nuts, sunflower seeds, mushrooms, asparagus, tofu
Allicin	Allicin can reduce atherosclerosis, or fatty deposits in the arteries, and normalizes lipoprotein balance.	Garlic
Phytosterols	Phytosterols lower LDL cholesterol and triglycerides by interfering with their absorption in the GI tract.	Vegetable oils, beans, nuts, whole grains, some fruits and veggies
Quercetin	Quercetin is a flavonoid antioxidant that appears to protect against the damage caused by LDL (bad) cholesterol, reduce arterial plaque buildup, and lower blood pressure.	Citrus, apples, onions, parsley, sage, buckwheat

IMMUNE SYSTEM

Nutrients	How Does It Work?	Plant Sources
Lycopene	Lycopene as a phytochemical seems to stimulate the immune system, slow the rate at which cancer cells grow, and prevent damage to DNA.	Tomato, watermelon, papaya, pink grapefruit, red carrot
Isoflavones (genistein and daidzein)	Isoflavones are a type of phytoestrogen, called selective estrogen receptor modulators (SERMS) in that they can modulate the effects of excess estrogen by binding to some of the same receptors as the hormone estrogen. Drugs used to treat breast cancer and osteoporosis are pharmaceutical-strength SERMS.	Soybeans
Isothiocyanates	Isothiocyanates are sulfur-containing elements that may prevent cancers by their toxin-neutralizing actions.	Broccoli, cauliflower, kale, Brussels sprouts, cabbage, watercress
Phytosterols	Phytosterols are known to halt the growth and spread of cancer cells.	Vegetable oils, beans, nuts, some fruits and veggies
Lignans	Lignans are phytoestrogens found inside seeds and several other plants, which may have a role in preventing hormone-associated cancers.	Flaxseeds, sesame seeds, soybeans, broccoli, cabbage, apricots, strawberries

Nutrients	How Does It Work?	Plant Sources
Lentinan	Now being used intravenously to treat malignant tumors and HIV, lentinan has been shown in lab research to reduce the growth of some cancer cells and even induce cancer cell death. The mushroom polysaccharide is also known to increase the activity of immune cells, such as T-cells, cytokines, monocytes, and tumor necrosis factor. It is showing promise in treating bacterial and viral infections.	Shiitake mushrooms
Vitamin C (ascorbic acid)	Vitamin C helps prevent and reduce the duration of colds and flu by directly stimulating cells' immune responses and increasing white blood cell activity.	Citrus fruits, papaya, Brussels sprouts, pineapple, peppers, tomatoes, broccoli, spinach, greens, cauliflower, strawberries
Omega-3 fatty acids	Omega-3 polyunsaturated fatty acids are important in steering anti-inflammatory pathways by reducing pro-inflammatory cytokines. This action also reduces anxiety and helps improve stress responses, further preventing both acute and chronic illness. Recent studies showed benefit in treating flu specifically by potentially shutting down viral replication at the cellular level.	Walnuts, flaxseeds, olive oil, chia seeds, hemp seeds
Allicin	Long known for its strong antibacterial, antifungal, antiviral, and antiparasitic activity, allicin has also been observed to inhibit the proliferation of human tumor cells and to interact with T-cells to down-regulate inflammatory reactions, such as those associated with autoimmunity and allergy.	Garlic
Zinc	Essential to keeping immune system function in balance, preventing immune overstimulation, which creates chronic inflammatory conditions that have been linked to degenerative disease processes.	Sesame seeds, pumpkin seeds, lentils, chickpeas, cashews, quinoa, almonds, peanuts, fortified cereals

METABOLIC–ENERGY PRODUCTION/CELL STRUCTURE AND FUNCTION

Carbohydrate	Carbohydrate is the primary source of quick and sustained fuel for cells.	Whole grains, vegetables, fruits, beans
Protein	After carbohydrate, protein is a backup source of fuel for the body. It also plays a role in the transport of oxygen in the body, essential for energy.	Nuts, flaxseeds, beans, brown rice, tofu, tempeh, miso, soy milk, brewer's yeast, quinoa, amaranth, chlorella, spirulina, sprouted seeds

Nutrients	How Does It Work?	Plant Sources
Vitamin B_1 (thiamine)	Thiamine helps the body's cells convert carbohydrates into energy. It creates the chemical that all cells use for energy, adenosine triphosphate (ATP).	Very small amounts are in virtually all foods. Good sources are sunflower seeds, flaxseeds, asparagus black beans, green peas, split peas, barley, lentils, oats, lima beans, brown rice, soybeans, pistachio, peanuts, Brazil nuts, pecans, raisins, blackstrap molasses.
Vitamin B_2 (riboflavin)	Riboflavin has a major role in energy production as a coenzyme component in glucose metabolism, corticosteroid production, and thyroid enzyme regulation.	Cremini mushrooms, asparagus, broccoli, spinach, greens, buckwheat, fortified cereals, soybeans, almonds
Vitamin B_3 (niacin)	Niacin transmits dietary carbohydrates into energy. It serves as a coenzyme for several major biochemical reactions, including detoxifying alcohol and utilizing carbohydrates, fats, and proteins, as well as in the synthesis of fatty acids.	Cremini mushrooms, lentils, tomatoes, bell peppers, sweet potatoes, peas, peanuts, beans, fortified cereals, beets, sunflower seeds, asparagus
Vitamin B_5 (pantothenic acid)	Pantothenic acid is essential for the synthesis and metabolism of protein and carbohydrates, which are the body's major energy sources. Its active form, coenzyme A, is involved in the Krebs cycle production of ATP, and is required for the health of the adrenal glands. It is also needed in the transmission of nerve impulses and the synthesis of hemoglobin.	Avocado, whole grains, legumes, broccoli, molasses, mushrooms, corn
Vitamin B_6 (pyridoxine)	B_6 breaks down proteins and sugars for the body and provides energy. It is also needed for protection of nerve fibers and required in the synthesis of neurotransmitters serotonin, norepinephrine, and histamine. It is a coenzyme in several processes, such as the formation of niacin from tryptophan, synthesis of intrinsic factor to absorb B_{12}, and formation of hemoglobin.	Spinach, bok choy, cabbage, peppers, garlic, cauliflower, potatoes, sweet potatoes, bananas, squash, broccoli, Brussels sprouts, greens, carrots
Vitamin B_9 (folate)	Folate converts food into energy and is essential for the formation and maturation of red and white blood cells. It is important in cell nuclear morphology, and therefore protective to tissues with rapidly multiplying cells, such as those of the stomach, intestines, vagina, and cervix.	Lentils, pinto beans, collard greens, chickpeas, asparagus, spinach, black beans, broccoli, cauliflower, parsley, beets
Vitamin B_{12} (Cobalamin)	B_{12} is needed as an essential cofactor in the synthesis of DNA. It is also involved in carbohydrate metabolism and prevention of neurological problems, because the nervous system is reliant on carbohydrates for fuel.	Fortified plant-based milks and cereals, nutritional yeast

Nutrients	How Does It Work?	Plant Sources
Chromium	Chromium helps to regulate levels of blood sugar, by aiding insulin monitor levels of carbohydrates, fats, and protein and turn them into energy.	Broccoli, oats, grapes, whole grains, mushrooms, tomatoes, asparagus, green beans, potatoes, bananas, molasses
Iodine	Iodine helps the body regulate energy production. It is necessary in the synthesis of thyroid hormone.	Sea vegetables such as kelp, arame, dulse, and nori, iodized salt, strawberries, cranberries, navy beans, potatoes
Magnesium	Magnesium creates energy and manufactures protein in the body. It works synergistically with B6 in biochemical pathways for prostaglandin and ATP production and is needed in high amounts for nerve impulse transmission.	Dark leafy greens, pumpkin seeds, almonds, sunflower seeds, sesame seeds, black beans, quinoa, Brazil nuts, cashews, soybeans, avocado, bananas, chocolate
Phosphorus	Phosphorus helps the body produce energy as a component of pathways that produce ATP.	Pumpkin seeds, sunflower seeds, Brazil nuts, tofu, lentils, peanuts, whole wheat, corn, broccoli, garlic
Potassium	Potassium is essential for the storage of glycogen in muscles, preventing cramping and spasms. It is part of the sodium potassium pump that regulates nerve and muscle cell function as well as acid/base balance.	White beans, leafy greens, baked potato, apricots, squash, avocado, mushrooms, bananas, sweet potato, soybeans, lentils.
Zinc	Zinc aids in protein and carbohydrate metabolism. It is concentrated in both red and white blood cells and stored in muscle, spleen, bone marrow, and liver.	Sesame seeds, pumpkin seeds, lentils, chickpeas, cashews, quinoa, almonds, peanuts, fortified cereals
Aspargine	Aspargine increases stamina and helps with resistance to fatigue.	Asparagus, potatoes, nuts, seeds, soy, whole grains
Carbohydrate	Carbohydrate is the primary source of quick and sustained fuel for cells. Complex carbohydrates offer sustained energy and avoid the peaks and valleys in energy from simple carbs.	Almost all plants have some amount of carbohydrate. This includes grains, beans, fruits, vegetables, nuts, and seeds.
Fiber	Fiber helps the body absorb carbohydrates more slowly, sustaining energy.	All plant foods contain some amount of fiber. Vegetables, fruits, whole grains, and beans have more concentrated amounts.
Protein	Protein regulates the release of energy in the body. Some proteins are enzymes, which are crucial in certain biochemical actions, such as the digestion of carbohydrates or the synthesis of cholesterol by the liver. Some proteins are hormones, created in one organ and essential to carry messages to other organs for proper functioning.	Almost all plants have some amount of protein. Concentrated sources include beans, nuts, and seeds.

COMPREHENSIVE NUTRIENT REFERENCE GUIDE

Nutrients	How Does It Work?	Plant Sources
Iron	Iron manufactures hemoglobin, which helps red blood cells carry oxygen throughout the body.	Dark leafy greens, prunes, raisins, dates, beans, lentils, chickpeas, soybeans, artichokes, pumpkin seeds, chocolate, thyme, blackstrap molasses, apricots, potatoes, quinoa, tempeh, tofu, tahini, broccoli
Vitamin A	Vitamin A contributes to the development and growth of cells through its effect on protein synthesis as well as cell differentiation.	Dark orange vegetables, such as carrot, pumpkin, squash, and sweet potato; green leafy vegetables, such as kale, collards, bok choy, and spinach; orange fruits, such as melon, peach, papaya, and mango; red pepper; fortified cereals

HAIR AND NAILS

Nutrients	How Does It Work?	Plant Sources
Essential amino acids	Amino acids are essential for nail repair as the basis for the proteins keratin and collagen.	Nuts, flaxseeds, beans, brown rice, tofu, tempeh, miso, soy milk, brewer's yeast, quinoa, amaranth, chlorella, spirulina, sprouted seeds
Vitamin B_3 (niacin)	Niacin dilates blood vessels, allowing for better circulation of blood to nourish your scalp and hair follicles.	Cremini mushrooms, lentils, tomatoes, bell peppers, sweet potatoes, peas, peanuts, beans, fortified cereals, beets, sunflower seeds, asparagus
Iodine	Iodine's importance in thyroid function makes it essential for hair and nail health, since the thyroid is responsible for tissue growth and its deficiency can lead to brittle, dry nails and loss of hair.	Sea vegetables. such as kelp, arame, dulse, and nori; iodized salt, strawberries, cranberries, navy beans, potatoes
Sulfur	Sulfur aids in the production of collagen for skin, nail, and hair health.	Nuts, flaxseeds, sunflower seeds, durian fruit, garlic, onions, asparagus, cabbage, Brussels sprouts, broccoli, kale, turnips

IMMUNE FUNCTION

Nutrients	How Does It Work?	Plant Sources
Protein	Proteins make up the structure of antibodies, a necessary part of the body's immune responses and essential amino acids, which are precursors to histamine, a compound that's involved in local immune responses.	Nuts, flaxseeds, beans, brown rice, tofu, tempeh, miso, soy milk, brewer's yeast, quinoa, amaranth, chlorella, spirulina, sprouted seeds

Nutrients	How Does It Work?	Plant Sources
Vitamin A	Vitamin A enhances immunity, especially against acute viral infections by increasing T lymphocytes and helping to maintain the integrity of mucous membranes to guard against pathogens. It contains carotenoids, which color orange and red foods and have proven helpful in the prevention and adjunctive treatment of cancers.	Dark orange vegetables, such as carrot, pumpkin, squash, and sweet potato; green leafy vegetables, such as kale, collards, bok choy, and spinach; orange fruits, such as melon, peach, papaya, and mango; red pepper; fortified cereals
Vitamin D (calciferol)	Calciferol regulates the immune system, making it important in preventing autoimmune conditions by direct communication with immune cells.	Vitamin D is manufactured by exposure to sunlight, but is also found in store-bought fortified plant-based milks and orange juice.
Vitamin E (tocopherol)	Vitamin E contributes to robust immunity and helps protect cells from free radicals.	Sunflower seeds, almonds, vegetable oils, greens, olives, avocado, peanuts, asparagus
Copper	Copper is important in immune function by its role in the regulation of neutrophils (white blood cells), its potent antioxidant properties, and its role in mobilizing iron from the liver. It is important to have a healthy ratio of copper to zinc for optimal immunity benefit.	Sesame seeds, cashews, soybeans, shiitake mushrooms, sunflower seeds, tempeh, chickpeas, lentils, walnuts
Iron	Iron helps the body monitor temperature and bolsters the immune system.	Dark leafy greens, prunes, raisins, dates, beans, lentils, chickpeas, soybeans, artichokes, pumpkin seeds, chocolate, thyme, blackstrap molasses, apricots, potatoes, quinoa, tempeh, tofu, tahini, broccoli
Zinc	Zinc helps optimize T-cell functions and support the thymus gland in its immune activity. It is well known for its role in treating acute viral infections as well as allergies and pharyngitis. Zinc sensitizes tissues to thyroid hormone and helps release vitamin A from the liver.	Sesame seeds, pumpkin seeds, lentils, chickpeas, cashews, quinoa, almonds, peanuts, fortified cereals
Rosmarinic acid	Rosmarinic acid has antioxidant, anti-inflammatory, and antimicrobial activities. It helps prevent cell damage caused by free radicals, said to reduce the risk for cancer and atherosclerosis. It is the phytochemical in certain plants historically used to treat peptic ulcers, arthritis, cataract, cancer, rheumatoid arthritis, and asthma.	Basil, rosemary, oregano, sage, thyme, mint

Nutrients	How Does It Work?	Plant Sources

Nutrients	How Does It Work?	Plant Sources
Omega-3 fatty acids	Omega-3s are important in all of the anti-inflammatory actions of the immune pathway. They work in balance with omega-6 healthy fats to ensure a balanced immune system.	Walnuts, flaxseeds, olive oil, chia seeds, hemp seeds
Omega-6 fatty acids	Omega-6s are important in the pro-inflammatory pathway in helping the immune system to respond appropriately. A healthy ratio of omega-6s to omega-3s helps keep the immune system in balance.	Sunflower oil, corn oil, soybean oil, avocado oil, walnuts, Brazil nuts, sesame seeds, pumpkin seeds
Allicin	Allicin is a sulfur compound known for its ability to reduce the secretion of inflammatory factors so as to reduce pain and curb infections.	Garlic
Quercetin	Quercetin prevents immune cells from releasing histamines, which are chemicals that cause allergic reactions. Therefore quercetin may help reduce symptoms of allergies, including runny nose, watery eyes, hives, and swelling of the face and lips.	Citrus, apples, onions, parsley, sage, buckwheat, berries, green tea
Bromelain	Bromelain is an enzyme that reduces joint pain and inflammation. It has a powerful effect in reducing swelling from injury as well as allergy/sinus infections.	Pineapple
Eugenol	Eugenol is a plant sterol oil that provides potent anti-inflammatory action.	Cloves, basil, cinnamon, oregano, nutmeg, turmeric
Lignan	Lignans provide healthy polyunsaturated essential fatty acids that help regulate immune responses and balance inflammatory pathways.	Flaxseeds, sesame seeds, soybeans, broccoli, cabbage, apricots, strawberries

REPRODUCTIVE/ SEXUAL

Nutrients	How Does It Work?	Plant Sources
Isoflavones (genistein and daidzein)	Isoflavones offer protection from both menopausal symptoms and osteoporosis by helping to modulate estrogen as natural SERMS (selective estrogen receptor modulators).	Soybeans
Folate	Folate is most important during rapid cell division during pregnancy. Folate also prevents damage to DNA.	Lentils, pinto beans, collard greens, chickpeas, asparagus, spinach, black beans, broccoli, cauliflower, parsley, beets
Vitamin D (calciferol)	Adequate vitamin D is necessary to help the body create sex hormones. It also plays a role in ovulation and proper hormonal balance, helping with symptoms of both PMS and menopause.	Vitamin D is manufactured by exposure to sunlight, but is also found in store-bought fortified plant-based milks and orange juice.

Nutrients	How Does It Work?	Plant Sources
Zinc	Important for sperm composition, motility, and quantity. It improves sperm motility by preventing oxidative stress, sperm death, and DNA fragmentation of the sperm.	Sesame seeds, pumpkin seeds, lentils, chickpeas, cashews, quinoa, almonds, peanuts, fortified cereals
Selenium	Selenium plays a role in sperm quality and count. It is also significant to the synthesis and health of sex hormones through its connection to the thyroid and its importance in adrenal health.	Brazil nuts, sunflower seeds, mushrooms, asparagus, tofu.
Essential fatty acids	Sufficient amounts of healthy fats are necessary for the synthesis of sex hormones in the adrenal gland.	Walnuts, flaxseeds, olive oil, chia seeds, hemp seeds
Vitamin E (tocopherol)	Vitamin E is an antioxidant that protects the prostate from inflammation and also has been used to help treat impotency.	Sunflower seeds, almonds, vegetable oils, greens, olives, avocado, peanuts, asparagus
Vitamin C (ascorbic acid)	Vitamin C plays an important role in the male reproductive system, helping to increase sperm count, improve sperm motility and maintain sperm morphology. It also concentrates in the adrenal glands, making it important in the production of sex hormones.	Citrus fruits, papaya, Brussels sprouts, pineapple, peppers, tomatoes, broccoli, spinach, greens, cauliflower, strawberries
Vitamin B_2 (riboflavin)	Riboflavin supports the function of the adrenal glands, small glands that produce hormones you can't live without (including sex hormones and cortisol, involved in stress management).	Cremini mushrooms, asparagus, broccoli, spinach, greens, buckwheat, fortified cereals, soybeans, almonds
Vitamin B_6 (pyridoxine)	Vitamin B_6 may be used as a hormone regulator. It also helps regulate blood sugars, alleviates PMS, and may be useful in relieving symptoms of pregnancy morning sickness. B6 has been shown to help with luteal phase defect, which affects fertility.	Spinach, bok choy, cabbage, peppers, garlic, cauliflower, potatoes, sweet potatoes, bananas, squash, broccoli, Brussels sprouts, greens, carrots
Vitamin B_{12} (cobalamin)	Vitamin B_{12} has been shown to improve sperm quality and production. It also may support pregnancy by helping to boost the endometrium lining in egg fertilization.	Fortified plant-based milks and cereals, fortified nutritional yeast (Red Star is a recommended brand)

MUSCULOSKELETAL

Protein	Protein is responsible for the structure and repair of muscle and tissue.	Nuts, flaxseeds, beans, brown rice, tofu, tempeh, miso, soy milk, brewer's yeast, quinoa, amaranth, chlorella, spirulina, sprouted seeds

Nutrients	How Does It Work?	Plant Sources
Vitamin B_6 (pyridoxine)	Pyridoxine helps facilitate the way the brain communicates with the body.	Spinach, bok choy, cabbage, peppers, garlic, cauliflower, potatoes, sweet potatoes, bananas, squash, broccoli, Brussels sprouts, greens, carrots
Essential amino acids	Amino acids are essential for muscle repair and growth.	Nuts, flaxseeds, beans, brown rice, tofu, tempeh, miso, soy milk, brewer's yeast, quinoa, amaranth, chlorella, spirulina, sprouted seeds
Vitamin D (calciferol)	Calciferol directs calcium into bones and regulates the neuromuscular system. It is needed to prevent rickets in infants—a malformation of the bones due to decreased deposition of calcium; and in adults, osteomalacia, a skeletal demineralization of the spine, pelvis, and lower extremities. Vitamin D deficiency is often seen in neuromuscular diseases, such as multiple sclerosis, myasthenia gravis, and Parkinson's.	Vitamin D is manufactured by exposure to sunlight, but is also found in store-bought fortified plant-based milks and orange juice.
Copper	Copper helps the body form connective tissue and facilitate muscle functioning.	Sesame seeds, cashews, soybeans, shiitake mushrooms, sunflower seeds, tempeh, chickpeas, lentils, walnuts
Magnesium	Magnesium regulates the absorption of calcium and is involved in the structural integrity of bones and teeth. It has the important job of regulating the contractility of smooth muscles, resulting in prevention of heart disease, improving asthma, lowering blood pressure, relieving tension headaches, and decreasing menstrual cramping.	Dark leafy greens, pumpkin seeds, almonds, sunflower seeds, sesame seeds, black beans, quinoa, Brazil nuts, cashews, soybeans, avocado, bananas, chocolate
Manganese	Manganese makes and maintains connective tissues and bones. It works on bone remodeling with vitamin K in helping to bind calcium ions to bone.	Hazelnuts, pumpkin seeds, whole wheat, tofu, spinach, kale, black tea, cloves, oats, chickpeas, brown rice, pineapple
Phosphorus	Phosphorus is essential in its structural role in bones and teeth. It also aids tissue repair and muscle maintenance.	Pumpkin seeds, sunflower seeds, Brazil nuts, tofu, lentils, peanuts, whole wheat, corn, broccoli, garlic
Potassium	Too little potassium, calcium, or magnesium in the body can contribute to leg cramps. Potassium especially is needed in balance to maintain proper electrical activity in nerves and muscles, including heart muscle. It also is essential for glycogen storage in muscles, preventing muscle fatigue.	White beans, leafy greens, baked potato, apricots, squash, avocado, mushrooms, bananas, sweet potato, soybeans, lentils

NERVOUS SYSTEM		
Essential amino acids	Amino acids both protect nerve cell structure and support the nervous system functioning through messaging. Methionine, phenylalanine, threonine, and tryptophan all have specific nervous system actions, such as boosting mood, memory, and learning, and helping to relieve depression, anxiety, and migraine headaches. Asparagine helps maintain equilibrium in the nervous system, with a calming effect.	Nuts, flaxseeds, beans, brown rice, tofu, tempeh, miso, soy milk, brewer's yeast, quinoa, amaranth, chlorella, spirulina, sprouted seeds
Vitamin B1 (thiamine)	Required B1 is required for the biochemical actions of methionine, threonine, serotonin, and other nervous system supportive amino acids. It is involved in carbohydrate metabolism in the brain. B1 is helpful in treating sensory neuropathy, trigeminal neuralgia, insomnia, depression, and anxiety. It serves as a cofactor in the metabolism of alcohol, and is therefore helpful in treating hangover symptoms.	Very small amounts are in virtually all foods. Good sources are sunflower seeds, flaxseeds, asparagus black beans, green peas, split peas, barley, lentils, oats, lima beans, brown rice, soybeans, pistachio, peanuts, Brazil nuts, pecans, raisins, blackstrap molasses
Vitamin B2 (riboflavin)	Riboflavin helps maintain the nervous system by activating B6, playing a role in glucose metabolism and utilization in the brain, and helping with thyroid enzyme regulation necessary for mood stabilization.	Cremini mushrooms, asparagus, broccoli, spinach, greens, buckwheat, fortified cereals, soybeans, almonds
Vitamin B3 (niacin)	Niacin contributes to the smooth functioning of the nervous system. It acts as an anti-anxiety treatment with similar effect to anxiety drugs. It has shown benefit in multiple sclerosis, Bell's palsy, trigeminal neuralgia, and migraines, and helps with circulation in such complaints such as Raynaud's syndrome.	Cremini mushrooms, lentils, tomatoes, bell peppers, sweet potatoes, peas, peanuts, beans, fortified cereals, beets, sunflower seeds, asparagus
Vitamin B5 (pantothenic acid)	B5 helps the central nervous system communicate with the brain. It is required for the production on steroid hormones in the adrenal glands. B5 helps with adaptation to environmental stress along with other B vitamins.	Avocado, whole grains, legumes, broccoli, molasses, mushrooms, corn
Vitamin B6 (pyridoxine)	Pyridoxine enables a healthy nervous system. It is needed to combat the exposure to environmental toxins that may affect the nervous system. It helps relieve PMS symptoms. B6 has been useful in carpal tunnel syndrome, infant seizures, rheumatism, dyskinesia/tremors, and diabetic neuropathy. It helps with depression as a cofactor in the conversion of tryptophan to serotonin. It is potentially beneficial in dementia and early Alzheimer's by supporting dopamine receptors.	Spinach, bok choy, cabbage, peppers, garlic, cauliflower, potatoes, sweet potatoes, bananas, squash, broccoli, Brussels sprouts, greens, carrots

Nutrients	How Does It Work?	Plant Sources
Calcium	Nerves use calcium to carry messages from the brain throughout the body.	Kale, broccoli, spinach, fortified cereals and plant-based milks, seaweeds, pistachios, sesame seeds, almonds, beans, and tofu.
Magnesium	As a mild muscle relaxant, magnesium helps relieve minor anxiety and nervous tension.	Dark leafy greens, pumpkin seeds, almonds, sunflower seeds, sesame seeds, black beans, quinoa, Brazil nuts, cashews, soybeans, avocado, bananas, chocolate
Phosphorus	Phosphorus helps the body maintain nerve cells as a key component of phospholipids, which protect cell membranes.	Pumpkin seeds, sunflower seeds, Brazil nuts, tofu, lentils, peanuts, whole wheat, corn, broccoli, garlic
Sodium	Sodium moderates the functioning of nerves and muscles through electrolyte balance.	Beets, celery, carrots, spinach, chard, most fruits
Lecithin	Lecithin is a source of phosphatidylcholine, which is important in nerve signaling and proper neurotransmitter functioning.	Brussels sprouts, leafy greens, legumes, peanut butter, soybeans

SKIN

Nutrients	How Does It Work?	Plant Sources
Essential amino acids	Amino acids serve in the production of hemoglobin and help wounds heal. Lysine protects skin, helpful in preventing HPV outbreaks. Methionine is helpful in wound healing and supporting growth hormone for tissue maintenance.	Nuts, flaxseeds, beans, brown rice, tofu, tempeh, miso, soy milk, brewer's yeast, quinoa, amaranth, chlorella, spirulina, sprouted seeds
Vitamin A	Vitamin A promotes healthy skin through retinoic action on the epithelial cells to maintain cilia to mucous membranes and create a protective barrier, which prevents infection and other skin reactions.	Dark orange vegetables, such as carrot, pumpkin, squash, and sweet potato; green leafy vegetables, such as kale, collards, bok choy, and spinach; orange fruits, such as melon, peach, papaya, and mango; red pepper; fortified cereals
Vitamin B3 (niacin)	Niacin contributes to maintenance of healthy skin by maintaining healthy circulation.	Cremini mushrooms, lentils, tomatoes, bell peppers, sweet potatoes, peas, peanuts, beans, fortified cereals, beets, sunflower seeds, asparagus

Nutrients	How Does It Work?	Plant Sources
Vitamin C (ascorbic acid)	Vitamin C helps with the healing of wounds and forms collagen in the body.	Citrus fruits, papaya, Brussels sprouts, pineapple, peppers, tomatoes, broccoli, spinach, greens, cauliflower, strawberries
Vitamin E (tocopherol)	Vitamin E contributes to healthy skin and eyes as a powerful antioxidant. It also relieves dry skin and helps maintain mucous membrane integrity.	Sunflower seeds, almonds, vegetable oils, greens, olives, avocado, peanuts, asparagus
Sulfur	Sulfur aids in the production of collagen for skin, nail, and hair health.	Nuts, flaxseeds, sunflower seeds, durian fruit, garlic, onions, asparagus, cabbage, Brussels sprouts, broccoli, kale, turnips
Beta-carotene	Beta-carotene protects skin from photoaging effects.	Broccoli, sweet potato, pumpkin, carrots, apricots, asparagus, grapefruit
Lutein	Lutein improves skin hydration and elasticity.	Kale, spinach, other greens, peas, corn
Zeaxanthin	Zeaxanthin helps prevent skin photoaging.	Green vegetables, citrus
Rutin	Rutin helps with the production of collagen.	Kasha, black tea, apple peels, onion, citrus
Phytosterols	Phytosterols maintain collagen in the skin.	Vegetable oils, beans, nuts, some fruits and veggies
Zinc	Zinc helps with the healing of wounds by increasing cell growth and repair in epithelial tissue. It is also involved as a cofactor in the metabolic pathway that lowers inflammation, helping to relieve eczema and other reactive skin issues.	Sesame seeds, pumpkin seeds, lentils, chickpeas, cashews, quinoa, almonds, peanuts, fortified cereals
Manganese	Manganese is necessary for all connective tissue function, including skin integrity. It also may help control skin inflammations.	Hazelnuts, pumpkin seeds, whole wheat, tofu, spinach, kale, black tea, cloves, oats, chickpeas, brown rice, pineapple

Notes

How to Use This Book

1. http://www.mayoclinic.org/healthy-lifestyle/stress-management/in-depth/positive-thinking/art-20043950.

Chapter 1:
Preventable Health Challenges

1. S. Y. Yang et al., "Growth Factors and Their Receptors in Cancer Metastases," *Frontiers in Bioscience* 16 (2011): 531–38; Y. Zhang et al., "Mechanisms of Breast Cancer Bone Metastasis," *Cancer Letters* 292, no. 1 (2010): 1–7; D. L. Kleinberg et al., "Growth Hormone and Insulin-like Growth Factor-I in the Transition from Normal Mammary Development to Preneoplastic Mammary Lesions," *Endocrine Review* 30, no. 1 (2009): 51–74; T. J. Key et al., "Insulin-like Growth Factor 1 (IGF1), IGF Binding Protein 3 (IGFBP3), and Breast Cancer Risk: Pooled Individual Data Analysis of 17 Prospective Studies," *The Lancet Oncology* 11, no. 6 (2010): 530–42; M. A. Rowlands et al., "Circulating Insulin-like Growth Factor Peptides and Prostate Cancer Risk: A Systematic Review and Meta-analysis," *International Journal of Cancer* 124, no. 10 (2009): 2416–29.

2. "A multicenter randomized controlled trial of a nutrition intervention program in a multi-ethnic adult population in the corporate setting reduces depression and anxiety and improves quality of life: the GEICO study." http://www.ncbi.nlm.nih.gov/pubmed/24524383.

3. G. Danaei et al., "The Preventable Causes of Death in the US: Comparative Risk Assessment of Dietary, Lifestyle and Metabolic Risk Factors," *PLoS Medicine* 6, no. 4 (2009): e1000058.

4. K. M. Narayam et al., "Lifetime Risk for Diabetes in the U.S.," *JAMA* 290, no. 14 (2003): 1883–90.

5. K. M. Narayam et al., "Diabetes: A Common, Growing, Serious, Costly and Potentially Preventable Public Health Problem," *Diabetes Research and Clinical Practice* 50, suppl. 2 (2000): 577–84.

6. Centers for Disease Control and Prevention, "Overweight and Obesity" (2012), accessed September 1, 2015, www.csc.gov/obesity/data/adult.html.7.

7. F. F. Marvasti and R. S. Stafford, "From Sick Care to Health Care—Reengineering Prevention into the U.S. System," *New England Journal of Medicine* 367 (2012): 889–91; G. Anderson, "Chronic Care: Making the Case for Ongoing Care," Robert Wood Johnson Foundation (2010), accessed September 1, 2015, www.rwjf.org/content/dam/farm/reorts/reports/2010/rwjf5483.

8. T. C. Campbell and T. M. Campbell, *The China Study* (Dallas, TX: Benbella Books).

9. D. Kessler, *The End of Overeating: Taking Control of the Insatiable American Appetite* (New York: Rodale, 2010); M. Moss, *Salt, Sugar, Fat: How the Food Giants Hooked Us* (New York: Random House; 2013).

10. Campbell and Campbell, *The China Study*; D. E. Sellmeyer et al., "A High Ratio of Dietary Animal to Vegetable Protein Increases the Rate of Bone Loss and the Risk of Fracture in Postmenopausal Women," *American Journal of Clinical Nutrition* 73 (2001): 118–22.

11. T. C. Campbell, *Whole: Rethinking the Science of Nutrition* (Dallas, TX: Benbella Books, 2013); N. D. Barnard, *Dr. Neal Barnard's Program for Reversing Diabetes* (New York: Rodale, 2007); H. A. Diehl and A. Ludington, *Health Power* (Hagerstown, MD: Review and Herald Publishing Assn., 2011).

12. J. Stamler, "George Lyman Duff Memorial Lecture: Lifestyles, Major Risk Factors, Proof and Public Policy," *Circulation* 58 (1978): 3–19.

13. D. Ornish et al., "Intensive Lifestyle

Changes for Reversal of Coronary Heart Disease," *JAMA* 280 (1998): 2001-7; D. Ornish et al., "Changes in Prostate Gene Expression in Men Undergoing Intensive Diet and Lifestyle Intervention," *Proceedings of the National Academy of Sciences* 102 (2008): 8369-75.

14. C. B. Esselstyn, *Prevent and Reverse Heart Disease* (New York: Penguin Group, 2007).

15. Barnard, *Dr. Neal Barnard's Program for Reversing Diabetes*.

16. P. Rankin et al., "Effectiveness of Volunteer-Delivered Lifestyle Modification Program for Reducing CVD Risk Factors," *American Journal of Cardiology* 109 (2012): 82-86.

17. "CHIP Program: Clinical Results Bibliography," accessed September 1, 2015, www.CHIP health.com/AboutCHIP/ScientificPublications.

18. Ibid.; Diehl and Ludington, *Health Power*.

Chapter 2: A Cornucopia of Nutritional
Theories—Which Is Right for You?

1. C. Orian Truss, "Tissue Injury Induced by *Candida albicans*: Mental and Neurologic Manifestations," *Journal of Orthomolecular Psychiatry* 7np. 1 (1978), 17-37.

2. S. N. Cheuvront, "The Zone Diet Phenomenon: A Closer Look at the Science Behind the Claims," *Journal of the American College of Nutrition* 22, no. 1 (February 2003): 9-17, PMID 12569110.

3. Jack Norris, "Vitamin K," VeganHealth.org. http://veganhealth.org/articles/vitamink.

Chapter 3: The Pillars of the
Plant Kingdom—Nutrient-Dense Foods
for Optimal Health

1. P.V. Rao, and S. H. Gan, "Cinnamon: a Multifaceted Medicinal Plant," PMC. US National Library of Medicine, National Institutes of Health. PMC4003790. http://www.ncbi.nlm.nih.gov/pmc /articles/PMC4003790/.

2. Michael Greger, "Increasing Muscle Strength with Fenugreek," Dr. Greger's Medical Nutrition Blog. http://nutritionfacts.org/2013/04/23/in creasing-muscle-strength-with-fenugreek/.

Clinical Wellness Programs Utilizing a Whole Food, Plant-Based Diet

Some of the leading doctors in the preventative medicine community oversee programs that successfully demonstrate the healing powers of a plant-based diet. Here are just a few of these programs, in case you want to seek one out to support you on your own journey to wellness.

The Complete Health Improvement Program (CHIP)
www.chiphealth.com

The Complete Health Improvement Program (CHIP) is a research tested lifestyle medicine intervention education program, designed to prevent, stop, and reverse chronic disease. Founded in the United States in 1998, CHIP has impacted over sixty thousand participants and generated twenty-plus published scientific papers. CHIP is a community-based intervention program that uses behavioral change principles in a group setting, education in an entertaining style, and modern adult learning tools to help participants make radical lifestyle changes that are proven to lower key risk factors in as little as thirty days.

CHIP is a powerful disease-reversal tool for health practitioners, community organizations, and workplaces, to address the rising chronic disease rates in a highly effective manner. A cornerstone of the CHIP program is an optimal way of eating so as to lose weight by eating more; embrace the importance of fiber; understand how diabetes, heart disease, and blood pressure are affected by food choices; optimize bone health and protein intake, and prevent cancer occurrence or reoccurrence— all with a whole food, plant-based diet.

The Complete Health Improvement Program takes participants through an intensive educational program with eighteen sessions running over three months. Throughout the program, participants are guided through the various stages of lifestyle change, helping to show them the benefits of an optimal lifestyle and giving them the tools to maintain positive lifestyle change. CHIP does not just focus on the way people eat and the way people move, but takes a whole-of-life perspective including stress management, sleep, self-worth, emotional well-being, and happiness. CHIP is designed to encourage participants' self-management, teaching them to take control of their own health through wiser choices.

The group setting provides a supportive environment to help reinforce positive lifestyle behaviors and build lasting friendships.

Through the use of entertaining, educational video sessions and the supporting text *Learn More*, participants are given the wealth of knowledge needed to make positive lifestyle changes. This information is greatly supported by the *Live More* workbook and CHIP facilitators, who challenge participants to live the best life possible, while providing invaluable support and encouragement throughout the journey.

Physicians Committee for Responsible Medicine (PCRM) Food for Life Programs
www.pcrm.org

Food for Life is an award-winning Physicians Committee for Responsible Medicine (PCRM) program designed by physicians, nurses, and registered dietitians that offers cancer, diabetes, weight management, employee wellness, and kids' classes that focus on the lifesaving effects of healthful eating. Each class includes information about how certain foods and nutrients work to promote health, along with cooking demonstrations of simple and nutritious recipes that can be recreated easily at home. Dr. Neal Barnard, president of PCRM, also offers a 21-day program for a smooth transition to what he calls the new four food groups: grains, legumes, vegetables, and fruits in his book, *Food for Life*. The Barnard Medical Center in Washington, DC, is the first plant-based state-of-the-art medical facility in the United States. You can learn more on its website.

TrueNorth Health Center
www.healthpromoting.com

TrueNorth Health Center was founded in 1984 by Drs. Alan Goldhamer and Jennifer Marano. The integrative medicine approach they established offers participants the opportunity to obtain evaluation and treatment for a wide variety of problems. The staff at TrueNorth Health Center includes medical doctors, osteopaths, chiropractors, naturopaths, psychologists, research scientists, and other health professionals. The Center is now the largest facility in the world that specializes in medically supervised water-only fasting. For over thirty years, the Center has helped over ten thousand people regain their health. Dr. Michael Klaper serves as a staff physician at TrueNorth.

Early in his career Dr. Klaper noticed that the diseases his patients presented with were made worse, or actually caused, by the high-fat, overly processed standard American diet (SAD). This prompted him to study the link between diet and disease, and to then implement nutritionally based therapies in his practice. He improved his own health substantially by following his 12-week program, and continues to enjoy a very active life and practice thirty years later.

Nearly all of his patients who followed his dietary, exercise, and stress-reduction programs soon became leaner and more energetic, while their elevated blood pressures and cholesterol levels returned to safer values. Many of them were able to resolve chronic diseases completely and/or reduce or discontinue their medication entirely.

Dr. McDougall's Health and Medical Center
www.drmcdougall.com

Dr. McDougall's Health and Medical Center offers a 10-day live-in program at the Flamingo Resort and Spa in Santa Rosa, California. During the program, all medical care is provided to each participant personally by John McDougall, MD. Dramatic improvements are simply the result of a highly nutritious diet, exercise, a focus on better daily habits, and gaining freedom from the unpleasant side effects of medication. Mary McDougall also takes participants to the market and out to lunch at local restaurants to help with incorporating new habits into life back home. In addition to John and Mary, the professional teaching staff provides cooking instruction, supervised exercise, and an in-depth education on the psychology behind successful change.

Over 90 percent of participants are able to stop their medications for hypertension, type 2 diabetes, arthritis, indigestion, and constipation. Those who must stay on medications are often able to switch to simpler, safer, more effective, and less expensive ones.

Hippocrates Health Institute
www.hippocratesinst.org

The Hippocrates Health Institute (HHI) is a nonprofit organization located in a tropical 50-acre setting in West Palm Beach, Florida, directed by Brian and Anna Maria Clement. It was first inspired by visionary and humanitarian Ann Wigmore half a century ago as an expression from Hippocrates, the father of modern medicine, nearly 2,500 years ago: "Let food be thy medicine and medicine be thy food." Ms. Wigmore and Viktoras Kulvinskas created this comprehensive institute that encourages people to transform the quality of their health and life. The goal of the institute is to assist people in taking responsibility for their life. Guests from all over the world benefit from health and nutritional counseling, noninvasive remedial and youth-enhancing therapies, state-of-the-art spa services, inspiring talks on life principles, and a tantalizing daily buffet of enzyme-rich, organic meals.

The Hippocrates Life Transformation Program includes a medical team and professional care servers who support guests as they transform their lives in an encouraging environment, along with others who are recovering from similar challenges. HHI alumni are people from all walks of life who share stories of recovery that are considered miraculous by some, but that are actually quite typical of people who

have embraced the Hippocrates lifestyle. After graduating, alumni are afforded the privilege of periodic, lifelong, written counsel.

Tree of Life Center Diabetes Reversal Program
www.treeoflifecenterus.com

The Tree of Life Center in Arizona was founded by Gabriel Cousens, MD, MD(H) to support and inspire holistic lifestyle through education and experience. The center's spiritual guidance, lifestyle education, and medical programs are complemented with panoramic mountain views and 100 percent organic, live food, which have drawn guests from over one hundred countries since 1995.

The Diabetes Recovery Program is a three-week plan that includes green juice fasting and a 100 percent organic, nutrient-dense, vegan, low-glycemic, low-insulin-scoring, and high-mineral diet of living foods. The revolutionary plan is also described in the book called *There Is a Cure for Diabetes: The Tree of Life 21-Day+ Program* by Gabriel Cousens.

Additional Resources

Further Reading

Want to learn more? Explore this section to deepen your knowledge of the information touched upon in *Healing the Vegan Way*.

Health and Wellness

Barnard, Neal, MD. *Dr. Neal Barnard's Program for Reversing Diabetes: The Scientifically Proven System for Reversing Diabetes without Drugs.*

_____. *Power Foods for the Brain: An Effective 3 Step Plan to Protect Your Mind and Strengthen Your Memory.*

Brazier, Brendan. *Thrive: The Whole Food Way to Lose Weight, Reduce Stress, and Stay Healthy for Life.*

Campbell, Colin T., and Howard Jacobson. *Whole: Rethinking the Science of Nutrition.*

Campbell, Colin T., and Thomas M. Campbell II. *The China Study: The Most Comprehensive Study of Nutrition Ever Conducted and the Startling Implications for Diet, Weight Loss, and Long-Term Health.*

Esselstyn, Caldwell. *Prevent and Reverse Heart Disease.*

Fuhrman, Joel, MD. *The End of Diabetes: The Eat to Live Plan to Prevent and Reverse Diabetes.*

_____. *Eat to Live: The Revolutionary Formula for Fast and Sustained Weight Loss.*

Greger, Michael, and Gene Stone. *How Not to Die: Discover the Foods Scientifically Proven to Prevent and Reverse Disease*

Hever, Julieanna. *The Complete Idiot's Guide to Plant-Based Nutrition.*

_____. *The Vegiterranean Diet.*

Klaper, Michael, MD. *Vegan Nutrition: Pure and Simple.*

Ornish, Dean. *Dr. Dean Ornish's Program for Reversing Heart Disease: The Only System Scientifically Proven to Reverse Heart Disease Without Drugs or Surgery.*

Pierre, John. *The Pillars of Health.*

Rebhal, Sayward. *Vegan Pregnancy Survival Guide.*

Pitchford, P. *Healing with Whole Foods.*

Fitness

Cheeke, Robert. *Vegan Bodybuilding & Fitness.*

Frasier, Matt, and Matthew Ruscigno. *No Meat Athlete: Run on Plants and Discover Your Fittest, Fastest, Happiest Self.*

Lifestyle

Adams, Carol J., Patti Breitman, and Virginia Messina. *Never Too Late to Go Vegan: The Over-50 Guide to Adopting and Thriving on a Plant-Based Diet.*

Barnard, Neal, MD. *Breaking the Food Seduction: The Hidden Reasons Behind Food Cravings—and 7 Steps to End Them Naturally.*

Davis, Brenda, RD, and Vesanto Melina, MS, RD. *The Complete Guide to Adopting a Healthy Plant-Based Diet.*

Hicks, J. Morris. *Healthy Eating, Healthy World.*

Jacobson, Michael, PhD. *Six Arguments for a Greener Diet: How a Plant-Based Diet Could Save Your Health and the Environment.*

Joy, Melanie. *Why We Love Dogs, Eat Pigs, and Wear Cows: An Introduction to Carnism.*

Jurek, Scott. *Eat & Run: My Unlikely Journey to Marathon Greatness.*

Krizmaniac, Judy. *A Teen's Guide to Going Vegetarian.*

Lyman, Howard. *Mad Cowboy: Plain Truth from the Cattle Rancher Who Won't Eat Meat.*

Marcus, Erik. *Vegan: The New Ethics of Eating.*

Messina, Virginia, and J. L. Fields. *Vegan for Her: The Woman's Guide to Being Healthy and Fit on a Plant-Based Diet.*

Norris, Jack, and Virginia Messina. *Vegan for Life: Everything You Need to Know to Be Healthy and Fit on a Plant-Based Diet.*

Robbins, John. *Diet for a New America.*

_____. *Healthy at 100.*

_____. *The New Good Life: Living Better than Ever in an Age of Less.*

_____. *No Happy Cows: Dispatches from the Frontlines of the Food Revolution.*

Roll, Rich. *Finding Ultra: Rejecting Middle Age, Becoming One of the World's Fittest Men, and Discovering Myself.*

Stone, Gene. *Forks Over Knives: The Plant-Based Way to Health.*

Stuart, Tristram. *The Bloodless Revolution: A Cultural History of Vegetarianism from 1600 to Modern Times.*

Tuttle, Will, PhD. *World Peace Diet: Eating for Spiritual Health and Social Harmony.*

Cookbooks

Esselstyn, Ryp. *The Engine 2 Diet: the Texas Firefighter's 28-Day Save-Your-Life Plan that Lowers Cholesterol and Burns Away the Pounds.*

Liddon, Angela. *O She Glows Every Day: Quick and Simply Satisfying Plant-Based Recipes.*

Nixon, Lindsay. *The Happy Herbivore Guide to Plant-Based Living.*

Prussack, Steven, and Bo Rinaldi. *The Complete Idiot's Guide to Juice Fasting.*

Reinfeld, Mark. *The 30-Minute Vegan's Soups On!*

_____. *The 30-Minute Vegan's Taste of Europe.*

Reinfeld, Mark, and Bo Rinaldi. *Vegan Fusion World Cuisine.*

Reinfeld, Mark, Bo Rinaldi, and Jennifer Murray. *The Complete Idiot's Guide to Eating Raw.*

Reinfeld, Mark, and Jennifer Murray. *The 30-Minute Vegan.*

_____. *The 30-Minute Vegan's Taste of the East.*

Rinaldi, Bo. *The Complete Idiot's Guide to Green Smoothies.*

Online Resources

Here are some of the more popular websites and blogs promoting a vegan and sustainable way of life. We also list some go-to sites for kitchen equipment and to stock up your veggie pantry.

Vegan Health and Wellness Websites

plantbaseddietitian.com/blog The Plant-Based Dietitian gives info on nutrition, social and environmental issues, recipes, and Q&A about plant-based eating.

wtfveganfood.com Will Travel for Vegan Food offers reviews and menu tips from restaurants around the United States and the world. Its author spent more than a year on the road with the objective of visiting every vegan restaurant.

www.chiphealth.com The Complete Health Improvement Program is an affordable, lifestyle enrichment program designed to reduce disease risk factors through the adoption of better health habits and appropriate lifestyle modifications.

www.happycow.net Happy Cow is a searchable dining guide to vegetarian restaurants, natural and health food stores, information on vegetarian nutrition, raw foods, and vegan recipes.

www.ivu.org The World Union of Vegetarian/Vegan Societies has been promoting vegetarianism worldwide since 1908.

www.ourhenhouse.org A nonprofit organization with a weekly podcast about vegan and other animal issues. Produces resources for people who want to take a role in changing the world for animals and vegan education.

www.pcrm.org The Physicians Committee for Responsible Medicine (PCRM) is a nonprofit organization that promotes preventive medicine, conducts clinical research, and encourages higher standards for ethics and effectiveness in research.

www.theveganrd.com A dietitian's perspective on being vegan. Tips on becoming a vegan RD, a copy of the "Plant Plate," and nutrition resources.

www.veganbodybuilding.com Vegan Body Building and Fitness is the website of vegan bodybuilder Robert Cheeke and features articles, videos, products, and a forum for the active vegan.

www.veganfitness.net Vegan Fitness is a community-driven message board seeking to provide a supportive, educational, and friendly environment for vegans, vegetarians, and those seeking to go vegan.

www.veganhealth.org A project of Vegan Outreach (a nonprofit organization working to end violence toward animals), this site is maintained by a registered dietician and goes into great nutritional detail, providing info by disease, by vitamin, by mineral, and by condition.

www.vegan.org Vegan Action is a nonprofit grassroots organization dedicated to educating people about the many benefits of a vegan lifestyle.

www.vrg.org The Vegetarian Resource Group (VRG) is a nonprofit organization dedicated to educating the public on vegetarianism, including information on health, nutrition, ecology, ethics, and world hunger.

Vegan Food and Lifestyle Websites

wtfveganfood.com Will Travel for Vegan Food offers reviews and menu tips from restaurants around the United States and the world, as its author spent more than a year on the road with the objective of visiting every vegan restaurant.

www.happycow.net Happy Cow is a searchable dining guide to vegetarian restaurants, natural and health food stores, information on vegetarian nutrition, raw foods, and vegan recipes.

www.vegan.com The popular site of Erik Marcus, geared toward the aspiring and long-term vegan that features articles, interviews, product evaluations, book reviews, and more.

www.vegan.meetup.com Meet up with other vegans in your town!

www.veganpet.com.au Veganpet provides nutritionally complete and balanced pet food and information on raising vegan pets.

www.vegetarianteen.com An online magazine with articles on vegetarian teen lifestyle, activism, nutrition, social issues, and more.

www.vegfamily.com Comprehensive resource for raising vegan children, including pregnancy, vegan recipes, book reviews, product reviews, message board, and more.

www.vegsource.com Features over ten thousand vegetarian and vegan recipes, discussion boards, nutritionists, medical doctors, experts, authors, articles, newsletter, and the vegetarian community.

www.vegweb.com A vegetarian mega site with recipes, photos, articles, online store, and more.

Raw Food Lifestyle Websites

www.gliving.tv The G Living Network is a hip and modern green lifestyle network with videos and articles on living in an earth-friendly way, including raw recipes, sustainable fashion, technology, and household design.

www.goneraw.com Gone Raw is a website created to help people share and discuss raw, vegan food recipes from around the world.

www.rawfoods.com Living and Raw Foods is the largest raw online community with appliances for the raw foodist, chat rooms, blogs, articles, classified ads, and recipes.

Specialty Foods and Products

www.amazon.com Amazon.com is perhaps the world's largest superstore. Check it out to order any kitchen equipment or specialty food items, including immersion blenders, gnocchi boards, Microplane zesters, spiralizers, and more.

www.foodfightgrocery.com Food Fight! Grocery is an all-vegan convenience store located in Portland, Oregon, with an online market that emphasizes junk foods, imports, and fun stuff.

www.goldminenaturalfood.com An online source for a vast selection of organic, raw, macrobiotic, vegan, gluten-free, Asian, gourmet, and specialty foods as well as natural cookware and home products.

www.livesuperfoods.com   The go-to site for all of your raw food needs, from food and supplements to appliances, such as juicers, blenders, dehydrators, and spiralizers.

www.veganessentials.com   The ultimate vegan superstore with everything from cosmetics, to clothing, to household products, supplements, and more. When it comes to vegan—you name it, they have it.

Eco-friendly Products and Services

www.877juicer.com   This website carries way more than juicers, including everything kitchen related, plus air purifiers, books, and articles.

www.greenpeople.org   Green People provides a directory of eco-friendly products and services.

www.kidbean.com   Organic, earth-friendly, and vegan products for families.

www.vitamix.com   Find the latest Vitamix blenders here on the official site, including factory-reconditioned models that still come with a seven-year warranty. For free shipping in the continental United States, enter code 06-002510.

Vegan Organizations

www.animalconcerns.org   Animal Concerns Community serves as a clearinghouse for information on the Internet related to animal rights and welfare.

www.earthsave.org   Founded by John Robbins, EarthSave is doing what it can to promote a shift to a plant-based diet. It posts news, information, and resources and publishes a magazine.

www.farmusa.org   Farm Animal Reform Movement (FARM) is an organization advocating a plant-based diet and humane treatment of farm animals through grassroots programs.

www.ivu.org   The World Union of Vegetarian/Vegan Societies has been promoting vegetarianism worldwide since 1908.

www.ourhenhouse.org   A nonprofit organization with a weekly podcast about vegan and other animal issues. Produces resources for people who want to take a role in changing the world for animals and vegan education.

www.vegan.org   Vegan Action is a nonprofit grassroots organization dedicated to educating people about the many benefits of a vegan lifestyle.

www.veganoutreach.com   Amazing resource for aspiring vegans. Vegan outreach is a wonderful organization dedicated to pamphleting and other educational activities.

Organic & Gardening Websites

www.avant-gardening.com   A site advocating organic gardening with information on composting, soil building, permaculture principles, botany, companion and intensive planting, and more.

www.biodynamics.com   The Biodynamic Farming and Gardening Association supports and promotes biodynamic farming, the oldest nonchemical agricultural movement.

www.extension.org   Managed by the University of Illinois, eXtension is a conglomeration of information from a network of US universities on almost any garden-related forum.

www.gefoodalert.org   GE Food Alert Campaign Center is a coalition of seven organizations committed to testing and labeling genetically engineered food.

www.kgi.org   Kitchen Gardeners International is a nonprofit community of people looking to empower one another by encouraging self-reliance by growing their own food in the backyard or sustainably in the community.

www.kidbean.com   Organic, earth-friendly, and vegan products for families.

www.nongmoproject.org   The Non-GMO Project is a nonprofit that practices third-party verification and labeling of non-GMO foods, striving to increase non-GMO product availability and education.

www.organicconsumers.org   The Organic Consumers Association is an online, grassroots, nonprofit organization dealing with issues of food safety, industrial agriculture, genetic engineering, corporate accountability, and environmental sustainability.

www.ota.com The Organic Trade Association website will tell you anything you want to know about the term organic, from food to textiles to health-care products. The OTA's mission is to encourage global sustainability through promoting and protecting the growth of diverse organic trade.

www.veganorganic.net Organic growing, green, clean, cruelty-free articles and information.

Environmental & Sustainability Websites

www.childrenoftheearth.org Children of the Earth United is a children's environmental education website that educates the public on ecological concepts and aims to provide a forum for people to share knowledge and ideas.

www.conservation.org Conservation International is involved in many conservation projects worldwide. On their site you can calculate your carbon footprint based on your living situation, car, travel habits, and diet.

www.dinegreen.com The Green Restaurant Association (GRA) is a national nonprofit organization that provides a convenient way for all sectors of the restaurant industry, which represents 10 percent of the US economy, to become more environmentally sustainable.

www.meetthegreens.org An educational site for kids about green living and sustainability, plus ecology, environmental care, and social equity by way of games, videos, carbon calculators, and other activities.

www.nrdcwildplaces.org Natural Resources Defense Council (NRDC) is an environmental action group with over 1 million members working to safeguard the American continents' natural systems.

www.ran.org Rainforest Action Network is working to protect tropical rainforests around the world and the human rights of those living in and around those forests.

www.sustainabletable.org Producers of the animated short *The Meatrix* and well-used *Eat Well Guide* with twenty-five thousand locally grown listings (just type in your zip code), Sustainable Table encourages and educates about sustainable food related issues.

www.treehugger.com Large variety of articles about green living: news, products, and solutions.

Recommended Movies and Documentaries

Blackfish (2013)
Director: Gabriela Cowperthwaite
Blackfish tells the story of Tilikum, a performing orca that killed several people at SeaWorld while in captivity, with footage and exploration of incidences of cruel treatment in captivity.

The Cove (2009) Director: Louie Psihoyos
The Cove follows a mission in a remote and hidden cove in Taiji, Japan, exposing ecological crimes happening worldwide.

Cowspiracy: The Sustainability Secret (2014)
Directors: Keegan Kuhn and Kip Anderson
An environmental documentary, *Cowspiracy* follows a filmmaker who seeks to expose animal agriculture as the most destructive industry facing our planet, and why the big environmental nonprofits are not facing up to this inconvenient truth.

Crazy Sexy Cancer (2007) Director: Kris Carr
Crazy Sexy Cancer looks at Kris Carr's battle with a rare vascular cancer in her liver and lungs and how plants helped her kick it.

Earthlings (2005) Director: Shaun Monson
Earthlings is a groundbreaking documentary about all the ways humans use animals for economic purposes, ranging from puppy mills to circuses to farm animals and then some.

Eating Alaska (2010)
Director: Ellen Frankenstein
Eating Alaska shows Alaskan natives and nonnatives trying to balance buying industrial processed foods with growing their own and living off the land in the twenty-first century, and the difficulties encountered by one vegetarian there.

Fast Food Nation (2006): Richard Linklater
A burger exec examines scientific findings that cow manure is contaminating the meat used in the company's top-selling hamburger and discovers the unsavory aspects of feedlots and slaughterhouses.

Fat, Sick & Nearly Dead (2010)
Directors: Joe Cross and Kurt Engfehr
When Joe Cross wakes up to the fact that he is overweight and suffering from an autoimmune disease, he documents his mission to drink only fruit and vegetable juice on the road traveling the United States for sixty days to get back in shape and return to vibrant health.

Fat, Sick & Nearly Dead 2 (2014)
Director: Kurt Engfehr
Part 2 of Joe's documentation revisits his journey by looking at ways to make healthy habits long-term for sustainability in health and wellness.

Fed Up (2014) Director: Stephanie Soechtig
with Katie Couric
Fed Up looks at how marketing, branding, and our additions, especially with sugar, run counter-intuitively to our resulting disparity in health and wellness.

Food Fight (2008) Director: Christopher Taylor
Food Fight looks into agribusiness policy and food culture in the context of how the California food movement has developed a lifestyle alternative to American agribusiness.

Food Inc. (2008) Director: Robert Kenner
The US food industry is examined in *Food, Inc.*, looking into what's been hidden from the American consumer in the large-scale systemic agribusiness industry.

Food Matters (2008) Directors: Carlo Ledesma
and James Colquhoun
In this documentary you'll hear interviews with some of the big health experts who talk about health, showing what works, what doesn't, and what you don't know about that might be harmful to your health and wellness.

Forks over Knives (2011) Director: Lee Fulkerson
Forks Over Knives is a groundbreaking documentary that takes a look at the proposal that most or all diseases of affluence, or degenerative diseases, which are part of our health crisis nowadays can be prevented and reversed by a plant-based diet.

Hungry for Change (2012)
Directors: Carlo Ledesma, Laurentine ten Bosch, James Colquhoun
Focusing on the diet and weight-loss industries, *Hungry for Change* looks at the deceitfulness present that actually keep you craving the foods that are not ideal for health and wellness.

The Meatrix (2003) Director: Louis Fox
The Meatrix is a four-minute, widely viewed short flash animation critical of factory farming and industrial agricultural practices, and is modeled on *The Matrix.*

Meat the Truth (2008) Director: Shaun Monson
Meat the Truth looks at one of the leading causes of climate change, which is intensive livestock production, which it shows to create more greenhouse gases than all modes of transport combined.

Plastic Planet (2009) Director: Werner Boote
Plastic Planet explores the heavy dependency on plastics since the 1950s, looking at the ubiquity of plastic and its industry.

Speciesism (2013) Director: Mark Devries
This film looks at what modern factory farms are hiding and how difficult it is to find them, much less access them, and features some difficult encounters with their owners.

Supersize Me (2004) Director: Morgan Spurlock
Watch what happens when a young healthy man takes on an experiment to eat only at McDonald's for an entire month—and sees his health capsize.

Sustainable Table: What's on Your Plate (2006)
Director: Mischa Hedges
Hear interviews of farmers, ag specialists, nutritionists, and activists that expose how our food system does not take environmental or

human health costs into consideration, and their alternatives.

Unity (2015) Shaun Monson

Unity is the sequel to *Earthlings* and explores humanity's transformation in five chapters: "Cosmic," "Mind," "Body," "Heart," and "Soul."

Vegucated (2011)
Director: Marisa Miller Wolfson

Vegucated follows three meat- and cheese-loving New Yorkers in their journey to keep to a vegan diet for six weeks, and who discover the dark sides of animal agriculture and how it affects health and environment as well.

Acknowledgments

This book would not be possible without the dedication and loving contributions from so many others. Big thanks go to the amazing Jessica Spain for her impeccable research, and work that can be seen throughout the book. Deep thanks and love go to my wife, Ashley Boudet, ND, for her substantial contributions to the content of the book, and invaluable support in editing.

I am deeply grateful to the contributing medical doctors and nutritionists who are tirelessly educating members of their profession, and the world at large on the imperative nature of a plant-based cuisine for the healing of our bodies and the planet. You are all true pioneers. Thanks go to Dr. Michael Klaper, Dr. Michael Greger, Dr. Hans Diehl, Dr. Joel Kahn, Julieanna Hever RD, Brenda Davis RD, Dr. Rosina Pellerano, and Dr. Bill Harris.

I live with continual gratitude for the support and love of my family and friends.

Thanks go to my mother, Roberta Reinfeld, and sisters Dawn and Jennifer Reinfeld. Also to Roger Vossler, Richard Slade, Bill Townsend, Cody Martin Townsend, and Sierra Molly Townsend.

A hearty thanks goes to my stellar recipe testers: Lisa Parker, Roland Barker, Suzanne Rudolph, Lisa Portnoff, Jennifer Mennuti, and Elizabeth Arraj. Thank you to Erik Rudolf, Ami Lawson, and Elizabeth Arraj for their incredible food photography.

Thanks to my dear friends, and partners in Vegan Fusion, Bo and Star Rinaldi, for their years of guidance, support, and love.

Final shout outs go to my amazing literary agent Marilyn Allen, and to my friend Daniel Rhoda who introduced me to her. Also to my editors at Da Capo, Claire Ivett and Renée Sedliar, for their insightful edits and major contributions to the structure and content of the book.

Mahalo (thank you) to you all!

About the Experts

Brenda Davis, registered dietitian, is a leader in her field and an internationally acclaimed speaker. She has worked as a public health nutritionist, clinical nutrition specialist, nutrition consultant, and academic nutrition instructor. Brenda is the lead dietitian in a diabetes research project in Majuro, Marshall Islands. She is a featured speaker at nutrition, medical, and health conferences throughout the world.

Brenda is coauthor of nine award-winning, best-selling books: *Becoming Vegan: Comprehensive Edition* (2014), *Becoming Vegan: Express Edition* (2013), *Becoming Vegan* (2000), *The New Becoming Vegetarian* (2003), *Becoming Vegetarian* (1994, 1995), *Becoming Raw* (2010), *The Raw Food Revolution Diet* (2008), *Defeating Diabetes* (2003), and *Dairy-Free and Delicious* (2001). She is also a contributing author to a tenth book, *The Complete Vegetarian* (2009). Her books are vegetarian/vegan nutrition classics, with over 750,000 copies in print in eight languages. Brenda has authored and coauthored several articles for peer-reviewed medical and nutrition journals and magazines.

Hans Diehl, DrHSc, MPH, FACN, is the program founder and clinical professor of preventive medicine at the School of Medicine at Loma Linda University at Loma Linda, California. He is the founder of CHIP (Complete Health Improvement Program) and the Lifestyle Medicine Institute in Loma Linda. His pioneering efforts with Nathan Pritikin and Denis Burkitt, MD, have shown that many of today's chronic diseases can be powerfully influenced through adapting simple lifestyle changes. Dr. Diehl is a best-selling author, researcher, and motivator.

More than thirty peer-reviewed clinical articles show the efficacy of his lifestyle medicine approach to these lifestyle-related common chronic diseases.

Michael Greger, MD, is a physician, author, and internationally recognized professional speaker on a number of important public health issues. Dr. Greger has lectured at the Conference on World Affairs, the National Institutes of Health, and the International Bird Flu Summit, among countless other symposia and institutions; testified before Congress; has appeared on shows such as *The Colbert Report* and *The Dr. Oz Show*; and was invited as an expert witness in defense of Oprah Winfrey at the infamous "meat defamation" trial. Currently, Dr. Greger proudly serves as the director of public health and animal agriculture at the Humane Society of the United States. He is well known for NutritionFacts.org, a completely nonprofit service updated yearly to provide free updates on the latest in nutrition research via bite-size videos. There are now hundreds of videos on more than a thousand topics, with new videos and articles uploaded every day.

Julieanna Hever, MS, RD, CPT, also known as the Plant-Based Dietitian, is a passionate advocate of the miracles associated with following a whole food, plant-based diet—the established effects of which provide positive healthful benefits. Julieanna is the host of Veria Living Network's *What Would Julieanna Do?*, author of the best-selling book *The Complete Idiot's Guide to Plant-Based Nutrition* and the brand-new book *The Vegiterranean Diet*, and the nutrition columnist for *VegNews Magazine*. She is the coauthor of the *Complete Idiot's Guide to Gluten-Free Vegan Cooking*. Julieanna has been featured on numerous television and radio shows, and lectures extensively throughout the United States and internationally. www. plantbaseddietitian.com

Joel Kahn, MD, is an interpreventional cardiologist and author of the best-selling book *The Whole Heart Solution*. He has been one of the top doctors in the fields of invasive, interventional, and preventative cardiology for over fifteen years, and was given the title of "America's Holistic Heart Doc" by *Reader's Digest*. His holistic practice focuses on educating clients that there are many options for preventing and reversing heart disease, including plant-based diets, exercise, and mind-body practices that are noninvasive, safer, and more affordable than many of the common surgical procedures available today. Dr. Kahn also serves as a clinical professor of medicine in cardiology at the Wayne State University School of Medicine, and associate professor of medicine at Oakland University Beaumont School of Medicine.

Michael Klaper, MD, is a gifted clinician, internationally recognized teacher, and sought-after speaker on diet and health. He has practiced medicine for more than forty years, and is a leading educator in applied plant-based nutrition and integrative medicine. Dr. Klaper is also the author of *Vegan Nutrition: Pure and Simple* (2002), *Pregnancy, Children, and the Vegan Diet* (1991), as well as numerous health videos.

He currently serves on the staff of the True-North Health Center in Santa Rosa, California, a nutritionally based medical clinic specializing in therapeutic fasting and health improvement through a whole food, plant-based diet.

Sharon Palmer, RDN, the Plant-Powered Dietitian, is an award-winning plant-based nutrition expert, editor, and author. Her books include *The Plant-Powered Diet: The Lifelong Eating Plan for Achieving Optimal Health Beginning Today* and *Plant-Powered for Life: Eat Your Way to Lasting Health with 52 Simple Steps & 125 Delicious Recipes*. In addition, Share writes every day for her popular *Plant-Powered* blog. Living in the chaparral hills overlooking Los Angeles with her husband and two sons, Sharon enjoys visiting the local farmers' market every week and cooking for friends and family.

Rosina Pellerano, MD, specializes in the medical care of disordered eating, from anorexia to obesity. She received medical training in Bridgeport Hospital and Yale New Haven Hospital in Connecticut, as well as an Adolescent and Young Adult Medicine Fellowship at George Washington University in DC. Dr. Pellerano was a George Mason University Student Health Center physician and has been a University of Miami Student Health Center physician for nine years. Through her clinical nutrition training at the Integrative Medicine Department of the University of Miami, she approaches her patients through nutritional healing. Dr. Pellerano has seen firsthand how the food you eat is a direct expression of well-being. Culinary medicine is her passion. She assists with meal support at the Jeremiah 29:11 Eating Disorder support group every week.

About the Contributors

Jessica Spain, research assistant. A green-living advocate and reformed globetrotter, Jessica is currently all about sharing the joys of a vegan diet through awareness and education. She tables at health fairs, leaflets at events, and collaborates with groups from EarthSave to the Humane League, showing people how a vegan lifestyle is a win-win-win for health, animal welfare, and the planet. Formerly working with refugees and asylum seekers, Jessica has traversed Brooklyn, East Africa, India, Sri Lanka, the United Kingdom, Los Angeles, and now—settled in Miami.

Ashley Boudet, ND, research and editing. Ashley Boudet is a naturopathic doctor who trained in primary care medicine at the National College of Natural Medicine in Oregon. Her extensive study of wellness, yoga, nutrition, and plant medicine have all contributed to an expanded vision of health and compassion toward all beings. She is committed to promoting a connection to nature as the pathway to healing ourselves and our planet, and enjoys supporting others on their own personal quests. www.doctorandchef.com

Elizabeth Arraj, recipe tester and food photographer. Elizabeth Arraj has trained under award winning Vegan Fusion chef Mark Reinfeld. She has received the T. Colin Campbell Center for Nutrition Studies Certificate in Plant-Based Nutrition. She teaches plant-based culinary classes at her local community college where she loves to inspire people how to cook nutrient beneficial foods. etar73@hotmail.com

Roland Barker, recipe tester. Roland is inspired by nature's abundance and ability to nourish and heal us, and as a cook, he tries to add to that his intention for healing and joy in the preparation of natural, whole foods. Xnau Web design: www.xnau.com

Jennifer Mennuti, recipe tester. Jennifer is an animal advocate focused on education and inspiration. She hosts monthly vegan events and parties to share her passion for delicious plant based foods and coordinates an outreach table weekly to raise awareness for nonprofit animal advocacy organizations.

Lisa Parker, recipe tester. An alchemist at heart, Lisa loves plants, colors, flavors, textures, and smells. She loves measuring and stirring and filling the kitchen with delectable fragrances. These days she cooks a lot for friends and family, has a botanical body product business, and works with her husband to create a tropical food forest and sanctuary at their home on Kaua'i. www.greensongbotanicals.com

Lisa Portnoff, recipe tester. Having eaten and cooked vegetarian, vegan, and raw foods for many years, Lisa finally devoted herself to the culinary world after a long, successful career as a ceramic and textile artist. She completed the New School Culinary Program in NYC, studied at the Natural Gourmet Institute, the Institute of Culinary Education, and is a proud Certified Vegan Fusion Chef. She has worked as a chef, caterer, personal chef, cooking instructor, and recipe tester and developer, and is now studying to become a holistic nutrition therapist. lisaportnoff@hotmail.com

Suzanne Rudolph, recipe tester. Suzanne is an avid world traveler with a lifelong passion for food. Her palate has been strongly influenced by the cuisines she has eaten while on trips to over thirty countries. Suzanne divides her time between catering and teaching classes for home cooks at the Auguste Escoffier School of Culinary Arts in Boulder, Colorado. www.rudy mademeals.com and http://www.examiner .com/user-suzannerudolph

Ami Lawson, food photographer. Ami is an artist and photographer with over twenty years' experience exploring animal friendly land-scapes of edible plants and gourmet cuisine through her camera lens. As an educator and advocate, she creates adventures and shines her light for others to see life simply through nature. www.EarthAngelOutreach.org

Erik Rudolph, food photographer. Erik Ru-dolph is a traveler, photographer, and glutton for good food. He currently resides in Boulder, Colorado, with his wife and culinary goddess, Suzanne.

Vegan Fusion Culinary Immersions

Hungry for more? Consider attending an immersion or workshop with Mark Reinfeld. Interested in teaching vegan and raw food classes in your community? Beginning courses as well as advanced teacher training courses are offered internationally and online at www.veganfusion.com.

Prepare to transform your life as you immerse yourself in the world of vegan and raw food cuisine!

Whether you are a trained chef, foodie, novice, or homemaker, we guarantee that you will learn the skills to create a lifetime of health:

- Experience greater confidence in the kitchen.
- Learn new tips and tricks that will greatly enhance your culinary abilities.
- Connect with others who share a similar interest in vegan and raw foods.

- Deepen your knowledge of the healing qualities of vegan foods.
- Discover new ideas for presentation that will transform an ordinary meal into a gourmet experience.

Topics include Vegan Soups; Salads & Dressings; the World of Grains and Beans; Tofu, Tempeh & Seitan Dishes; Casseroles and Sauces; Wraps, Spreads, Sandwiches and Rolls; Vegan Desserts; Raw Cuisine 1-Smoothies, Pâtés, Pasta and Pudding; Raw Cuisine 2-Elixirs, Soups, Plant Cheeses, Ravioli, Lasagna, Parfaits, and Ice Cream; Raw Cuisine 3-Nut and Seed Milks, Granola, Pizza, Tacos, and Live Pies.

The 5-day and 10-day Vegan Fusion Culinary Immersion includes daily gourmet vegan feasts and the Vegan Fusion Cuisine Chef Training manual , and is level one in Vegan Fusion Chef Certification process.

Index

A

Academy of Nutrition and Dietetics (American Dietetic Association), 22, 41, 43
Açai
  Açai Power Bowl/variations, 120
  Açai Spritzer/variations, 142–143
Addiction and food industry, xii, 20, 25, 35–36, 37
Advanced glycation end-products (AGEs), 34
Adventist Health Study, 15
Advertising and diet, 20
Adzuki (aduki) beans
  cooking, 98
  Simple One-Pot Meal, 266–267
Agatston, Arthur, 30
Agave nectar
  description/controversy, 89
  sugar replacement amount, 89
AGEs (advanced glycation end-products), 34
Alcohol consumption, 3, 4, 68, 74, 75–76
Alkaline diet, 26
Almonds
  Almond Butter Chocolate Chip Cookies, 310–311
  Almond Dipping Sauce/variations, 233–234
  Cauliflower Steak with Ethiopian-Spiced Almonds/variations, 200–201
  nutrition, 51–52
Amaranth
  cooking, 96
  nutrition, 53
  Quinoa Amaranth Cakes/variations, 168–169
American Cancer Society, 11
American College of Cardiology, 8
American Diabetes Association, 7, 29
American Dietetic Association (Academy of Nutrition and Dietetics), 22, 41, 43
American Heart Association, 8, 41–42
American Journal of Clinical Nutrition, 12
American Journal of Health Promotion, 17

Anasazi beans, cooking, 98
Anatomy of Hope, The (Groopman), xviii
Ancho Chile Sauce/variations, 232–233
Angiogenesis inhibitors, 10
Anti-Candida diet, 27
Anti-inflammatory (wellness) diet, 26
Antiaging components, 10
Antibiotics
  dietary and, 34
  use consequences, 27
Antioxidants
  plant-based diet and, 9, 10, 11, 12–13, 41, 43
  See also specific foods
Appetizers. See Snacks, savory/appetizers
Apples
  apple seeds toxicity, 134
  nutrition, 49
  overview/types, 302
  Raw Apple Crumble/variations, 300–301
Apricots
  Apricot Oat Bars/variations, 308
  nutrition, 43
  Raw Apricot Fennel Granola/variations, 121–122
Arame
  Edamame Arame Salad/variations, 198–199
  nutrition, 86
Art of Prolonging Human Life, The (Hufeland), 32
Artichoke
  Broiled Artichoke Fritters/variations, 155
  Grilled Artichoke, 154
  how to eat, 152
  Lemon Garlic Steamed Artichokes with Simple Dipping Sauce/variations, 153–154
  White Bean Artichoke Dip with Arugula/variations, 155–156
Artificial sweeteners, 38, 76
Arugula, White Bean Artichoke Dip with Arugula/variations, 155–156

Asparagus
  Chili Lime Grilled Asparagus with
    Mushrooms and Bell Pepper/variations,
    193–194
  Creamy Asparagus Soup with Corn/
    variations, 250
Atkins diet, 29, 30
Atkins, Robert C., 30
Avocado
  Avocado Mousse-Stuffed Tomatoes/variation,
    152–153
  Glorious Guacamole/variation, 151–152
  Oil-Free Avocado Dressing, 225
  Tomato Avocado Salad/variations, 183–184
Ayurvedic diet/recommendations, 26–27, 139

B.
Bacon, Coco Bacon/variation, 112
Baking/dessert pantry ingredients, 84
Baking sheets, 83
Balsamic Reduction, 109
Bananas
  Banana Date Breakfast Muffins/variations,
    122–123
  Banana Mango Ice Cream/variations, 298
  Crazy Good Banana Chocolate Treat, 306
Bariatrics, 13
Barley
  barley malt syrup, 89
  cooking, 96
  nutrition/types, 53
  Pearled Barley with Mushrooms and Corn/
    variations, 210
Barnard, Neal, 7, 14, 21
Basil
  Basil Rose Lemonade/variations, 141–142
  Fire-Roasted Tomato Sauce/variations,
    239–240
BBQ
  BBQ Roasted Tofu with Collards/variations,
    278–279
  Smoky BBQ Sauce, 231–232
Beans
  Collards and Red Beans, 191
  Curried Broccoli Soup with Great Northern
    Beans/variations, 253–254

Green Beans with White Bean Fennel Sauce/
  variations, 217–218
Mexican Two-Bean Soup/variations, 256–
  257
Roasted Veggies and Beans/variations,
  267–268
White Bean Artichoke Dip with Arugula/
  variations, 155–156
See also specific types
Beet greens nutrition, 45
Beets nutrition, 44–45
Berbere/Ethiopian Spice Mix, 106
Berries
  Berry Green Smoothie, 147
  nutrition overview, 49
  See also specific types
Beverages
  meal plans and, 70–73
  overview/recipes, 132–149
  quicker and easier, 140, 141
  recommendations/water and, 76, 132
  starting your day and, 132, 140
  Ultimate Hangover Cure, 135
  See also Elixirs; Juices/juicing; Smoothies;
    Teas
Biology of Belief, The (Lipton), xviii
Black beans
  Black Bean and Corn Salad, 189
  Black Bean Grits/variations, 272–273
  Black Bean Tostones/variations, 167–168
  cooking, 98
  Fruit-Sweetened Black Bean Brownies/
    variations, 312–313
  Millet Black Bean Veggie Burgers/variations,
    269–270
  nutrition, 55
Black-eyed peas, cooking, 98
Blackburn, Elizabeth, 15
Blackstrap molasses, 43, 89
Blender, 82
"Bliss point" term and food industry, 20, 35
Blood types and diet, 39
Blue Zone, 74
Blueberries, Lemon Blueberry Pancakes/
  variations, 123–124
BMI (body mass index), 13

Bok choy
    nutrition, 45
    Steamed Italian Baby Bok Choy/variations,
        196–197
Bone health and diet, 42
Brand-Miller, Jennie, 29
Brazil nuts
    Brazil Nut Milk, 104
    nutrition, 52, 104, 111
    Raw Brazil Nut Parmesan, 111
    Raw Carrot Brazil Nut Soup, 245–246
Bread recommendations, 84
Breakfast
    meal plans and, 70–73
    overview/recipes, 117–131
    quick breakfasts, 117
    See also specific recipes
Breastfeeding and vitamins, 23
British Medical Journal, 18
Broccoli
    Broccoli Dill Quiche/variation, 274–276
    Curried Broccoli Soup with Great Northern
        Beans/variations, 253–254
    Millet and Butternut Squash with Broccoli/
        variations, 284–285
    nutrition, 45
    Spaghetti Squash with Broccoli/variations,
        207–208
Broccoli Rabe Penne Pasta with Oil-Free Cream
        Sauce/variations, 292–293
Broth, Healing Broth/variations, 243
Brown rice
    cooking, 96
    Golden Rice/variations, 204–205
    Maca Horchata/variations, 147–148
    nutrition, 53
    Unfried Rice/variations, 205–206
Brown rice syrup, 89
Brownies, Fruit-Sweetened Black Bean
        Brownies/variations, 312–313
Bruschetta, Okra Bruschetta/variations, 162–
        163
Brussels Sprouts, Broasted Brussels Sprouts/
        variations, 194
Buckwheat
    cooking, 96

Crunchy Chocolate Buckwheat Clusters/
        variations, 299–300
    Mushroom Kasha/variations, 213–214
    nutrition, 53
Bulgur, cooking, 97
Burgers. See Veggie burgers

C
Cabbage (green/red) nutrition, 45
Cacao nutrition, 57–58
Cacao powder
    Choco-Chia Pudding/variations, 295–296
    Raw Chocolate Pudding/variations, 296–297
Caesar Dressing/variation, 225
Caesar Salad/variations, 181
Caesar's Restaurant, 181
Cake, Raw Carrot Ginger Cake/variations,
        309–310
Calcium sources, 42
Campbell, T. Colin, 7, 12, 19
Campbell, Thomas M., 12, 19
Cancer
    as chronic disease, 19
    definition/description, 9–10, 11
    overview, 9–13
    plant-based diet and, 10, 11, 12–13
    treatment, 11
Candida albicans, 27
Capers, 84
Cardini, Caesar, 181
Cardiovascular disease. See Heart disease
Carrots
    Raw Carrot Brazil Nut Soup, 245–246
    Raw Carrot Ginger Cake/variations, 309–310
    Sunrise Carrot Juice/variations, 137
Casein protein, 13
Cashews
    Cashew Cream Frosting, 309
    Cashew Ricotta Cheese, 283
    nutrition, 52
    Raw Cashew Sour Cream/variation, 113
    Strawberry Cashew Cream/variations, 297
    Truffled Cashew Cheese/variation, 159–160
Casserole dishes, 83
Cast-iron skillets, 43
Catsup, Homemade, 110–111

Cauliflower
   Broiled Cauliflower with Sun-Dried Tomatoes/
      variations, 194–195
   Buffalo Cauliflower/variations, 163–164
   Cauliflower Casserole/variations, 285–286
   Cauliflower Steak with Ethiopian-Spiced
      Almonds/variations, 200–201
   Mushroom Cauliflower Tacos/variations,
      277–278
   Smashed Roasted Cauliflower and Parsnip/
      variations, 202
Cayenne pepper nutrition, 56
CDC. *See* Centers for Disease Control (CDC)
Celiac disease, xvi, 28
Centers for Disease Control (CDC)
   on cancer, 11
   on diabetes, 6
   on heart disease, 4–5
Chard
   Ginger Rainbow Chard/variations, 189–190
   nutrition, 45–46
   Three Greens with Tomato Sauce/variations,
      197
Cheese, commercial Parmesan cheese, 111
Cheese (vegan)
   Cashew Ricotta Cheese, 283
   Easy Cheezy Sauce/variations, 233
   pantry and, 87–88
   Raw Brazil Nut Parmesan, 111
   Soft Plant-Based Cheeses template recipe, 160
   Truffled Cashew Cheese/variation, 159–160
Chewing importance, 139
Chia seeds
   Chia Pudding template recipe, 117
   Choco-Chia Pudding/variations, 295–296
   nutrition, 50
   Simple Breakfast Chia Pudding, 117
Chickpeas. *See* Garbanzo beans (chickpeas)
Chiffonade described, 95
Childhood obesity, 13
Chimichurri, Zesty Chimichurri Sauce/
      variation, 231
China Study, The (Campbell and Campbell)
   description, 12–13
   diseases of affluence/poverty and, 19
   healing story, 7

Chinese cuisine spices, 85–85
CHIP (Complete Health Improvement Program),
   xiv, xix, 21
Chipotle chili powder, 85
Chlorella nutrition, 58
Chocolate chips (vegan)
   Almond Butter Chocolate Chip Cookies,
      310–311
   Chocolate Dipping Sauce, 304
   Chocolate Pecan Dipped Fruit/variations,
      304–305
   Crazy Good Banana Chocolate Treat, 306
   Crunchy Chocolate Buckwheat Clusters/
      variations, 299–300
   melting, 300
Cholesterol
   diet and, 5, 8–9, 21, 23, 42
   functions, 8
   healing story, 9
   high cholesterol health risks, 8, 9, 21
   high cholesterol treatment, 8–9
   overview, 8–9
   types, 8
Chop described, 95
Chronic diseases description/examples, 19
Chutney
   Cilantro Mint Chutney/variations, 229–230
   Gold Bar Squash Chutney/variations, 161–
      162
Cilantro
   Cilantro Lime Vinaigrette/variations, 221–
      222
   Cilantro Mint Chutney/variations, 229–230
Cinnamon nutrition, 56
Citrus fruits
   nutrition overview, 49–50
   See also specific types
Citrus juicer, 82
Citrus Magic/variations, 137–138
"Clean 15"/"Dirty Dozen," 61, 216
Clinical Wellness Programs, 341–343
Cleansing
   Galactic Green Juice, 135
   Green Master Cleanse/variations, 138
   juices and, 139
   overview, xix–xx

Cobbler
    Fruit Cobbler Template recipe, 312
    Fruit-Sweetened Pistachio Peach Cobbler, 311
Coco Bacon/variation, 112
Cocoa powder, Choco-Maca Elixir/variations,
    145
Coconut
    coconut crystals, 89
    coconut milk, 85
    coconut oil, 85
    Pecan Coconut Topping, 304
    Raw Coconut Curry Sauce/variations, 237–238
    Raw Coconut Curry Vegetables, 268–269
Collards
    BBQ Roasted Tofu with Collards/variations,
        278–279
    Collards and Red Beans, 191
    nutrition, 46
    Raw Collard Veggie Rolls/variations, 260
    Three Greens with Tomato Sauce/variations,
        197
Color
    phytonutrients and, 13, 17
    selecting in diet, 75
Colorectal cancer, 11, 13, 40–41, 53
Community/socializing importance, xvii–xviii,
    xx, 14, 74
Community-supported agriculture programs
    (CSAs), xvii
Complete Health Improvement Program (CHIP),
    xv–xx, 21, 341
Complete Idiot's Guide to Eating Raw, The
    (Reinfeld), 63
Composting, 92
Condiments
    pantry and, 87, 108–115
    superfood condiments, 87
    transitional condiments, 88
Congees
    Congee with Fenugreek/variations, 247–249
    description, 242
Cookies/bars
    Almond Butter Chocolate Chip Cookies,
        310–311
    Cranberry Walnut Power Krispy Bars/
        variations, 305–306

Crunchy Chocolate Buckwheat Clusters/
    variations, 299–300
Simple Cookie template recipe, 310
Corn
    Black Bean and Corn Salad, 189
    Corn Casserole/variations, 286–287
    Creamy Asparagus Soup with Corn/
        variations, 250
    Pearled Barley with Mushrooms and Corn/
        variations, 210
    Roasted Zucchini and Corn/variations, 192
Cornmeal, cooking, 96
Couscous
    cooking, 96
    Israeli Couscous Tabouli/variations, 203
    nutrition, 53
Cousens, Gabriel, 6, 63
Cracked wheat, cooking, 97
Cranberry Walnut Power Krispy Bars/variations,
    305–306
Croutons, Herb Croutons/variations, 111–112
CSAs (community-supported agriculture
    programs), xvii
Cube described, 95
Cucumber
    Asian Cucumber Salad/variations, 175
    green juices and, 135–136
    hydration and, 135, 136
    Raw Cucumber Fennel Soup/variations,
        244–245
Cultured (fermented) food
    overview/nutrition, 58, 66–67
    raw foods and, 66–67
    tips, 178
    See also specific foods; specific recipes
Currants, Watercress with Pistachios and
    Currants/variations, 179
Curry
    Curried Broccoli Soup with Great Northern
        Beans/variations, 253–254
    Curried Crispy Chickpeas/variations, 154
    Curried Garbanzo Cakes with Poppy Seeds/
        variations, 164–165
    Curry Kale Salad/variations, 184–185
    Raw Coconut Curry Sauce/variations, 237–238
    Raw Coconut Curry Vegetables, 268–269

Curry (*continued*)

    Simple Curry Dressing, 185

    Thai Curry Vegetables/variations, 289–290

Cutting board recommendation, 81

D

Dairy myth, 42

Dash (dietary approaches to stop hypertension) diet, 32

Date sugar, 89

Date Syrup, 88

Dates

    Banana Date Breakfast Muffins/variations, 122–123

    Date Glazed Sweet Potatoes/variations, 208–209

    overview/types, 125

Davis, Brenda, 25, 74–77

Davis, William, 28

Dehydrated foods, 35, 68

Dehydrator, 82

Dessert/baking pantry ingredients, 84

Desserts/sweet snacks

    meal plans and, 70–73

    overview/recipes, 294–313

    See also specific recipes

Diabetes

    Barnard's program/outcomes, 7

    as chronic disease, 19

    description, 6, 19

    GEICO employees study/outcomes, 17

    healing stories, 7–8, 64–65

    overview, 6–8

    plant-based diet/lifestyle and, 6–7, 17, 21

    statistics, 6, 19

    Tree of Life program/outcomes, 6–7

Dice described, 95

Diehl, Hans, xiv, 14, 19–21

Diet composition

    advertising and, 20

    American diet changes over time/disease consequences, 20–21

    developing countries/changes over time, 19–20

    empty-calories and, 16, 20

    foods-as-grown and, 19–20

Diet for a New America, A (Robbins), 14

Diet industry, 37

Dietitians of Canada, 22–23

Diets

    low-carb diets, 30–32

    opinions and, 24

    overview, 25–36, 38–39

    See also specific diets

Digest Aid Juice/variations, 136–137

Dill, Broccoli Dill Quiche/variation, 274–276

Dinner

    meal plans and, 70–73

    See also Main dishes

Dipping sauces

    Almond Dipping Sauce/variations, 233–234

    Chocolate Dipping Sauce, 304

    Creamy Mexican Dipping Sauce/variations, 234–235

    Simple Artichoke Dipping Sauce/variations, 153–154

Dips, White Bean Artichoke Dip with Arugula/variations, 155–156

"Dirty Dozen"/"Clean 15," 61, 216

Diseases

    of dietary excess, 4

    preventable diseases and, xi–xiii, 3–21, 23, 34, 74

    preventable diseases and economics, 4, 19–20

    See also specific diseases

Disordered eating, 37

Dopamine, 36

Dressings

    Oil-Free Papaya Salad Dressing/variations, 176

    Oil-Free Provençal Dressing/variation, 183

    overview/recipes, 219–229

    Simple Balsamic Dressing, 179–180

    Simple Curry Dressing, 185

    Tahini Dijon Dressing, 187

    Waldorf Dressing/variations, 180–181

    See also specific recipes

Drinks. *See* Beverages; *specific types/recipes*

E

Eat to Live (Fuhrman), 6

Edamame, Edamame Arame Salad/variations, 198–199

Eggplant, Grilled Eggplant Towers with Cashew Ricotta/variations, 282–284
80/10/10 diet (low-fat raw vegan diet), 38–39
Elixirs
    Choco-Maca Elixir/variations, 145
    Flu Buster/variations, 140–141
    Ginger Turmeric Shooter/variations, 140
    Noni-Shot, 141
    See also Cleansing
Emotional health imbalances. *See* Mental/ emotional health imbalances
End of Overeating, The (Kessler), 35
Energy balls
    Raw Energy Balls template recipe, 299
    Raw Hemp Energy Balls, 298–299
Environmental impacts
    diet and, xii, xvii, 14, 22, 60, 61
    organic vs. nonorganic food, 60, 76
    See also Local foods importance
Environmental Working Group (EWG), 61, 76
Enzyme Nutrition (Howell), 65
Enzymes and raw (living foods) diet, 65–66
Epilepsy, refractory, 29
Erewhon Market, 32
Esselstyn, Caldwell, Jr., 5, 14, 15, 21, 34, 36
Ethiopian Spice Mix/Berbere, 106
Exercise
    benefits, xvii–xviii, 6, 10, 13
    diabetes and, 6
    IGF-1 levels and, 10
    overview, xvii–xviii

F

Factory farms, 20
Fajitas, Tempeh Fajitas/variations, 279–280
Falafel, Baked Falafel/variations, 262–263
Farro
    cooking, 96
    nutrition, 54
Fast foods, xii, 20, 25, 37, 64, 68
Fat types summary, 42
Fats, plant-based diets overview, 17
Fava beans nutrition, 55
Fennel/fennel seeds
    Green Beans with White Bean Fennel Sauce/ variations, 217–218

Raw Apricot Fennel Granola/variations, 121–122
Raw Cucumber Fennel Soup/variations, 244–245
Sun-Dried Tomato Fennel Breakfast Tart/ variations, 129–130
Fenugreek nutrition, 56–57
Fermented food. *See* Cultured (fermented) food
Fiber
    benefits/plant-based diet, xii, 9, 10, 13, 17, 19, 23, 25, 40–41, 42
    processing/refinement and, 20
    recommended amounts, 40
Figs, Sunflower Seed Fig Puree, 118–119
Flax oil, Simple Flax or Hemp Oil Dressing/ variations, 221
Flaxseeds
    Lemon Blueberry Pancakes/variations, 123–124
    nutrition, 50
    pantry and, 85
Flour
    Gluten-Free Flour Mix, 105
    recommendations, 84
Flu Buster/variations, 140–141
Food preparation tips, 91–92
Food processor, 82
Food relationship overviews, 37, 76–77
Fritters, Broiled Artichoke Fritters/variations, 155
Frosting, Cashew Cream Frosting, 309
Fructose consumption, 38
Fruit
    Chocolate Pecan Dipped Fruit/variations, 304–305
    daily servings/benefits, 18
    dried fruits for pantry, 85
    Fruit Cobbler template recipe, 312
    fruit syrup, 88, 89
    Grilled Fruit, 304
    Herb and Fruit Water, 140
    Mixed Fruit Kanten/variations, 301–302
    nutrition, 49–50
    Rainbow Fruit and Créme/variations, 118
    Raw Breakfast Seed and Fruit Puree template recipe, 119

Fruit (*continued*)
    Trifecta Stewed Dried Fruit/variations, 121
    See also Smoothies; *specific types*
Fuhrman, Joel, 6, 16

G

GAPS (Gut and Psychology Syndrome) Diet,
    27–28
Garbanzo beans (chickpeas)
    cooking, 98
    Curried Crispy Chickpeas/variations, 154
    Curried Garbanzo Cakes with Poppy Seeds/
        variations, 164–165
    Kalamata Rosemary Hummus/variations,
        157–159
    Moroccan Chickpea Stew/variations, 255–256
    nutrition, 55
    Quinoa Chickpea Pilaf/variations, 211
Garlic
    Garlicky Greens/variations, 191–192
    Lemon Garlic Steamed Artichokes with
        Simple Dipping Sauce/variations, 153–154
    nutrition, 57, 114
    Roasted Garlic Spread/variations, 114–115
    Wasabi Garlic Twice-Baked Potatoes/
        variations, 209–210
Garlic press, 82
Gazpacho, Watermelon Gazpacho/variation,
    243–244
GEICO employees study/outcomes, 17–18
Ginger
    Ginger Rainbow Chard/variations, 189–190
    Ginger Turmeric Shooter/variations, 140
    nutrition, 57
    Raw Carrot Ginger Cake/variations, 309–310
GL (glycemic load), 29
Global Burden of Disease Project, 12
Gluten
    celiac disease and, xvi, 28
    description, xvi
    health issues, 28
Gluten-free
    diet overview, xvi, 28
    Flour Mix, 105
    label meaning, 28
Glycemic index/diet, 28–29, 31

Glycemic load (GL), 29
GMO (genetically engineered/modified
    organism)
    assassin seeds, 60–61
    labeling and, 61–62
    overview, 60–62
    website, 62
Goji berries nutrition, 58
Graham, Doug, 38–39
Grain Brain (Perlmutter), 28
Grains
    cooking/charts, 95–97
    Grain Vegetable Dish template recipe, 213
    nutrition overview, 53–55
    pantry and, 85
    toasting, 101–102
    See also specific types
Granola
    Homemade Granola template recipe, 126
    Pepita Pecan Granola/variations, 124–125
    Raw Apricot Fennel Granola/variations,
        121–122
Gravy, Oil-Free Mushroom Gravy/variations,
    240–241
Great northern beans
    cooking, 98
    nutrition, 55
Green beans
    Green Beans with White Bean Fennel Sauce/
        variations, 217–218
    nutrition, 46
Green coffee, 50
Green juice
    fasting and, 6
    See also Juices/juicing
Greens
    Garlicky Greens/variations, 191–192
    nutrition overview, 45, 46, 47, 49
    Simple Green Sauté template recipe, 190
    Three Greens with Tomato Sauce/variations,
        197
    See also specific types
Greger, Michael, 10, 12, 23, 34, 57
Grilling
    Chili Lime Grilled Asparagus with Mushrooms
        and Bell Pepper/variations, 193–194

Grilled Artichoke, 154
Grilled Eggplant Towers with Cashew
    Ricotta/variations, 282–284
Grilled Fruit, 304
Grilled Mediterranean Vegetables and
    Quinoa/variations, 212–213
Grilled Plantain Kebabs/variations, 166–167
overview, 101
Grits
    Black Bean Grits/variations, 272–273
    Multigrain Grits/variation, 126–127
Groopman, Jerome, xviii
Guacamole, Glorious Guacamole/variation,
    151–152
Gut and Psychology Syndrome (GAPS) Diet,
    27–28
Gut flora
    ensuring healthy microbiome, 75–76
    overview, 75–76

H

Haas, Sidney Valentine, 27–28
Hangover Cure, Ultimate, 135
Hartzler, Geoffrey, 14
Hash, Purple Potato Tempeh Hash/variations,
    130–131
Hay, William Howard, 26
Healing stories
    arthritis (DISH), 64–65
    China Study, The, 7
    diabetes, 7–8, 64–65
    heart disease, 5–6
    high cholesterol, 9
    juices/juicing, 67–68
    obesity/overweight issues, 16
    raw (living foods) diet, 64–65, 67–68
Health behavior importance, 3–4
Health Via Food and Weight Control in the 1920s
    and '30s (Hay), 26
Healthy life
    precepts for (overview), xvii–xx
    See also Plant-based whole food diet
Heart disease
    CDC on, 4–5
    as chronic disease, 19
    cultures not having/diets, 5

examples of ailments, 4
healing story, 5–6
overview, 4–6
plant-based diet/lifestyle and, 5, 14–15, 21, 23
recommendations, 5
statistics, 4–5
website/blog resources, 14
Hearts of palm
    Quinoa Amaranth Cakes/variations, 168–169
    sustainable harvesting and, 169
Heavy metals, xix, 34
Hemp oil, Simple Flax or Hemp Oil Dressing/
    variations, 221
Hemp seeds (hearts)
    nutrition, 50–51
    Raw Hemp Energy Balls, 298–299
    Raw Hempseed Ranch Dressing/variations,
        224–225
    Sesame Hemp Revitalizer/variations, 145–146
Herbs
    Creamy Herbed Polenta/variations, 170–171
    dried/fresh herbs substitution, 85
    Herb and Fruit Water, 140
    Herb Croutons/variations, 111–112
    Herb-Roasted Potatoes/variations, 214–215
    Herbes de Provence Spice Mix, 106–107
    Herbs and Fruit Water, 140
    herbs/spices nutrition overview, 56–57
    pantry and, 85, 87
    See also specific types
Hever, Julieanna, 33, 40–43
Hierarchy of human needs, xx
Hippocrates, 50, 114, 221
Horseradish Dijon Dressing/variations, 226
Howell, Edward, 65–66
Hufeland, Christoph Wilhelm, 32
Hummus
    Hummus (Bean Puree) template recipe, 159
    Kalamata Rosemary Hummus/variations,
        157–159
Hyperlipidemia (high cholesterol), 8

I

IARC Group 1 meaning/examples, 11
IARC Group 2A meaning/example, 11
IARC Working Group, 11

Ice cream, Banana Mango Ice Cream/variations, 298

IGF-1
  cancer and, 10, 12
  diet and, 10, 12
  function, 10, 12

IGF-1 binding protein, 10, 12

Indian Spice Mix, 106

Infectious disease, 3

Inflammation
  problems/consequences, 26, 28
  role, 26

Instinct to Heal, The (Servan-Schreiber), xviii

Intensive therapeutic lifestyle change (ITLC)
  programs, 21

International Data Corporation, 3-4

Iodine, 23

Iron
  sources, 42-43
  summary, 42-43

Irritable bowel syndrome (IBS), 28, 31-32

Ital Roasted Squash and Sweet Potato Soup/
  variations, 251-252

Italian Spice Mix, 105

Italian Spring Vegetable Stew/variations,
  252-253

ITLC (Intensive therapeutic lifestyle change)
  programs, 21

J

Jalapeño peppers/Scoville scale, 109, 179

Jamaican Patties/variations, 280-281

Jenkins, David J., 29

Journal of Epidemiology & Community Health,
  18

Journal of the American Medical Association,
  13, 30

Juicers
  brands/recommendations, 65, 82
  citrus juicer, 82

Juices/juicing
  Citrus Magic/variations, 137-138
  cleanses and, 139
  Digest Aid Juice/variations, 136-137
  Galactic Green Juice, 135
  Green Juice template recipe, 136

healing story, 67-68
  peel and, 134
  raw foods and, 67
  smoothies vs., 139
  Sunrise Carrot Juice/variations, 137
  tips on, 134

Julienne described, 95

K

Kahn, Joel, 14-15

Kale
  Cream of Kale/variations, 201
  Curry Kale Salad/variations, 184-185
  Kale Kolada/variations, 143
  Kale Salad template recipes, 184
  Lemon Tempeh with Kale and Rice Noodles/
    variations, 276-277
  nutrition, 46
  Ranch Kale Salad/variations, 185-186
  Sesame Kale Salad/variations, 186-187
  Three Greens with Tomato Sauce/variations,
    197

Kamut, cooking, 96

Kasha, Mushroom Kasha/variations, 213-214

Kebabs, Grilled Plantain Kebabs/variations,
  166-167

Kelp granules/flakes, 59, 86

Ketogenic diet, 29-30

Ketosis, 29

Kidney beans
  cooking, 98
  nutrition, 55

Kimchi, Quick Kimchi/variations, 178

Kitchari/variations, 257-258

Kitchen gear overview, 81-83

Knife cuts, 95

Knives, 81

Kombu, 86

Kordich, Jay, 67

Kushi, Michio, 32

L

Lancet, The, 14

Lavender tips, 142

LDH cholesterol, 8

LDL cholesterol, 8

"Leaky gut," 27
Legumes
  benefits, 17
  cooking/chart, 97–98
  improving digestion/reducing gas, 97
  Legume and Vegetable Salad template recipe,
    188–189
  nutrition overview, 55–56
  pantry and, 85
  soaking, 97
  See also specific types
Lemon
  Creamy Lemon Tahini Dressing/variations,
    228–229
  Lemon Blueberry Pancakes/variations,
    123–124
  Lemon Dijon Marinade, 107
  Lemon Garlic Steamed Artichokes with
    Simple Dipping Sauce/variations, 153–154
  Lemon Tempeh with Kale and Rice Noodles/
    variations, 276–277
Lemonade, Basil Rose Lemonade/variations,
  141–142
Lentils
  cooking, 98
  Creamy Lentil Saag/variations, 290–291
  Lentil Walnut Loaf, 288
  nutrition, 55–56
Lettuce, Veggie Lettuce Boats/variations,
  160–161
Leukemia, 9, 11
LFD (low FODMAP diet), 28, 31–32
Lifestyle Heart Trial, 14
Lifestyle Medicine Institute, 21
Lima beans, cooking, 98
Lime
  Chili Lime Grilled Asparagus with
    Mushrooms and Bell Pepper/variations,
    193–194
  Cilantro Lime Vinaigrette/variations, 221–222
Lipton, Bruce, xviii
Liquid smoke, 85
Living foods diet. *See* Raw/living foods diet
Local foods importance, xvii, 33, 44, 48, 54, 60,
  74, 76, 77, 83, 269, 298
Love, Medicine, and Miracles (Siegel), xviii

Low-fat raw vegan (80/10/10) diet, 38–39
Low-fat Swank diet, 36
Low FODMAP diet (LFD), 28, 31–32
Low-sodium diet
  overview, xv–xvi, 32
  Salt-Free Seasoning, 108–109
  SOS (No salt, oil, sugar) diet, 35–36
Lucuma powder, 89
Lunch
  meal plans and, 70–73
  See also specific food types/recipes
Luo han, 38
Lustig, Robert, 38

       M
Maca
  Choco-Maca Elixir/variations, 145
  Maca Horchata/variations, 147–148
  nutrition, 58–59
Macadamia nuts, Oil-Free Macadamia Wasabi
    Dressing/variations, 226–227
McBride, Natasha Campbell, 27, 28
McDougall, John, 14, 36, 38
Macrobiotic diet, 32–33
Macronutrients summary, 40, 74
Magnesium/benefits, 17
Main dishes
  meal plans and, 70–73
  overview/recipes, 259–293
  See also specific recipes
Mango, Banana Mango Ice Cream/variations,
  298
Maple Baked Tempeh/variations, 262
Maple Balsamic Marinade, 107
Maple syrup, 89
Marinades
  about, 107
  for Chili Lime Grilled Asparagus with
    Mushrooms and Bell Pepper/variations,
    193–194
  Kebab Marinade/variations, 166
  Lemon Dijon Marinade, 107
  Maple Balsamic Marinade, 107
  recipes/pantry and, 107
Maslow, Abraham, xx
Mayo clinic, xviii

Mayonnaise
  pantry and, 88
  Vegan Mayonnaise/variation, 113–114
Meal plans
  fourteen day plan, 71–73
  overview, 70
Measurement conversions
  metric conversion chart, 318
  tablespoons/cup, 99
  tablespoons/teaspoons, 99
Measuring cups, 82
Measuring spoons, 82
Meat
  cancer and, 11–13, 34
  fat source/disease consequences, 20–21
  government subsidies and, 20
  processed meat/health problems, 11, 12
Medicare, 14, 23
Medicine
  nutritional counseling and, xi
  from plants, 23
Meditation, xix
Mediterranean diet, 33
Mental/emotional health imbalances
  overview, 16–18
  plant-based diet benefits, 16–18
Methionine, 10
Metric conversion chart, 318
Mexican Spice Mix, 106
Milk
  Brazil Nut Milk, 104
  Gold Milk/variations, 144–145
  High-Protein Vanilla Almond Shake/
    variations, 148–149
  nut-milk bags, 82
  for pantry, 85
  Plant-Based Milk template recipe, 104
  Quinoa Milk/variations, 143–144
Millet
  cooking, 96
  Millet and Butternut Squash with Broccoli/
    variations, 284–285
  Millet Black Bean Veggie Burgers/variations,
    269–270
  nutrition, 54

Mince described, 95
Mind-body types (Ayurvedic diet), 26–27
Mindful eating, 76–77
Minerals, trace, 17
Mint, Cilantro Mint Chutney/variations,
    229–230
Mirin, 85
Miso
  Miso Vegetable Soup/variations, 246–247
  overview, 248
  paste, 85, 248
Mixing bowls, 82
Monk Bowl, 94, 267
Moringa nutrition, 59
Moroccan Spice Mix, 106
Muffins, Banana Date Breakfast Muffins/
    variations, 122–123
Multiple sclerosis (MS) and diet, 36
Mung beans, cooking, 98
Mushrooms
  Chili Lime Grilled Asparagus with
    Mushrooms and Bell Pepper/variations,
    193–194
  Kentucky Baked Portobello Nuggets/
    variations, 165
  Magnificent Mushroom Burger/variation,
    270–271
  Mushroom Cauliflower Tacos/variations,
    277–278
  Mushroom Kasha/variations, 213–214
  nutrition, 46–47
  Oil-Free Mushroom Gravy/variations, 240–241
  Pearled Barley with Mushrooms and Corn/
    variations, 210
Mustard greens nutrition, 46

N
National Heart, Lung, and Blood Institute (US-
    based), 32
National Institutes of Health, 11, 17, 32
Navy beans, cooking, 98
Noncommunicable diseases (NCDs)
  examples of, 3
  healthy lifestyle and, 4
  statistics on, 3

WHO recommendations, 3
See also specific diseases
Noni fruit nutrition, 59
Noni-Shot, 141
Noodles
    Asian Noodle Soup/variations, 249
    Lemon Tempeh with Kale and Rice Noodles/
        variations, 276–277
    pantry and, 86
Nori
    Nori Rolls/variations, 263–265
    nutrition, 86
Norris, Jack, 41
Nut-milk bags, 82
Nutrient density
    description/benefits, 16, 44, 74–75
    importance in diet, 74–75
    nutrient-dense foods overview, 44–59
    Recommended Dietary Allowances (RDA)
        and, 44
    See also specific foods
Nutrient reference guide, 319–338
Nutrition
    labels importance, 32
    See also Nutrient density; *specific recipes*
Nutrition and Cancer, 12
Nutritional yeast, 86
Nuts
    Designer Seed and Nut Crust Pizzas/
        variation, 265–266
    nut butters for pantry, 85
    nutrition overview, 51–52
    pantry and, 85
    soaking chart, 105
    toasting, 101–102
    See also specific types

Oats
    Apricot Oat Bars/variations, 308
    cooking/by types, 96
    Overnight Oatmeal, 127–128
    Tahini Oat Sauce/variations, 238
Oats, steel-cut
    cooking, 96

Iron-Rich Morning Glory Steel-Cut Oats/
    variations, 127
    nutrition, 54
Obesity/overweight issues
    childhood obesity, 13
    disorders overview, 13
    GEICO employees study/outcomes, 17
    healing story, 16
    manufacturers supersizing and, 19
    overview, 13, 16
    statistics on, 13
    sugar and weight gain, 38, 88
    See also Weight loss
Oil-free diet
    description, 33–34
    SOS (No salt, oil, sugar) diet, 35–36
Oils, pantry and, 85, 86, 87
Okra
    Okra Bruschetta/variations, 162–163
    Pickled Okra, 181–182
Olives
    Kalamata Rosemary Hummus/variations,
        157–159
    overview/types, 158
Omega-3 fatty acids sources, 17, 42, 46, 50, 52,
    75, 76
One-pot meal
    Monk Bowl, 94, 267
    Simple One-Pot Meal, 266–267
    Template recipe, 267
Onions
    Caramelized Onions, 162
    nutrition, 47
Orange juice, Oil-Free Orange Tarragon
    Dressing/variations, 220
Organic foods
    environmental impacts/nonorganic foods vs.,
        60, 76
    overview/benefits, xvi, 60, 134
Ornish, Dean, 5, 14–15, 21
Oshawa, George, 32

Paleo diet, 34–35
Palmer, Sharon, 7

Pancakes, Lemon Blueberry Pancakes/
    variations, 123–124
Pantry basic foods
    overview, 103–115
    See also specific foods
Pantry, vegan pantry overview, 83–90
Papayas
    Green Papaya Salad/variations, 175–176
    nutrition, 50
    Oil-Free Papaya Salad Dressing/variations,
    176
Parsnips
    Parsnip Fries/variations, 199
    Smashed Roasted Cauliflower and Parsnip/
    variations, 202
Pastas
    pantry and, 86
    See also Noodles; *specific recipes*
Pâté
    Pecan Veggie Pâté, 169–170
    Raw Pâté template recipe, 170
Peaches, Fruit-Sweetened Pistachio Peach
    Cobbler, 311
Pears, Fruit-Sweetened Baked Pears/variations,
    303–304
Pecans
    Chocolate Pecan Dipped Fruit/variations,
    304–305
    nutrition, 52
    Pecan Coconut Topping, 304
    Pecan Veggie Pâté, 169–170
    Pepita Pecan Granola/variations, 124–125
Peeler, finger peeler, 82
Peeling tips, 110
Pellerano, Rosina, 37
Pennington, Alfred W., 30
Pepitas. *See* Pumpkin seeds (pepitas)
Peppers
    Ancho Chile Sauce/variations, 232–233
    Chili Lime Grilled Asparagus with
    Mushrooms and Bell Pepper/variations,
    193–194
    Mexican Seitan-Stuffed Peppers/variations,
    291–292
    red peppers nutrition, 47
    Roasted Red Pepper Sauce/variations, 235–236

Scoville scale, 109, 179
    See also specific types
Perlmutter, David, 28
Pesto Sauce, 215–216
Physicians Committee for Responsible
    Medicine, 7
Pickled Okra, 181–182
Pickled Veggies template recipe, 182
Pickling Spice Mix, 182
Pineapple
    about, 143
    Kale Kolada/variations, 143
Pinto beans
    cooking, 98
    Spicy Pinto Beans/variations, 206–207
Pistachios
    Fruit-Sweetened Pistachio Peach Cobbler, 311
    nutrition, 52
    Watercress with Pistachios and Currants/
    variations, 179
Pita Chips, Homemade/variation, 159
Pituitary gland, 10
Pizza, Designer Seed and Nut Crust Pizzas/
    variation, 265–266
Plant-based analogue products, 84
Plant-based whole food diet
    complete nutrition and, 22–24, 76
    diet design steps and, 74–77
    macronutrient sources and, 74
    meta-analysis research study, 18
    modern medicine vs., 19, 21
    myth/complete nutrition and, 22–24, 34, 40,
    41, 42–43
    myths overview, 40–43
    possible supplements and, 23, 41, 76
    preventable health challenges and, xi–xiii,
    3–21, 23, 34, 74
    transitioning to, xvii
    vitamins needed and, 23
Plant-Powered Diet, The (Palmer), 7
Plantains
    Black Bean Tostones/variations, 167–168
    Grilled Plantain Kebabs/variations, 166–167
    nutrition/working with, 166, 167
    Sweet and Spicy Baked Plantain/variations,
    306

Plastics and toxins, xix

Plums, nutrition, 50

Poblano pepper. *See* Ancho Chile Sauce/ variations

Polenta
cooking, 96
Creamy Herbed Polenta/variations, 170–171

Pollan, Michael, 35

Poppy seeds, Curried Garbanzo Cakes with Poppy Seeds/variations, 164–165

Positive attitude importance, xviii

Potatoes
Fingerling Potatoes with Pesto/variations, 215–217
Herb-Roasted Potatoes/variations, 214–215
overview/types, 216
Purple Potato Tempeh Hash/variations, 130–131
Wasabi Garlic Twice-Baked Potatoes/ variations, 209–210
See also Sweet potatoes

Pots/pans, 82

Prebiotics, 75

Pregnancy and vitamins, 23

Preparing food tips, 91–92

Prevent and Reverse Heart Disease (Esselstyn Jr.), 5, 34

Pritikin, Nathan, 14

Pritikin studies, 12

Probiotics
following antibiotic therapy, 76
food sources, 75
See also Cultured (fermented) food

Processed oils overview, xvi, 5

Produce, "Clean 15"/"Dirty Dozen," 61, 216

Program for Reversing Diabetes (Barnard), 7

Prostate cancer, 10, 11, 12, 15, 19, 21

Protein
RDUs, 40
summary, 40

Prussack, Steve, 67–68

Psychoendoneuroimmunology (PENI), xviii

Psychoneuroimmunology (PNI), xviii

Pudding
Choco-Chia Pudding/variations, 295–296
Pumpkin Pudding/variations, 307

Raw Chocolate Pudding/variations, 296–297
Simple Breakfast Chia Pudding, 117

Pumpkin Pudding/variations, 307

Pumpkin seeds (pepitas)
Creamy Pepita Dressing/variation, 227–228
nutrition, 51
Pepita Pecan Granola/variations, 124–125
Raw Pumpkin Seed and Sunseed Yogurt/ variations, 119–120

Q

Quiche
Broccoli Dill Quiche/variation, 274–276
Template recipe, 274

Quinoa
cooking, 96
Green Quinoa/variations, 203–204
Grilled Mediterranean Vegetables and Quinoa/variations, 212–213
nutrition, 54
pantry and, 86
Quinoa Amaranth Cakes/variations, 168–169
Quinoa Chickpea Pilaf/variations, 211
Quinoa Milk/variations, 143–144
Simple One-Pot Meal, 266–267
sprouting, 144

R

Radishes nutrition, 47

Ranch Sauce, 186

Rastafari culture, 251

Ratatouille/variations, 273–274

Raw (living foods) diet
adding to your diet, 66–67, 68, 76
benefits, 35, 63–65, 76
data on, 66
enzymes and, 65–66
healing stories, 64–65, 67–68
nutrients and cooking, 63–64, 66
overview/description, 35, 63–64
questions on, 66
sample program, 68–69
temperature maximums and, 35, 66

Raw Vegetable Juices: What's Missing in Your Body? (Walker), 65

Rice
    cooking/by types, 96
    See also Brown rice
Rice cooker, 97
Rinaldi, Bo, 94
Rose water tips, 142
Rosemary, Kalamata Rosemary Hummus/
    variations, 157–159
Rye, cooking, 97

S

Salads/Sides
    meal plans and, 70–73
    overview/recipes, 172–218
    See also specific recipes
Salsa, Smoky Salsa/variations, 151
Salt-Free Seasoning, 108–109
Salts
    overview, 32
    pantry and, 86
Saturated fat myth, 41
Sauces
    Green Beans with White Bean Fennel Sauce/
        variations, 217–218
    overview/recipes, 219, 230–241
    Pesto Sauce, 215–216
    Ranch Sauce, 186
    Simple Vegan Cream Sauce/template recipe,
        292–293
    Turmeric Hot Sauce/variations, 109–110
    See also Dipping sauces; *specific recipes*
Sauerkraut, Simple Sauerkraut/variations,
    176–177
Sautés
    Collards and Red Beans, 191
    Simple Green Sauté template recipe, 190
SCD (specific carbohydrate diet), 27–28
Scoville scale/heat units, 109, 179
Scoville, Wilbur, 179
Sea vegetables
    examples, 86
    nutrition, 59
    pantry and, 86–87
    See also specific types
Sears, Barry, 31

Seeds
    Designer Seed and Nut Crust Pizzas/
        variation, 265–266
    nutrition overview, 50–51
    pantry and, 85
    Raw Breakfast Seed and Fruit Puree template
        recipe, 119
    seed butters for pantry, 85
    soaking chart, 105
    toasting, 101–102
    See also specific seeds
Seitan
    Mexican Seitan-Stuffed Peppers/variations,
        291–292
    overview/working with, 100–101
Serotonin, 54, 122, 257, 312
Servan-Schreiber, David, xviii
Sesame seeds
    nutrition, 51
    Sesame Hemp Revitalizer/variations, 145–146
    Sesame Kale Salad/variations, 186–187
Seventh Day Adventists study, 15
Shakes, High-Protein Vanilla Almond Shake/
    variations, 148–149
SIBO (small intestinal bacterial overgrowth), 28
Sides. *See* Salads/Sides; *specific recipes*
Siegel, Bernie, xviii
Sleep-inducing effects, 220, 257
Sleep overview, xviii–xix
Slice described, 95
Sloppy Joes/variations, 281–282
Small intestinal bacterial overgrowth (SIBO), 28
Smoked paprika, 87
Smoothies
    Berry Green Smoothie, 147
    Green Smoothie template recipe, 147
    juices vs., 139
    recommendations, 76
    Tropical Smoothie/variations, 146
Snacks and meal plans, 70–73
Snacks, savory/appetizers
    meal plans and, 70–73
    overview/recipes, 150–171
    See also specific recipes
Soaking chart, nuts/seeds, 105

Socializing/community importance, xvii–xviii, xx, 14, 74
SOS (No salt, oil, sugar) diet, 35–36
Soup stock, 108
Soups/stews
    meal plans and, 70–73
    overview/recipes, 242–258
    See also specific recipes
Sour cream
    Raw Cashew Sour Cream/variation, 113
    Vegan Sour Cream, 112–113
South Beach diet, 29, 30
Soy
    myths on, 42
    substitute for, xvi
    summary/benefits, 42
    See also specific types
Soy sauce substitute, xvi
Soybeans
    cooking, 98
    nutrition, 56
Spatulas, 82–83
Specific carbohydrate diet (SCD), 27–28
Spectrum program, 5
Spelt
    cooking, 97
    overview/nutrition, xvi, 54
Spices
    herbs/spices nutrition overview, 56–57
    pantry and, 85, 87, 105–107
    spice blends, 105–107
    toasting, 101–102
Spinach
    Creamy Lentil Saag/variations, 290–291
    nutrition, 47–48
Spirulina nutrition, 59
Split peas
    cooking, 98
    nutrition, 56
    Smoky Split Pea Soup/variations, 254–255
Spread, Roasted Garlic Spread/variations, 114–115
Sprout bags, 82
Sprouts
    overview/nutrition, 48, 67, 173

raw foods, 67
    sprouting quinoa, 144
    Super Sprout Salad/variations, 173
Squash
    Gold Bar Squash Chutney/variations, 161–162
    Ital Roasted Squash and Sweet Potato Soup/variations, 251–252
    Millet and Butternut Squash with Broccoli/variations, 284–285
    nutrition, 48
    Simple Roasted Butternut Squash Sauce/variations, 236–237
    Spaghetti Squash with Broccoli/variations, 207–208
Standard American diet (SAD)
    cancer and, 12
    description/health consequences, 4, 25
    heart disease and, 4, 5
Star anise, 121
Starch solution diet, 36, 38
Starch Solution, The (McDougall), 36
Statin drugs, 8, 9, 64, 65
Steaming (water sautéing), 101
Stevia, 38, 89
Stews. *See* Soups/stews; *specific recipes*
Storing prepared foods, 94
Strawberries
    Strawberry Cashew Cream/variations, 297
    Strawberry Vinaigrette/variation, 222–223
Stress management importance, xviii, xix, 4, 5, 14, 16–17, 21, 51
Sucanat, 89
Sugar
    problems with, 38, 88
    weight gain/metabolism and, 38, 88
    See also Sweeteners
Sugar-free diet, 38
    See also SOS (No salt, oil, sugar) diet
Sunflower seeds
    nutrition, 51
    Raw Pumpkin Seed and Sunseed Yogurt/variations, 119–120
    Sunflower Seed Fig Puree, 118–119
Swank, Roy, 36
Sweet-and-Sour Sauce, 236

Sweet potatoes
  Date Glazed Sweet Potatoes/variations,
    208–209
  Ital Roasted Squash and Sweet Potato Soup/
    variations, 251–252
  nutrition, 48
  Oil-Free Creamy Sweet Potato Dressing/
    variations, 229
  yams vs., 48
Sweeteners
  healthy/unhealthy substitutes, 38
  natural sweeteners chart/replacement
    amounts, 89–90
  pantry and, 87, 88–90
Symbols/sidebars explained, xv, 93

T

Tabouli, Israeli Couscous Tabouli/variations, 203
Taco
  Mushroom Cauliflower Tacos/variations,
    277–278
  Walnut Taco Salad, 187–188
Tamari, wheat-free, 88
Tamarind
  Raw Tamarind Sauce/variations, 230–231
  tamarind paste, 87
Tapenade, Sun-Dried Tomato Tapenade/
    variations, 156–157
Tarragon, Oil-Free Orange Tarragon Dressing/
    variations, 220
Tarts, Sun-Dried Tomato Fennel Breakfast Tart/
    variations, 129–130
Teas
  Digestive Tea/variations, 133
  Warming Herbal Chai/variation, 133–134
Teff, cooking, 97
Tempeh
  description/types, 99–100
  grilling, 101
  Lemon Tempeh with Kale and Rice Noodles/
    variations, 276–277
  Maple Baked Tempeh/variations, 262
  pantry and, 87
  Purple Potato Tempeh Hash/variations,
    130–131
  roasting, 100

storing, 100
tempeh cutlets, 100
Tempeh Fajitas/variations, 279–280
working with, 99–100
Template recipes
  Chia Pudding, 117
  Creamy Dressings, 228
  Creamy Vegan Soup, 251
  description/example, 93–94
  Fruit Cobbler, 312
  Garden Scramble, 128
  Grain Vegetable Dish, 213
  Green Juices, 136
  Green Smoothie, 147
  Homemade Granola, 126
  Hummus (Bean Puree), 159
  Kale Salad, 184
  Legume and Vegetable Salad, 188–189
  Monk Bowl (one-pot meal), 94, 267
  Pickled Veggies, 182
  Plant-based Milk, 104
  Quiche, 274
  Raw Breakfast Seed and Fruit Puree, 119
  Raw Energy Balls, 299
  Raw Pâté, 170
  Raw Vegetable Soup, 246
  Simple Cookie recipe, 310
  Simple Green Sauté, 190
  Simple Vegan Cream Sauce, 293
  Soft Plant-Based Cheeses, 160
  Superfood Trail Mix, 295
  Ultimate Salad, 174
  Vegan Loaf, 287
  Veggie Burgers, 272
  Vinaigrette, 223
Thai Curry Vegetables/variations, 289–290
Thai food essentials and pantry, 87
There Is a Cure for Diabetes (Cousens), 6
Thyroid function and diet, 46, 52, 86, 104
Toaster oven
  benefits, 82
  tips on using, 82, 101
Toasting overview, 101–102
Tofu
  BBQ Roasted Tofu with Collards/variations,
    278–279

forms of, 97, 99
Garden Veggie Scramble, 128–129
grilling, 101
pantry and, 87
pressing, 99
roasting, 100
Simple Baked Tofu/variations, 260–261
storing, 99
tofu cutlets/cubes, 99
working with, 99
Tomatoes
  Avocado Mousse-Stuffed Tomatoes/variation,
    152–153
  Broiled Cauliflower with Sun-Dried Tomatoes/
    variations, 194–195
  Fire-Roasted Tomato Sauce/variations,
    239–240
  nutrition, 49–50
  Provençal Salad/variations, 183
  Sun-Dried Tomato Fennel Breakfast Tart/
    variations, 129–130
  Sun-Dried Tomato Tapenade/variations,
    156–157
  Tomato Avocado Salad/variations, 183–184
Toxin exposure
  cleansing and, xix–xx
  diet and, 34
  environment and, xix
Trail mix
  Superfood Trail Mix, 295
  Template recipe, 295
Tree of Life Center, Arizona, 6
Triclosan, xix
Triticale nutrition, 55
Truffle oil
  buying tips, 159
  pantry and, 87
  Truffled Cashew Cheese/variation, 159–160
Truss, C. Orian, 27
Tryptophan, 17
Turmeric
  Ginger Turmeric Shooter/variations, 140
  Golden Turmeric Dressing/variation, 223–224
  nutrition, 57
  Turmeric Hot Sauce/variations, 109–110
  turmeric paste, 144

Turnip greens nutrition, 46

U
Umeboshi vinegar, Oil-Free Asian Umeboshi
    Dressing/variations, 220–221
US Department of Agriculture (USDA), 22, 23, 48

V
Vanilla beans, 87
Variety in diet, 75
Vegan Fusion description, 92–93, 314–317
Vegan Loaf
  Lentil Walnut Loaf, 288
  template recipe, 287
Vegetables
  daily servings/benefits, 18
  Garden Veggie Scramble, 128–129
  Grain Vegetable Dish template recipe, 213
  Legume and Vegetable Salad template recipe,
    188–189
  nutrition overview, 44–49
  Simple Chop Salad/variations, 174–175
  Veggie Lettuce Boats/variations, 160–161
  See also specific recipes; specific types
Veggie burgers
  Magnificent Mushroom Burger/variation,
    270–271
  Millet Black Bean Veggie Burgers/variations,
    269–270
  Template recipe, 272
Veggie rolls, Raw Collard Veggie Rolls/
    variations, 260
Vegiterranean Diet, The (Hever), 33
Vinaigrette
  Cilantro Lime Vinaigrette/variations, 221–222
  Strawberry Vinaigrette/variation, 222–223
  Template recipe, 223
Vinegars and pantry, 88, 109
Vitamin B_6/B_9 benefits, 17
Vitamin B_{12} importance, 23
Vitamin D importance, 23
Vitamin K, 41
Vitamix, 82

W
Wakame, 86

Waldorf Dressing/variations, 180–181

Waldorf Salad, 180

Walker, Norman, 65

Walnuts

    Cranberry Walnut Power Krispy Bars/
        variations, 305–306

    Lentil Walnut Loaf, 288

    nutrition, 52–53

    Raw Walnut Crumble, 188

    Walnut Taco Salad, 187–188

Wasabi

    Oil-Free Macadamia Wasabi Dressing/
        variations, 226–227

    Wasabi Garlic Twice-Baked Potatoes/
        variations, 209–210

Watercress

    nutrition, 49

    Watercress with Pistachios and Currants/
        variations, 179

Watermelon

    Rehydrating Watermelon Chiller/variations,
        136

    Watermelon Gazpacho/variation, 243–244

Weight loss

    diabetes and, 6

    dieting/cycle and, 16

    See also Obesity/overweight issues

Wellness (Anti-inflammatory) diet, 26

Wheat Belly (Davis), 28

Wheat, cooking, 97

World Health Organization (WHO)

    on noncommunicable diseases (NCDs), 3

    processed meat label, 11

X

Xylitol, 90

Y

Yacón, 90

Yams vs. sweet potatoes, 48

Yeast syndrome, 27

Yogurt, Raw Pumpkin Seed and Sunseed
    Yogurt/variations, 119–120

Z

Zester, 82

Zone diet, 30–31

Zone, The: A Dietary Road Map (Sears), 31

Zucchini, Roasted Zucchini and Corn/
    variations, 192

About the Author

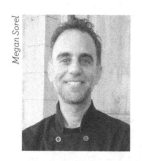

"The male equivalent to a vegan Rachael Ray—Mark Reinfeld's recipes are flavorful and approachable and certainly have the same potential for mass appeal." — *Publishers Weekly*

Mark Reinfeld has over twenty years of experience preparing creative vegan and raw food cuisine. Mark was the executive chef for the North American Vegetarian Society's 2012–2016 Summerfest, one of the largest vegetarian conferences in the world. He is the winner of Vegan.com's Recipe of the Year Award and is described by VegCooking.com as being "poised on the leading edge of contemporary vegan cooking." He is the founding chef of the Blossoming Lotus Restaurant, winner of *Honolulu Advertiser*'s Ilima Award for Best Restaurant on Kaua'i. Mark is also the recipient of a Platinum Carrot Award for living foods—a national award given by the Aspen Center of Integral Health to America's top "innovative and trailblazing healthy chefs."

Mark received his initial culinary training from his grandfather Ben Bimstein, a renowned chef and ice carver in New York City. He developed his love for world culture and cuisine during travel journeys through Europe, Asia, and the Middle East. In 1997, Mark formed the Blossoming Lotus Personal Chef Service in Malibu, California. To further his knowledge of the healing properties of food, he received a master's degree in holistic nutrition.

His first cookbook, *Vegan World Fusion Cuisine*, coauthored with Bo Rinaldi and with a foreword by Dr. Jane Goodall, has won several national awards, including Cookbook of the Year, Best New Cookbook, Best Book by a Small Press, and a Gourmand Award for Best Vegetarian Cookbook in the USA. In addition, Mark coauthored *The Complete Idiot's Guide to Eating Raw* and the four books in the *30-Minute Vegan* series.

Mark specializes in vegan recipe development and offers chef trainings and certification as well as consulting services internationally. He conducts online vegan culinary lessons at veganfusion.com as well as vegan and raw food workshops, teacher trainings, immersions, and retreats worldwide.

The 30-Minute Vegan Series

If you have enjoyed *Healing the Vegan Way*, please check out the books in the 30-Minute Vegan Series.

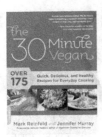

The 30-Minute Vegan, by Mark Reinfeld and Jennifer Murray

Paperback: 978-0-7382-1327-9
Ebook: 978-0-7867-4814-3

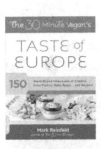

The 30-Minute Vegan's Taste of Europe, by Mark Reinfeld

Paperback: 978-0-7382-1433-7
Ebook: 978-0-7382-1616-4

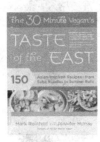

The 30-Minute Vegan's Taste of the East, by Mark Reinfeld and Jennifer Murray

Paperback: 978-0-7382-1382-8
Ebook: 978-0-7382-1416-0

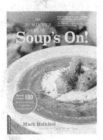

The 30-Minute Vegan's Soups On! by Mark Reinfeld

Paperback
ISBN-10: 0-7382-1673-9
ISBN-13: 978-0-7382-1673-7